Natural Antimalarial Drug Discovery and Development in the Global South

Odangowei Inetiminebi Ogidi
https://orcid.org/0000-0002-9961-893X
Bayelsa Medical University, Nigeria

IGI Global
Scientific Publishing
Publishing Tomorrow's Research Today

Vice President of Editorial Melissa Wagner
Director of Acquisitions Mikaela Felty
Director of Book Development Jocelynn Hessler
Production Manager Mike Brehm
Cover Design Jose Rosado

Published in the United States of America by
IGI Global Scientific Publishing
701 East Chocolate Avenue
Hershey, PA, 17033, USA
Tel: 717-533-8845 | Fax: 717-533-7115
Website: https://www.igi-global.com E-mail: cust@igi-global.com

Library of Congress Cataloging-in-Publication Data

Names: Ogidi, Odangowei, 1983- editor
Title: Natural antimalarial drug discovery and development in the Global South / edited by Odangowei Ogidi.
Description: Hershey, PA : IGI Global Scientific Publishing, [2026] | Includes bibliographical references and index. | Summary: "This book aims to highlight regional case studies and successful integrations of traditional medicine into modern drug discovery pipelines"-- Provided by publisher.
Identifiers: LCCN 2025046638 (print) | LCCN 2025046639 (ebook) | ISBN 9798337358215 hardcover | ISBN 9798337358222 paperback | ISBN 9798337358239 ebook
Subjects: LCSH: Antimalarials--Development--Developing countries | Malaria--Homeopathic treatment | Medicinal plants--Developing countries | Materia medica, Vegetable--Developing countries
Classification: LCC RC159.A5 N38 2026 (print) | LCC RC159.A5 (ebook)
LC record available at https://lccn.loc.gov/2025046638
LC ebook record available at https://lccn.loc.gov/2025046639
British Cataloguing in Publication Data
A Cataloguing in Publication record for this book is available from the British Library.

Table of Contents

Detailed Table of Contents

Malaria continues to be a significant global health challenge in the 21st century, disproportionately impacting populations in the Global South. This chapter "Global Burden of Malaria in the 21st Century" provides a comprehensive overview of malaria's epidemiology, socio-economic impact, and the evolving challenges in control efforts. The discussion covers current trends in incidence and mortality, highlights regional disparities, and examines the intricate interplay of biological, environmental, and social factors that drive transmission. This chapter examines the ways in which drug and insecticide resistance, climate change, and inadequate healthcare infrastructure are transforming malaria patterns. Ultimately, it highlights the importance of policy intervention and research, particularly regarding the development of natural antimalarial drug research platforms in endemic countries. By placing malaria within a multidisciplinary framework, we aim to guide and promote efforts to connect the gaps between burden, innovation, and justice solutions in the Global South.

Phytochemicals, the bioactive secondary metabolites produced by plants as part of their defense mechanisms, have gained significant attention for their multifaceted role in plant-based therapeutics. These compounds—mainly alkaloids, flavonoids, and terpenoids—not only ensure plant survival under biotic and abiotic stresses but also provide numerous health-promoting effects in hum, phytochemicals contribute to

Phytochemicals are plant derived bioactive compounds that have emerged as potential contenders in the battle against malaria owing to their versatile mechanisms of action against *Plasmodium* parasites. This chapter discusses the diverse roles of phytochemicals in interfering with the lifecycle of the parasite, especially at the erythrocytic stages, which are accountable for the clinical presentation of malaria. These include the inhibition of heme polymerization, disruption of parasite invasion and adhesion, induction of apoptosis, and manipulation of the host immune system. Moreover, a number of phytochemicals exhibit synergy when combined with traditional antimalarial drugs, providing new hope for the reversal of drug resistance. In contrast to the issues associated with bioavailability and standardization, current research is still discovering new plant based compounds with significant antiplasmodial activity. This chapter presents a detailed review of these mechanisms and describes the therapeutic potential of phytochemicals and their use in the design of next generation antimalarial strategies.

The transition from laboratory research to clinical application in the realm of natural products represents a critical juncture in the development of novel therapeutics. The integration of natural products into modern medicine remains a cornerstone of pharmaceutical innovation. This process involves not only the meticulous isolation and classification of bioactive compounds but also the rigorous assessment of their efficacy and safety through a series of preclinical and clinical trials. There is the need to address the public health threat of malaria, and the invaluable contributions of natural products to clinical candidates is inevitable. This chapter discusses various kinds of natural products with evidence-based antimalarial activity, along with their potential clinical candidacy. It covers the challenges at the preclinical and clinical developmental level in translating natural products to clinical candidates and future prospects.

In this context, computational tools are not just auxiliary assets—they are becoming indispensable engines of innovation in pharmaceutical sciences.

Preface

Malaria remains one of the most persistent public health challenges of the twenty-first century, disproportionately burdening populations in the Global South. Despite major advances in vector control and chemotherapeutic interventions, the rise of resistance to existing antimalarial drugs underscores the urgent need for innovative and sustainable therapeutic solutions. In this context, nature's pharmacopoeia rooted in the traditional medicinal practices of indigenous communities offers an invaluable, yet underexplored, reservoir of bioactive compounds. ***Natural Antimalarial Drug Discovery and Development in the Global South*** was conceived as an interdisciplinary response to this global health imperative. The book bridges ethnomedicine, phytochemistry, pharmacology, computational science, and policy to illuminate how natural products research can drive next-generation antimalarial therapies. It highlights the pivotal role of scientists, traditional healers, and local communities across Africa, Asia, and Latin America, whose knowledge systems and biodiversity resources continue to shape the frontier of global drug discovery.

This volume is organized to guide readers along the full continuum of discovery from ethnobotanical documentation and phytochemical screening to bioassay-guided isolation, mechanism elucidation, and translational research. The chapters collectively emphasize methodological rigor, ethical collaboration, and equitable benefit-sharing as foundational principles for research in the Global South. In addition, the integration of artificial intelligence, omics technologies, and sustainable cultivation practices underscores the growing synergy between traditional wisdom and modern innovation.

CHAPTER OVERVIEW

Chapter 1: Global Burden of Malaria in the 21st Century

Odangowei Ogidi and Uchechi Enenebeaku

This opening chapter establishes the epidemiological and socio-economic context of malaria today. It explores the evolving global burden, regional disparities, and the complex interactions among biological, environmental, and structural determinants of malaria transmission. The authors critically examine how resistance, climate change, and weak health systems are reshaping the malaria landscape, while advocating for natural product research platforms and policy reforms to drive innovation in endemic regions.

Chapter 2: The Science of Phytochemicals—An Introduction to Plant-Based Therapeutics

Aamir Abdullah, Abdullah Khan, R. Somasundaram, and Sana Rais

This chapter introduces the biochemical and pharmacological foundations of plant-based therapeutics. It examines the roles of alkaloids, flavonoids, and terpenoids—the primary phytochemical classes with antimalarial potential—highlighting their biosynthetic origins, mechanisms of action, and contributions to nutraceutical and pharmaceutical development. The discussion lays the groundwork for understanding how natural compounds transition from traditional use to modern therapeutic frameworks.

Chapter 3: Amazon Ethnomedicine and Malaria Control in Latin America—Field-Based Plant Surveys and Partnerships with Indigenous Communities

Aman Suresh Tharayil et al.

Drawing on field research in the Amazon basin, this chapter explores how indigenous knowledge and ethnomedicine contribute to malaria control. Through participatory surveys and phytochemical validation, the authors document medicinal plants used by riverine and indigenous communities and discuss their pharmacological promise and cultural significance. The chapter advocates for policy frameworks that recognize indigenous health systems, ensure equitable benefit-sharing, and promote sustainable biodiversity management.

Chapter 4: Mechanisms of Action of Phytochemicals Against *Plasmodium* Parasites

Rahul Kumar

Focusing on molecular pharmacology, this chapter delves into how phytochemicals target *Plasmodium* parasites. It details mechanisms such as inhibition of heme polymerization, interference with parasite invasion, and modulation of immune responses. The author also discusses the synergistic effects of combining phytochemicals with standard drugs, offering new strategies to combat resistance and enhance therapeutic efficacy.

Chapter 5: From Lab to Field—Translating Natural Products into Clinical Candidates

Chinyere Ezeanya-Bakpa et al.

This chapter bridges the gap between laboratory discovery and real-world application. It traces the pathway from natural compound isolation to clinical trials, emphasizing challenges in standardization, safety evaluation, and regulatory approval. The authors highlight successful case studies and the potential of natural antimalarial compounds to serve as viable clinical candidates, particularly within resource-limited settings.

Chapter 6: Indigenous Knowledge and Antimalarial Enema Therapies—An Ethnobotanical Survey from Cross River State, Nigeria

Peggy Willie et al.

Through an ethnobotanical survey among the Efik and Qua peoples, this chapter documents traditional enema-based therapies for malaria. It identifies key medicinal plant species and discusses their known phytochemical constituents and pharmacological relevance. The findings reinforce the significance of indigenous practices as reservoirs of scientific insight and potential leads in antimalarial drug discovery.

Chapter 7: AI and Computational Chemistry in Phytochemical Drug Discovery

Selvakumar P., Manjunath T.C., and Mythili R.

The concluding chapter situates natural product research within the digital revolution of drug discovery. It explores how artificial intelligence, machine learning, and computational chemistry are transforming phytochemical screening, molecular modeling, and lead optimization. The authors argue that these technologies democratize innovation, enabling Global South researchers to accelerate discovery pipelines and reduce research costs.

Beyond its scientific contributions, this book advances a vision of health equity and scientific sovereignty. By empowering regional researchers, institutions, and communities, it seeks to reposition the Global South not merely as a site of disease burden, but as a leader in biomedical innovation and discovery. We hope that this work serves as a reference for researchers, students, clinicians, and policymakers committed to the eradication of malaria and to the sustainable advancement of natural product sciences. May it also inspire a renewed appreciation for the enduring partnership between nature and humanity in the ongoing fight against this ancient disease.

Odangowei Inetiminebi Ogidi
Bayelsa Medical University, Nigeria

Chapter 1
Global Burden of Malaria in the 21st Century

Odangowei Inetiminebi Ogidi
https://orcid.org/0000-0002-9961-893X
Bayelsa Medical University, Yenagoa, Nigeria

Uchechi Emmanuela Enenebeaku
https://orcid.org/0000-0002-2349-9890
University of Agriculture and Environmental Sciences, Umuagwo, Nigeria

ABSTRACT

Malaria continues to be a significant global health challenge in the 21st century, disproportionately impacting populations in the Global South. This chapter "Global Burden of Malaria in the 21st Century" provides a comprehensive overview of malaria's epidemiology, socio-economic impact, and the evolving challenges in control efforts. The discussion covers current trends in incidence and mortality, highlights regional disparities, and examines the intricate interplay of biological, environmental, and social factors that drive transmission. This chapter examines the ways in which drug and insecticide resistance, climate change, and inadequate healthcare infrastructure are transforming malaria patterns. Ultimately, it highlights the importance of policy intervention and research, particularly regarding the development of natural antimalarial drug research platforms in endemic countries. By placing malaria within a multidisciplinary framework, we aim to guide and promote efforts to connect the gaps between burden, innovation, and justice solutions in the Global South.

DOI: 10.4018/979-8-3373-5821-5.ch001

INTRODUCTION

Malaria remains one of the most incapacitating infectious illnesses of the 21st century, continuing to impose a significant toll on international public health despite decades of progress in prevention, treatment, and control (WHO, 2024). In 2023 alone, a staggering 263 million new malaria cases and nearly 597,000 malaria-attributable deaths were reported, emphasizing the disease's enduring burden—the largest proportion of which were in sub-Saharan Africa (WHO, 2025; WHO, 2024). Children under the age of five remain disproportionately affected, with the majority of deaths happening among them (WHO, 2024). These figures reflect longstanding challenges such as inadequate healthcare infrastructure, low coverage of preventive measures, and socioeconomic disparities across endemic regions (WHO, 2024).

Innovations in the early 2000s brought dramatic reductions in malaria infections and deaths by widespread utilization of insecticide-treated bed nets, rapid diagnostics, and artemisinin-based medications. Between 2000 and 2023, interventions have been calculated to avert over 2.2 billion malaria infections and 12.7 million deaths. Nonetheless, since approximately 2015, advancement has plateaued, indicating steady challenges to sustained progress. The COVID-19 pandemic was a severe setback for malaria control, as supply chains and health services were interrupted in 2020, and an estimated 55,000 additional malaria deaths occurred (WHO, 2024). Beyond pandemics, mounting threats such as climate change and armed conflict are expanding unfavorable environmental conditions and decreasing access to care, driving the transmission of malaria.

Fragile health systems torn apart by conflict in countries like Yemen and Sudan have also derailed prevention and treatment efforts, with millions more displaced and out of reach of basic services. These crises are exacerbated by extreme inequities in access to preventive interventions—almost half of all children under the age of five years in sub-Saharan Africa did not sleep under insecticide-treated bed nets in 2023, despite mass distribution campaigns. Growing resistance to frontline malaria instruments compounds these challenges. Resistance to artemisinin has been confirmed in East Africa, threatening the efficacy of the most potent antimalarial drugs. Meanwhile, resistance to pyrethroids, which undermines the deployment of insecticide-treated bed nets, is rapidly expanding across the continent.

In spite of these difficulties, two malaria vaccines (RTS,S (Mosquirix) and R21/Matrix-M) have emerged as game-changing tools. WHO recommended both vaccines in October 2023 for use in children in moderate- to high-transmission settings under a four-dose schedule beginning at about five months of age (WHO, 2025). Rollout has begun: through late 2024, more than 12 million doses had been shipped to 17 African countries for subnational introductions, with an additional eight countries planning to introduce them in 2025 (WHO, 2024).

Uganda launched the largest vaccine rollout to date in April 2025, vaccinating 1.1 million children under two in high-transmission districts with the R21/Matrix-M formulation (WHO, 2025). Mozambique also launched R21 in August 2024 in 22 districts in Zambézia province, with plans to vaccinate around 300,000 children (WHO, 2024). In Ghana, the rollout continues to expand: more than 1 million doses of RTS,S have been administered and R21 is rolling out to additional districts.

Both vaccines also have favorable safety profiles, as supported by MVIP and clinical trial safety data. No such safety concerns as increased cerebral malaria or sex-specific mortality were reported for RTS,S in implementation (WHO, 2025). Safety follow-up of R21, including in the VAC078 trial, has reported manageable adverse events, although continued surveillance remains very important (WHO, 2025).

Financial strategies are evolving to make vaccines more accessible. GSK and Bharat Biotech announced plans to reduce the cost of RTS,S to below US $5 per dose by 2028. This will involve the transfer of manufacturing to Bharat, with GSK supplying adjuvant components. Concurrently, Gavi's model supports vaccine procurement and rollout, aiming to immunize millions of children—if adequately funded. Global financing mechanisms remain crucial. Planned recent budget cuts to the U.S. President's Malaria Initiative (PMI) risk reversing prevention; full funding of PMI would avert up to 14 million cases and save over 100,000 lives in 2025 (WHO, 2025). The cuts underscore the fragility of progress against malaria control and the need for sustained global investment. This chapter explores the malaria burden in the 21st century, emphasizing the ongoing congruence between remarkable advances and obstinate challenges to disease control. It analyzes how epidemiologic trends, continued interventions, and new innovations specifically the arrival of vaccines such as RTS,S and R21/Matrix-M which are revolutionizing the global malaria campaign. In addition to the scientific advancement, the chapter also sheds light on how efforts in vaccination are to be linked with strengthened health systems, secure funding, engaged community, and continued research.

EPIDEMIOLOGICAL TRENDS

The global burden of malaria in the 21st century has shown a complex pattern of initial decline followed by stagnation in recent years. Between 2000 and 2015, substantial progress was achieved, with malaria incidence falling by approximately 27% and mortality rates declining by 37%, largely due to the scale-up of insecticide-treated nets (ITNs), indoor residual spraying (IRS), and the widespread adoption of artemisinin-based combination therapies (ACTs) (WHO, 2015). However, since 2017, progress has slowed, and in some regions, reversed, with an estimated 249 million malaria cases and 608,000 deaths globally in 2023 (WHO, 2023). Sub-Saharan Africa continues to carry the heaviest burden, accounting for over 90% of global cases and deaths, with children under five years of age disproportionately affected (Snow et al., 2021). Challenges including drug and insecticide resistance, inadequate health system capacity, and disruptions caused by the COVID-19 pandemic, have further constrained progress (Ogidi, 2022; Bhatt et al., 2015; WHO, 2021). Despite these obstacles, significant milestones such as the pilot implementation of the RTS,S vaccine and recent approval of R21/Matrix-M represent major advances in malaria prevention and may offer new opportunities to reduce the disease burden in endemic countries (Datoo et al., 2021; WHO, 2023). Nonetheless, the global community remains off-track to achieve the WHO target of reducing malaria incidence and mortality by 90% by 2030, underscoring the need for renewed investment, innovation, and coordinated action (WHO, 2021). Table 1 shows the epidemiological trends of the global burden of malaria in the 21st century.

Table 1. Epidemiological Trends – Global Burden of Malaria in the 21st Century

Indicator	2000	2010	2020	2023	Trend/Notes	References
Estimated malaria cases (global)	~245 million	~233 million	~241 million	~249 million	Overall decline between 2000–2015, but resurgence/stagnation since 2017 due to funding gaps, resistance, and COVID-19 disruptions.	WHO (2015, 2021, 2023)
Estimated malaria deaths (global)	~864,000	~627,000	~625,000	~608,000	Deaths declined by ~30% from 2000–2015, but progress has slowed; mortality remains high in sub-Saharan Africa.	WHO (2015, 2021, 2023)
Children <5 years deaths	>700,000 annually	~460,000	~475,000	~453,000	Children under five still account for ~80% of malaria deaths.	WHO (2023); Snow et al. (2021)
Regional distribution of cases	Africa: ~85%SE Asia: ~10%Others: <5%	Africa: ~90%SE Asia: ~7%	Africa: ~95%	Africa: ~94%	Sub-Saharan Africa remains disproportionately affected.	WHO (2021, 2023)
High-burden countries	Nigeria, DRC, India	Nigeria, DRC, India	Nigeria, DRC, Uganda, Mozambique	Nigeria, DRC, Uganda, Mozambique	Since 2018, WHO identified 11 high-burden, high-impact (HBHI) countries—10 in Africa + India.	WHO (2021, 2023)
Insecticide-treated net (ITN) coverage	<2%	~50% household	~68% households	~66% households	Major scale-up post-2000 contributed to declines in cases/deaths; coverage has plateaued.	Bhatt et al. (2015); WHO (2021, 2023)
Artemisinin-based combination therapy (ACT) access	Limited (<10%)	~45% of cases treated with ACTs	~70%	~72%	Scale-up of ACTs was central to mortality reduction; drug resistance is an emerging threat.	WHO (2015, 2021, 2023)

continued on following page

Table 1. Continued

Indicator	2000	2010	2020	2023	Trend/Notes	References
Vaccination	None	None	RTS,S pilot programs (Ghana, Kenya, Malawi)	RTS,S + R21 approved for wider rollout (2021–2023)	Vaccines mark a major new milestone in malaria prevention.	WHO (2023); Datoo et al. (2021)
Overall progress	High burden, rising deaths	Significant reduction in burden (2000–2015)	Plateau/stagnation	Mixed: some countries nearing elimination, others experiencing setbacks	Global target to reduce malaria incidence and mortality by 90% by 2030 is off-track.	WHO (2021, 2023)

Global Incidence and Mortality Over the Last Two Decades

For the last two decades, malaria has been the most enduring public health threat globally. In the year 2000, it is estimated that there were 226 million cases, and almost 896,000 died of the disease (WHO, 2024). These numbers represented extensive endemicity on several continents and led to intensified worldwide action for malaria control and elimination. Early in the 2000s, during a period of heightened intervention, mortality rates for malaria began to shift. As of 2015, deaths due to malaria had declined to around 562,000, a reduction of more than one-third since the year 2000. Deployment of insecticide-treated nets, rapid diagnostic tests, and artemisinin-based combination therapies was responsible for these advances.

Despite these developments, the recent years have witnessed foreboding reversals. In 2023, cases of malaria had risen to 263 million, up from nearly 37 million in 2000 (WHO, 2024). Mortality rates also rose, with malaria deaths standing at around 597,000 worldwide—an indicator that the world is no longer set to meet global elimination targets. Malaria incidence rates are equally symptomatic of these epidemiological shifts. In 2000, it was estimated at over 80 per 1,000 at-risk population. It fell to 58 per 1,000 in 2019, showing considerable progress. But the figure went up to 60.4 in 2023, which shows lost momentum in control (WHO, 2022; WHO, 2024). Yet, from 2000 to 2023, global malaria efforts were estimated to have prevented more than 2.2 billion cases and 12.7 million deaths. The statistics underscore the importance of continued intervention despite setbacks.

Regional Hotspots: Sub-Saharan Africa, South-East Asia, and Latin America

The world's burden of malaria is still extremely unequal, with the vast majority in sub-Saharan Africa. In 2023, 94% of all malaria and 95% of all malaria deaths took place in this area (WHO, 2024). The highest burden fell on children aged below five years, as they contributed to the bulk of all deaths globally. On the African continent, Nigeria, the Democratic Republic of Congo, Niger, and Tanzania accounted for more than half of all deaths from malaria worldwide, with Nigeria alone contributing more than 30% (WHO, 2024). This highlights the need to provide focused, country-specific interventions in high burden areas.

To respond to these disparities, WHO launched the High-Burden High-Impact (HBHI) initiative in 2018 in 11 countries responsible for two-thirds of cases and 68% of deaths worldwide. These countries, redoubled efforts notwithstanding, continued reporting increasing incidence and mortality during the years 2017-2023. In regions outside Africa, South-East Asia witnessed phenomenal progress. Between 2000 and 2020, deaths from malaria in the region were reduced by 75%, from about 35,000 to 9,000. The achievements have been credited to coordinated government action and greater availability of preventives and cures.

India, in particular, has made incredible strides. From 2017 to 2023, malaria cases fell by 69% in India, and deaths fell by 68%, leading the country to be dropped from the WHO high-burden list (WHO Regional Office, 2021). This indicates the scale of decline that can be achieved through sustained investment in treatment and surveillance. Latin America continues to face enormous challenges by comparison. Other nations such as Venezuela and Haiti, and portions of the Amazon Basin, remain malaria hotbeds due to political unrest, health system weaknesses, and environmental changes (Beat Malaria, 2024). The same applies to Myanmar in Southeast Asia, whose gains have been marred by conflict and weak governance (WHO, 2024).

Progress Since the Early 2000s and Stalling in the Mid-2010s

The early 21st century was a period of unparalleled progress toward controlling malaria. Investment in preventive interventions, access to therapeutic measures, and coordinated international policies paid dividends in terms of high incidence and mortality reductions worldwide. Successes were welcomed as proof that elimination of malaria was a feasible long-term goal (Reuters, 2024; WHO, 2024). A turning point was indicated in the mid-2010s. Although earlier momentum, international progress slowed down around 2015, with incidence and mortality rates stabilizing at mostly unchanged levels since then. This leveling off underscored the system-wide weaknesses in the form of drug resistance, financing gaps, and fragmentation in coverage of interventions (WHO, 2024).

The 2020 COVID-19 pandemic added to the issues as well. Disruptions to health systems led to some 11 million additional cases and 55,000 additional deaths of malaria, negating some of the improvement that was experienced before (WHO, 2024). Mortality rates, declining to 13 per 100,000 population in 2019, spiked again to nearly 15 in 2020 before improving only incrementally over the next years

(WHO, 2024). Climate change has also been a significant driver of malaria. Environmental shocks such as the destructive 2022 floods in Pakistan have ushered in a five-fold increase in malaria, documenting the vulnerability of endemic areas to environmental shocks (WHO, 2023). Rising temperatures and altered patterns of precipitation are likely to expand mosquito habitats, extend transmission seasons, and enhance caseloads.

Conflict and displacement add another dimension of complexity. Political upheaval in Ethiopia, Sudan, and Myanmar has disrupted malaria intervention programs, reduced treatment access, and triggered outbreak cycles. The crises illustrate how broader socio-political determinants directly impact malaria epidemiology. Global objectives remain far from realization. Incidence has reached 60.4 cases per 1,000 at-risk population and mortality 13.7 per 100,000 as of 2023—well above the WHO Global Technical Strategy targets of 21.3 and 5.5, respectively (WHO, 2024). The gap between targets and actuality serves to emphasize the urgency for new strategies.

However, a few countries have eliminated malaria. Cabo Verde and Egypt were recently certified as free of malaria, adding to the number of malaria-free countries to 44 by the year 2024 (Beat Malaria, 2024). These are examples of what can be achieved with unflinching commitment. Elimination is not, however, perpetual. Risk of reintroduction continues to be extremely high in countries with weak surveillance and prevention systems. Malaria-free status should be ensured by sustained surveillance with the focus that elimination is not the end of the fight (Beat Malaria, 2024). Past two decades' epidemiological trends tell a complex story of gains and setbacks. The achievement made in the early 2000s has come to a plateau, and new challenges due to climate change, conflict, and pandemics have undone gains in certain places. While huge mortality declines since 2000 are a success story, malaria remains a tremendous burden, particularly in Africa (WHO, 2024).

DETERMINANTS OF MALARIA BURDEN

The burden of malaria is shaped by a complex interplay of biological, environmental, socioeconomic, and health system determinants (Figure 1). Biologically, the distribution and efficiency of *Anopheles* mosquito, coupled with the genetic diversity and drug resistance of *Plasmodium* parasites, strongly influence transmission dynamics and disease severity. Environmental factors such as climate variability, rainfall, temperature, and land-use practices create favorable breeding habitats, particularly in tropical and subtropical regions. Socioeconomic conditions, including poverty, inadequate housing, limited access to preventive tools, and population mobility, further exacerbate vulnerability, especially among rural and marginalized communities. Weak health systems, which are characterized by poor surveillance, insufficient diagnostic capacity, inadequate treatment coverage, and reliance on external funding, undermine effective control and elimination efforts. Together, these determinants sustain malaria transmission and explain the disproportionate burden borne by sub-Saharan Africa, where structural, ecological, and systemic vulnerabilities converge.

Figure 1. Determinants of malaria burden

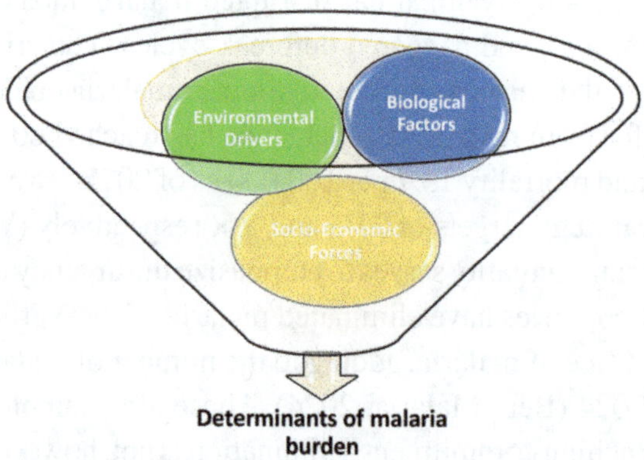

Biological Factors

Spread of malaria is determined primarily by biological factors, the foremost of which is the infecting *Plasmodium* species in humans. The four major species are *Plasmodium falciparum, P. vivax, P. ovale,* and *P. malariae,* with *P. knowlesi* added as a zoonotic species (Enenebeaku et al., 2022a; Centers for Disease Control and Prevention, 2024). Of these, *P. falciparum* is the most lethal, responsible for the majority of malaria deaths globally and particularly in sub-Saharan Africa (WHO, 2024). *Plasmodium vivax* offers a different scenario. While it never kills to any significant extent compared to *P. falciparum*, it is widespread elsewhere on the planet aside from Africa and is prone to relapse due to latent liver forms referred to as hypnozoites (Price et al., 2020). This biological feature makes control and elimination in Asia and Latin America specifically difficult. The other key determinant is the mosquito vector ecology. Malaria transmission depends on female *Anopheles* mosquitoes, which number over 400, but only about 40 are significant in human malaria (CDC, 2024). Distribution of the vectors, feeding habits, and resistance to insecticides influence local malaria epidemiology (Sherrard-Smith et al., 2022).

The main vector in Africa is Anopheles gambiae, which is highly anthropophilic (human-preference compared to animal-preference) and efficient at transmitting P.

falciparum (WHO, 2024). *Anopheles stephensi* and *A. darlingi* are major ones in Asia and the Latin Americas. Global distribution of *A. stephensi* into urban Africa is of special concern since it increases malaria risk in urban localities (Sinka et al., 2020). The emergence and spread of resistant strains of *Plasmodium falciparum* remain major obstacles to effective malaria control and elimination. Antimalarial drug resistance, particularly to artemisinin and its partner drugs, first appeared in Southeast Asia during the latter half of the 20th century and has since spread to parts of Africa, undermining the efficacy of artemisinin-based combination therapies (ACTs) (WHO, 2023). Partial artemisinin resistance in *P. falciparum*, characterized by delayed parasite clearance associated with mutations in the *kelch13* gene, has now been confirmed in East African countries such as Uganda and Rwanda (Uwimana et al., 2021). Similarly, insecticide resistance in *Anopheles* mosquito vectors poses a serious threat to vector control interventions. Pyrethroid resistance, the most widespread form, has been reported across Africa and Asia, reducing the effectiveness of long-lasting insecticidal nets (LLINs) (Hemingway et al., 2016). Although newer-generation nets combining pyrethroids with synergists or alternative insecticides have been developed, their high cost and limited availability continue to restrict coverage (WHO, 2024).

Environmental Drivers

Climatic variation is one of the principal environmental determinants of malaria transmission. Temperature, rainfall, and humidity are highly influential on mosquito growth and the development of parasites within mosquitoes. Even minimal increases in mean temperatures can accelerate the development of parasites and extend transmission seasons (Ogidi et al., 2025b; Ryan et al., 2020). Evidence exists that climate change is transforming the geographical pattern of malaria risk. African highland regions formerly considered safe from malaria have experienced increased incidence as temperatures have increased and allowed mosquitoes to survive at higher elevations (Siraj et al., 2014). Similarly, climate models project widespread expansion of malaria transmission potential in Asia and Africa by 2050 (Caminade et al., 2014).

Rainfall patterns also impact transmission. Anopheles mosquitoes are bred by heavy rains, while prolonged droughts can decimate mosquito populations but also cause migration, seeding vulnerability elsewhere (WHO, 2023). The catastrophic floods in Pakistan in 2022 that saw a five-fold increase in malaria cases are a stark example of climate shocks sparking epidemics (WHO, 2023). Land use changes also play a fundamental role. Agricultural expansion, irrigation schemes, and deforestation alter local ecosystems that in many situations offer optimal breeding places for malaria vectors. For example, irrigation projects in Africa have been linked with increased malaria transmission due to water pooling that is stagnant (Keiser et al., 2005).

Urbanization comes with its novel challenges. Although cities typically reduce the threat of malaria due to better-developed infrastructure, the invasion of African cities by *Anopheles stephensi* has reversed this assumption (Sinka et al., 2020). The urban-adapted mosquito breeds in water storage tanks, and as a result, malaria is emerging as a growing concern in rapidly developing cities. Environmental degradation also increases transmission. Mining, road-building, and human settlement expansion have a tendency to fragment natural landscapes, which forms new vector habitats. Deforestation in the Amazon Basin has been associated with increased malaria transmission, linking ecological disruption to public health expenses (Oliveira-Ferreira et al., 2010).

Socio-Economic Forces

Malaria remains a disease of poverty, and socio-economic conditions exert a strong influence on exposure, prevention, and treatment (Sachs & Malaney, 2002). Poorer households often do not have access to insecticide-treated bed nets, early diagnosis, or effective treatment and continue to be in cycles of illness and economic loss. Infrastructure shortages contribute significantly to the role of continued malaria. Weak health systems, poor laboratory capacity, and insufficient drug supplies thwart early diagnosis and treatment in the majority of endemic countries. In the sub-Saharan region of Africa, rural residents are worst affected due to geographical isolation and poor transport networks (WHO, 2024). Population displacement and migration also contribute to malaria risk. Internally displaced people and refugees are resettled in areas of malaria endemicity without adequate protection, and conflict undermines control programs (Martens & Hall, 2000). South Sudan and Myanmar civil wars, for example, have coincided with malaria rebound because of weakened health systems.

Armed conflict not only disrupts service delivery but also creates favorable breeding conditions for mosquitoes such as derelict agricultural land and sanitation in crowded camps (Rowe et al., 2009). Such humanitarian crises depict the intimate linkage between conflict and malaria transmission. Labor migration is also contributory. Seasonal agricultural laborers who travel between provinces can both acquire and spread malaria infections, creating border zones such as Cambodian-Thailand borders control issues (Carrara et al., 2013). This mobility typically undermines sub-regional elimination initiatives.

Socio-economic inequality among countries further decides malaria results. Treated beds and treatment will be more likely in affluent city residences, with less affluent rural homes more exposed and at higher risk of death (WHO, 2024).

The disparity points towards treating malaria as a disease of inequity along with infection. Educational status is yet another determinant. Socio-economically deprived communities lacking sound knowledge of malaria prevention and treatment tend to postpone seeking care, leading to increased mortality (WHO, 2023). Public health campaigns have been proven to have quantifiable impact in bridging this knowledge gap (WHO, 2023). Last but not least, long-term financing and political commitment are essential socio-economic determinants. In view of the estimated US$8.3 billion yearly requirement for malaria control, international investments were as low as just around US$4 billion in 2023 (WHO, 2024). Lacking adequate resources, the war against malaria cannot be properly extended evenly in all regions where it is most required.

CHALLENGES IN CONTROL AND ELIMINATION OF MALARIA

The control and elimination of malaria face numerous challenges that span biological, health system, socioeconomic, environmental, and political dimensions (Table 2). Biologically, the emergence of drug-resistant *Plasmodium* parasites and insecticide-resistant mosquito vectors undermines the efficacy of frontline treatments and vector control measures, while asymptomatic infections and parasite genetic diversity sustain hidden transmission reservoirs. Weak healthcare systems further complicate progress through inadequate diagnostic capacity, supply chain disruptions, insufficient surveillance, and heavy reliance on external funding (Afakwu-Adimoha & Ogidi, 2025; Ogidi et al., 2023). Socioeconomic barriers such as poverty, population mobility, and limited community acceptance of interventions like insecticide-treated nets exacerbate transmission risks. Environmental changes, including climate variability, urbanization, irrigation, and deforestation, create favorable conditions for mosquito breeding and extend transmission zones. In addition, political instability, conflict, and cross-border malaria spread hinder coordinated responses, while governance and policy gaps reduce the sustainability of interventions. Collectively, these interlinked challenges necessitate integrated, adaptive, and well-resourced approaches to achieve and sustain malaria elimination.

Table 2. Challenges in the Control and Elimination of Malaria

Category	Challenges	Description / Examples
Biological	Antimalarial drug resistance	Resistance of *Plasmodium falciparum* and *P. vivax* to artemisinin-based combination therapies (ACTs) and other antimalarials undermines treatment efficacy.
	Insecticide resistance	Increasing resistance of *Anopheles* mosquitoes to pyrethroids, carbamates, and organophosphates reduces the effectiveness of insecticide-treated nets (ITNs) and indoor residual spraying (IRS).
	Parasite genetic diversity	High variability of malaria parasites complicates vaccine development and reduces long-term effectiveness of immunization strategies.
	Asymptomatic and submicroscopic infections	Undetected carriers act as reservoirs of transmission, sustaining malaria in endemic communities.
Health System	Weak healthcare infrastructure	Limited diagnostic tools, inadequate laboratory capacity, and shortage of trained personnel hinder effective case management.
	Supply chain and logistics	Frequent stock-outs of medicines, rapid diagnostic tests (RDTs), and ITNs compromise program coverage.
	Inadequate surveillance	Weak disease reporting and monitoring systems delay detection of outbreaks and emergence of resistance.
	Insufficient and unsustainable financing	Heavy reliance on donor funding and inadequate domestic resource allocation limit program continuity.
Socioeconomic	Poverty and inequity	Poor housing, inadequate sanitation, and inability to afford prevention or treatment exacerbate malaria burden.
	Human migration and mobility	Seasonal labor migration, displacement due to conflict, and cross-border movement facilitate reintroduction of malaria into controlled or eliminated areas.
	Community acceptance and adherence	Misconceptions about malaria, reluctance to use ITNs or IRS, and poor adherence to treatment regimens reduce intervention impact.
Environmental	Climate variability and change	Shifting rainfall patterns and rising temperatures expand vector habitats and transmission seasons.
	Urbanization and poor planning	Unplanned settlements with poor drainage create mosquito breeding grounds.
	Agricultural and development projects	Irrigation schemes, dams, and deforestation alter ecosystems, enhancing vector breeding sites.
Political and Operational	Conflict and instability	Armed conflict and political unrest disrupt health service delivery and malaria control programs.
	Cross-border transmission	Malaria elimination is undermined in countries sharing porous borders with high-burden neighbors.
	Policy and governance gaps	Weak political commitment, fragmented coordination, and limited integration across sectors impede sustained progress.

Insecticide Resistance in Mosquitoes

Vector control remains one of the pillars of malaria prevention. Widespread dissemination of insecticide-treated nets (ITNs) and indoor residual spraying (IRS) has been credited with preventing millions of cases since the early 2000s (World Health Organization, 2024). However, the effectiveness of these interventions is progressively undermined by insecticide resistance. Mosquitoes, in this case, Anopheles gambiae in Africa, have developed resistance to the most common insecticides—pyrethroids (Hemingway et al., 2016). This is an issue because pyrethroids are the only class approved for use in ITNs, and thus widespread resistance poses a huge danger to malaria control programs.

Resistance is driven by genetic mutations in mosquito populations and by alterations in vector behavior. Some Anopheles species now bite at different times, shifting from night to early evening or morning, when humans are less apt to be under nets (Ranson & Lissenden, 2016). These adaptations severely compromise traditional interventions. WHO has recommended the use of next-generation ITNs that also treat with additional insecticides, such as piperonyl butoxide (PBO), to circumvent resistance (WHO, 2023). PBO-treated nets can restore efficacy partially at higher cost, according to field trials in Tanzania and Uganda, which discourages wide-scale deployment (Gleave et al., 2018). IRS is also faced with these issues. While alternative insecticides such as organophosphates and carbamates are available, their cost and logistical requirements restrict use in resource-constrained settings (Oxborough, 2016). As such, without new, affordable insecticide options, vector control programs remain under the specter of resistance.

Drug Resistance and Treatment Failure

Artemisinin combination therapies (ACTs) have been the first line of treatment for *Plasmodium falciparum* malaria since the early 2000s. They facilitated the reduction in mortality, but resistance to artemisinin is currently a significant threat (Uwimana et al., 2021). Initially confined to the Greater Mekong Subregion, artemisinin resistance has been observed in East Africa, including Uganda and Rwanda (WHO, 2023). This dissemination raises fears over treatment failure in those nations with the highest burden of malaria mortality.

Resistance is manifested as decreased parasite clearance following treatment. While ACTs remain largely effective due to the partner drugs, more and more evidence exists for decreased efficacy of these combinations (Balikagala et al., 2021). Decreased susceptibility to lumefantrine, piperaquine, and amodiaquine has also been documented, which further narrows treatment options (Ashley et al., 2018). These trends are similar to the dire 20th-century chloroquine resistance crisis that caused millions to die. Methods to delay the onset of resistance are cycling treatment regimens, increased surveillance of response to treatment, and designing new drugs. Possible contenders such as ganaplacide-lumefantrine and triple ACTs are in development, but deployment on a large scale is decades away (Burrows et al., 2017).

Weak Health Systems and Surveillance in Endemic Areas

Effective malaria control depends on well-functioning health systems and good surveillance, but poor infrastructure bedevils the majority of endemic countries. Rural and distant communities in sub-Saharan Africa face ongoing shortages in diagnostic tools, critical medicines, and qualified healthcare workers (Snow et al., 2017).

Weak diagnostic capacity leads to under-reporting and misdiagnosis, concealing the true burden of malaria and hindering treatment. Other febrile illnesses are presumptively treated for malaria, yet some confirmed cases are not treated due to stockouts of ACTs (WHO, 2024). Supply chain issues are another critical vulnerability. Inadequate storage and distribution facilities often result in stockouts of drugs or outdated medicine in health facilities, reducing trust in health systems and driving patients towards care from informal providers (Patouillard et al., 2017).

Surveillance gaps limit the timeliness of outbreak detection. In the majority of nations, data collection relies on incomplete facility-based reports rather than active community surveillance (WHO, 2023). This delays the response to localized spikes and handicaps efforts at tracking trends of resistance. Programs involving community health workers have helped bridge some gaps by delivering diagnosis and treatment at the household level. However, the majority of CHWs are subjected to inadequate training, poor remuneration, and lack of supervision, compromising the program's effectiveness (Haines et al., 2007). Strengthening health systems remains the cornerstone to malaria elimination sustainability.

Impact of Global Events

Pandemics, conflict, and mass migration have extensive implications for malaria control. The COVID-19 pandemic showed exactly how quickly progress can be undone when global health systems are weakened. In 2020 alone, 55,000 additional malaria deaths were registered due to service disruption (WHO, 2021). Travel restrictions and lockdowns disrupted supply chains for mosquito nets, drugs, and diagnostics. Health workers were redirected to COVID-19 response efforts, and community-level malaria programs were suspended in most countries (Weiss et al.,

2021). The pandemic demonstrated the fragility of malaria gains to broader global health crises (Ogidi et al., 2021).

Conflict is yet another determinant. In South Sudan, Democratic Republic of Congo, and Yemen, armed conflict has devastated health infrastructure, displaced communities, and increased malaria incidence. Refugee camps generally provide ideal breeding grounds for malaria vectors due to overcrowding and poor sanitation. Migration also affects malaria transmission dynamics. Seasonal labor migration in Southeast Asia has rendered elimination more difficult along border regions, with mobile populations carrying parasites across national boundaries (Carrara et al., 2013). The mobility also re-introduces malaria into areas that had previously been malaria-free zones. Environmental catastrophes brought about by climate change also worsen the control of malaria. The floods in Pakistan in 2022 caused a surge of over 5 million malaria cases that overburdened the country's health system (WHO, 2023). Such weather extremes are projected to happen with increased frequency, which complicates elimination strategies.

Financing trends globally also form a weakness. Despite the heavy burden of malaria, financing has leveled off, and global investment stood at US$4 billion in 2023—just half of the US$8.3 billion required annually (WHO, 2024). Funding gaps endanger the long-term viability of interventions and the creation of new tools. Generally, dangers to malaria control and elimination are multifaceted. Insecticide resistance undermines vector control interventions, and drug resistance threatens the effectiveness of treatment. Weak health systems and poor surveillance permit ongoing transmission, and global crises—from pandemics to conflict and climate crises—exacerbate underlying vulnerabilities. Collectively, these difficulties explain the stalling of progress against malaria since the mid-2010s after earlier success. Goals of malaria elimination will remain out of reach unless these are addressed through new investment, innovation, and political will. Enduring control and eventual eradication are only possible through an integrated approach using biological, environmental, and socio-political solutions.

SOCIO-ECONOMIC IMPACTS OF MALARIA

Burden on Households

The impact of malaria on households is immense, especially in endemic and impoverished regions. Direct healthcare cost includes charges for laboratory tests, medicine, hospitalization, and transport to the health centers (Sachs & Malaney, 2002). In the majority of sub-Saharan nations, the charges consume a sizable portion of household income. In addition to direct spending, families lose indirect economic amounts. Caregivers often miss time in the workplace to provide care for ailing children, and adult patients may miss working for days or even weeks. This results in reduced productivity and lost wages, supplementing already stretched home economies (Chima et al., 2003).

Households living in malaria-endemic regions spend disproportionately on prevention, i.e., purchasing insecticide-treated bed nets (ITNs) or indoor spraying services. Affordability remains a challenge, and the nets are sometimes diverted to other uses due to the economic requirements (Pulford et al., 2011). Repeated bouts of malaria also undermine household resilience. Households are forced to sell off their assets, withdraw children from school in order to cut costs, or reallocate resources away from food security and housing upgrading (Hailu et al., 2009). The disease thereby drives intergenerational cycles of poverty. Poor households, particularly female-headed households or those located in rural areas, are also disproportionately hit. Lack of access to formal employment, health facilities, and financial protection mechanisms makes the economic effects of malaria worse (WHO, 2024).

Lost Labor Productivity

The cost of malaria is seen most drastically in terms of lost productivity in labor. Malaria affects primarily working-age adults and school-going children, devaluing both present and future economic capital (Gallup & Sachs, 2001). Farmers, the source of strength of rural African communities, become frequently incapacitated during malarial attacks, resulting in reduced output from farming. It is most impairing during periods of peak agricultural seasonality, when availability of labor has direct implications for local food security (Ettling et al., 1994). Children who suffer from recurrent malaria episodes exhibit persistent cognitive impairment and reduced educational attainment (Holding & Snow, 2001). This limits their future work productivity and generates poverty traps in the endemic regions.

Malaria absenteeism also affects formal employment. Malaria may lead to the loss of several days of work annually by workers in the construction, manufacturing, and mining industries. Employers incur additional costs in terms of lost productivity and absenteeism (Shepard et al., 2013). Macroeconomically, the net effect of malaria productivity losses significantly contributes to national economic subpar performance, particularly in high-transmission countries (Gallup & Sachs, 2001).

National Economic Estimates

The financial impact of malaria goes beyond individual families to national economies. Malaria has been estimated to lower GDP growth in epidemic nations by as much as 1.3% per year (Gallup & Sachs, 2001). This loss accumulates over the years and accounts for chronic income differentials between malaria-endemic and non-endemic nations. National exchequers are further saddled with heavy healthcare expenditure on malaria. Malaria is responsible for as much as 40% of sub-Saharan countries' public health expenditures, diverting resources away from other high-priority services such as maternal and child health (WHO, 2023).

Tourism, which is one of the major economic drivers in most African countries, is also adversely affected. Countries with a high rate of malaria transmission lose foreign visitors, who may perceive malaria as a public health threat (Wangdi et al., 2021). Loss of tourism revenues erodes overall economic growth. Foreign investment is also restricted due to malaria. Investors are able to avoid malaria-endemic regions due to concerns regarding the health of labor, insurance costs, and disruption of activities (Bloom & Sachs, 1998). Such lost opportunities further perpetuate underdevelopment. Conversely, malaria elimination has been shown to generate economic gains. Those countries that have eliminated malaria, such as Sri Lanka, have experienced improved investment climates and tourism growth (Feachem et al., 2019). This highlights the economic advantage of sustained malaria control.

Regional Disparities and Vulnerability Factors

Socio-economic effects of malaria are not evenly distributed. Sub-Saharan Africa bears the majority of the disease, accounting for 94% of cases and 95% of deaths in 2023 (WHO, 2024). Concentration of this disease worsens economic inequality between the rest of the world and Africa. Inequalities within regions are determined by socio-economic and geographical factors. Rural communities are more at risk of malaria due to inadequate shelter, lower levels of access to healthcare, and greater exposure to mosquito breeding sites (Tusting et al., 2017). Urban communities, although comparatively protected, are increasingly vulnerable with the spread of Anopheles stephensi in urban African cities (Sinka et al., 2020).

Poverty generates and is generated by malaria. Poor households have less ability to afford preventive gear, early treatment, or protective housing, making them more vulnerable. On the other hand, repeated malaria infections maintain poverty through health costs and missed income (Sachs & Malaley, 2002). Migration and displacement exacerbate the problem. Refugees and internally displaced individuals settle in populations with high transmission and inadequate protection, while wars bring about disruption to control operations. This has been witnessed in South Sudan, Yemen, and Myanmar.

Climate change widens regional disparities. Warmer temperatures and shifts in the patterns of rainfall will expand the areas for malaria transmission, making previously low-risk districts more economically exposed (Ryan et al., 2020). Poor nations with weakly developed health systems will struggle to adapt. Malaria, on the other hand, generates a disease-poverty cycle that slows down development at all tiers. Reducing its socio-economic burden requires biomedical interventions together with investments in education, infrastructure, and poverty alleviation (WHO, 2024).

CURRENT INITIATIVES & POLICY FRAMEWORKS

Roll Back Malaria Partnership

Roll Back Malaria (RBM) Partnership came into being in 1998 as a global mechanism for collaborative action against malaria. It brought together governments, multilateral agencies, private sector actors, and civil society to form a common platform for advocacy, mobilization of resources, and technical assistance (Roll Back Malaria, 2020). RBM played a key role in putting malaria onto the global health agenda. It helped in the fulfillment of global commitments that resulted in mass scale-up of interventions such as insecticide-treated nets (ITNs), rapid diagnostic tests, and artemisinin-based combination therapies (WHO, 2023).

This collaboration also enabled biennial Global Malaria Action Plans (GMAPs) that provided strategic blueprints for the control and elimination of malaria. The first GMAP (2008–2015) aimed to reduce malaria deaths globally to near-zero levels by 2015, while the next GMAP2 (2016–2030) aligned with the Sustainable Development Goals (SDGs) (Roll Back Malaria, 2020). RBM advocacy and communication have ensured the maintenance of political will. For instance, World Malaria Day campaigns raised public attention and sustained donor investment in malaria financing (WHO, 2024). However, RBM has been faced with inconsistent implementation of its strategies across the countries and dependence on unreliable donor support. Despite these, it is still a central convening platform for partnerships to end malaria worldwide (Roll Back Malaria, 2020).

The Global Fund to Fight AIDS, Tuberculosis, and Malaria

The Global Fund was established in 2002 as a financing mechanism to support country-led programs aimed at fighting malaria, HIV/AIDS, and tuberculosis. The Global Fund then grew into the largest multilateral financier of malaria control (Global Fund, 2023). Between 2002 and 2022, the Global Fund disbursed more than US $16 billion for malaria programs, accounting for over 50% of all worldwide financing for malaria (Global Fund, 2023). These investments have funded ITN distribution, diagnostics, treatment, and community health worker programs.

Support from the Global Fund has immensely increased access to lifesaving interventions. As of 2022, Global Fund-supported programs had delivered more than

230 million ITNs and administered 1.3 billion malaria treatments across the world (Global Fund, 2023). The performance-based financing mechanism of the Global Fund enforces accountability by linking disbursements to quantifiable outcomes. This model has enhanced program effectiveness in most recipient countries (Atun & Kazatchkine, 2010). Yet, the Global Fund remains beset by persistent funding shortfalls. The gap between available resources and the estimated demands of the globe persists, particularly with drug and insecticide resistance increasing program costs (WHO, 2024).

WHO Strategies and Global Technical Frameworks

The World Health Organization (WHO) plays a pivotal role in setting global standards for malaria control. WHO launched the Global Technical Strategy for Malaria (GTS) 2016–2030 in 2015, setting ambitious goals for reducing malaria incidence and mortality by 90% by 2030 and malaria elimination in at least 35 countries (WHO, 2015). The GTS is based on three pillars: universal access to malaria prevention, diagnosis, and treatment; intensified drive toward elimination in chosen nations; and innovation in tools and methods of implementation (WHO, 2015). The progress under the GTS has been combined. Despite the prevention of millions of cases and deaths since its introduction, the 2023 targets for incidence and mortality were not achieved, and global incidence remains three times greater than the optimum level (WHO, 2024).

WHO launched the High Burden to High Impact (HBHI) strategy in 2023, aiming at the 11 highest malaria-burdened countries. The approach emphasizes data-driven strategies, political engagement, and country ownership for accelerated progress (WHO, 2023). WHO further prequalifies malaria medicines and vaccines, ensuring safety and efficacy. Its prequalification of the RTS,S and R21/Matrix-M vaccines in 2021 and 2023, respectively, were record milestones for malaria prevention (WHO, 2024).

National Malaria Control Programmes

National Malaria Control Programmes (NMCPs) are the operational field strength for malaria response. NMCPs are national programmes implementing global strategy at the country level with substantial external donor support from organisations such as the Global Fund, PMI, and WHO (Snow et al., 2017). In sub-Saharan Africa, NMCPs have implemented mass ITN distribution campaigns that underpin malaria prevention. For example, Nigeria's NMCP distributed more than 30 million ITNs in a single year alone in 2021 (WHO, 2023). Rwanda and Ethiopia have demonstrated political will through the integration of malaria services into community health worker programs, significantly improving access to diagnosis and treatment in rural areas (Whitty et al., 2021).

In Asia, Sri Lanka and China eliminated malaria with strong NMCPs that focused on surveillance, cross-border coordination, and continued government support (Feachem et al., 2019). National leadership is key to elimination, as these experiences point out. Though good progress has been made, capacity is a problem for most NMCPs, with inadequate surveillance systems, low funding, and shortages of skilled staff. Maintaining strong NMCPs is crucial to meeting elimination goals (Snow et al., 2017).

Strategic plan summaries from other high-burden countries:

Nigeria: Nigeria's National Malaria Strategic Plan (2021-2025) is a case in point. Under this plan: The goal is to reduce parasite prevalence to below 10% and lower mortality attributable to malaria to fewer than 50 deaths per 1,000 live births by 2025. Key objectives include achieving ≥80% access to vector control interventions, ensuring diagnosis, chemoprevention, and treatment for 80% of at-risk populations, strengthening malaria data reporting from health facilities, and increasing funding through predictable and innovative sources (Whitty et al., 2021).

Uganda: Under the Uganda Malaria Reduction and Elimination Strategic Plan (UMRESP) 2021–2025, Uganda's goals are to reduce malaria morbidity by 50% and malaria-related mortality by 75%, using 2019 levels as baseline. Key strategic objectives include accelerating access to preventive and curative malaria services; improving quality of services in both public and private sectors; promoting behaviour change and community engagement; using robust data and evidence for malaria programming; moving targeted districts from control to elimination phases; and strengthening coordination, multisectoral collaboration, and political commitment at all levels. Core interventions emphasise vector control, case management, chemoprevention and vaccine deployment in high-risk groups, surveillance & operational research, plus advocacy, social mobilisation, and private sector partnerships (Snow et al., 2017).

Ghana: Ghana's National Malaria Elimination Strategic Plan (2024–2028) targets a 90% reduction in malaria mortality and a 50% reduction in malaria incidence by 2028, using 2022 as baseline. Alongside this, Ghana aims to eliminate malaria in 21 districts with very low burdens by 2028. Major strategic emphases include strengthening active and passive surveillance and monitoring & evaluation systems; ensuring all confirmed cases are treated quickly and completely (within 72 hours); expanding vaccine coverage; maintaining mass distributions of long-lasting insecticide-treated nets; indoor residual spraying; and focusing on high-risk populations (especially children under five and pregnant women) and vulnerable regions (WHO, 2024).

Democratic Republic of the Congo (DRC): The DRC's National Malaria Strategic Plan 2024–2028 aims to reduce malaria morbidity by 70% and malaria mortality by

50% from 2021 levels. Its strategic pillars include protecting at least 90% of people exposed to malaria risk through adequate measures by 2028 (e.g. mass and routine distribution of ITNs, targeted indoor residual spraying, entomological surveillance and insecticide resistance management), improved case management using rapid diagnostics and artemisinin-based therapies, preventive treatment for pregnant women and infants, community engagement, and multisectoral collaboration. Strengthening governance, supply chains, surveillance systems, human resource capacity, and prioritization of vulnerable populations are central dimensions (WHO, 2023).

Integration with Broader Health and Development Goals

Malaria control is increasingly understood to be integral to overall health and development policy. Malaria control has a direct contribution towards the achievement of Sustainable Development Goal (SDG) 3 of having healthy lives and well-being for all people at all ages (United Nations, 2015). Malaria control interventions also advance Universal Health Coverage (UHC) as it expand access to priority health care services such as diagnostics, treatment, and preventive interventions. Malaria services are integrated into primary health systems to enhance resilience against other health risks (WHO, 2024).

Investment in malaria control also contributes to economic development through the prevention of healthcare costs and improvement in labor productivity, thus complementing SDG 1 on poverty elimination and SDG 8 on economic growth (Sachs & Malaney, 2002). Malaria programs also intersect with education outcomes. Malaria reduction improves school attendance and cognition, complementing SDG 4 on quality education (Holding & Snow, 2001).

Furthermore, gender equality comes as a result of controlling malaria. Women are typically expected to take care of family members who have fallen ill and get disproportionately affected during pregnancy, when malaria causes serious complications. Successful malaria interventions consequently promote SDG 5 on gender equality (WHO, 2023). Integration with the greater health frameworks also improves efficiency. For instance, malaria programs might converge with maternal and child health programs, immunization campaigns, and nutrition programs in a manner where they utilize common infrastructure and resources (Atun et al., 2010). International and country-level malaria action has recorded unprecedented gains since the early 2000s. The RBM Partnership, Global Fund, and WHO frameworks have mobilized resources, expressed strategic priorities, and supported national programs. But durable challenges—like resistance, weak health systems, and financing gaps—threaten to return progress to zero.

Aligning malaria control with broader development goals, namely the SDGs and UHC, offers a means to ensure continued progress. Linking malaria interventions with economic growth, education, and gender equality makes malaria control both an imperative for health as well as an agent of social and economic transformation. Finally, prolonged political will, creative funding, and inter-sectoral partnership will be required in order to realize the lofty target of malaria elimination by 2030. In their absence, the globe will lose the gains of the last twenty years (Afakwu-Adimoha & Ogidi, 2025).

ROLE OF NATURAL PRODUCT-BASED DRUG RESEARCH

Historical Perspective: Plant-Derived Antimalarials

The historical trajectory of malaria control and treatment is deeply intertwined with the use of natural products. One of the oldest and most effective antimalarials was possibly, the quinine derived from the bark of the Cinchona tree, native to South America (Achan et al., 2011). The use of Cinchona bark to cure fevers by the native population precedes its incorporation into European medicine. Quinine was first isolated in 1820 by French chemists Pierre Joseph Pelletier and Joseph Caventou, revolutionizing the treatment of malaria in the 19th and 20th centuries (Butler & Newman, 2008). Quinine remained the gold standard treatment for decades and was central to the reduction of malaria mortality in colonial areas (Enenebeaku et al., 2021, 2022b).

The discovery of chloroquine, a man-made derivative of quinine, in the 20th century was another milestone. Chloroquine was cheap, very effective, and widely spread from the 1940s onwards (Slater, 2009). It was the backbone of global malaria eradication efforts for several decades. However, the emergence of chloroquine resistance in Southeast Asia and Africa during the 1950s–60s was a tremendous blow for malaria control (Payne, 1987). Resistance spread globally and eroded decades of progress, underlining vulnerability in reliance on one class of drugs. The second natural product revolution was the isolation of artemisinin from Chinese medicinal plant Artemisia annua. In the 1970s, Chinese scientist Tu Youyou isolated artemisinin, which was the foundation of the most effective antimalarial drugs to date (Tu, 2011).

Gains and Limitations of Past Successes

Artemisinin and its derivatives have been the biggest assets to modern malaria management. In combination therapies (ACTs), they reduced mortality due to malaria globally from the early 2000s significantly (WHO, 2024). Their rapid action against blood-stage parasites rendered them more effective than the older drugs. The success of artemisinin-driven drugs also highlighted the importance of ethnopharmacology and traditional medicine in drug discovery. Tu Youyou's work demonstrated that centuries-old remedies could yield modern breakthroughs when studied with rigorous scientific methods (Tu, 2011).

Drugs derived from natural products are limited as well. Quinine and chloroquine, for all their early promise, were eventually undermined by widespread resistance. The same pattern has been repeated with artemisinin, where partial resistance has emerged in Southeast Asia and Africa (Uwimana et al., 2021). Drug resistance points to an inherent limitation of natural product-based drugs: parasites will always evolve under selective pressure. Without sustained innovation, even the most potent compounds are diminished over time (Dondorp et al., 2009).

Another limitation lies in supply and production. Quinine had to be extracted from the bark of Cinchona, and artemisinin production depends upon the cultivation of *A. annua*, which is susceptible to agricultural variability and long growth cycles (van Agtmael et al., 1999). This renders large-scale, cheap production problematic. Semi-synthetic processes have partially overcome this constraint. For instance, synthetic biology has been used to engineer yeast to produce artemisinin precursors, which increases scalability (Paddon et al., 2013). However, these kinds of technologies are costly and not yet widely used in low-income settings.

Renewed Interest in Biodiversity-Rich Regions of the Global South

Given the growing risk of resistance, researchers are once more turning to natural products as a source of new antimalarial prospects. Biodiversity hotspots of the Global South, and in particular tropical forests in Africa, Asia, and Latin America, are being regarded as treasure chests of prospective therapeutic compounds (Graziose et al., 2010). The traditional medicine systems of Africa alone have identified hundreds of plant species with antimalarial activity. As an example, extracts of *Cryptolepis sanguinolenta* (West Africa) and *Azadirachta indica* (neem tree, India) have shown promising activity in preclinical studies (Willcox et al., 2011; Ogidi et al., 2025c, 2020).

Marine organisms represent another new frontier in antimalarial drug discovery. Secondary metabolites of sponges, cyanobacteria, and algae have been discovered to possess antiplasmodial activity in the laboratory (Martins et al., 2019). These sources are even less investigated than terrestrial plants. The revival of interest in natural products is also motivated by the global push for bioprospecting with equity. The Nagoya Protocol on Access and Benefit Sharing provides for equitable sharing of benefits from genetic resources, which encourages research and development partnerships at the local level (Convention on Biological Diversity, 2014).

Sub-Saharan African nations are also putting more money into research on local medicinal plants. Each of Nigeria, Ghana, and South Africa has established national institutes for researching herbal medicines in the hope of developing standardized, clinically tested remedies (Chinsembu, 2016). Latin America is also leveraging its own biodiversity. Screening programs at research institutes in Brazil have tested plants from the Amazon region for antimalarial activity and identified potential candidates such as Aspidosperma alkaloids for future development (Oliveira-Ferreira et al., 2010).

In Asia, the ancient Ayurvedic and Chinese systems of medicine still inform drug discovery pipelines. Besides A. annua, other plants such as Swertia chirata and Tinospora cordifolia are also being explored for antimalarial activity (Chirangi et al., 2018). The integration of ethnopharmacology with contemporary screening technologies has accelerated the discovery process. High-throughput screening, metabolomics, and computer-assisted drug design allow researchers to identify promising leads more efficiently than in the past (Harvey et al., 2015). Though progress has been achieved, significant challenges remain. Natural product leads frequently fail during clinical development due to toxicity, poor bioavailability, or lack of efficacy in vivo (Graziose et al., 2010). Rigorous standardization and validation remain crucial to success.

Partnerships between international consortia and Global South institutions are closing these gaps. Initiatives like the Medicines for Malaria Venture (MMV) foster natural product research while ensuring accessibility and affordability of resulting therapies (MMV, 2023). Renewed interest in natural products is not only a scientific necessity but also a political and economic opportunity. By investing in traditional knowledge and biodiversity, Global South countries can lead global drug discovery (Chinsembu, 2016).

At the same time, ethical concerns must be resolved. Historical cases of biopiracy—where firms extracted knowledge and materials without reciprocity have fueled suspicion. Equitable benefit-sharing agreements must be in place to avoid a repeat of earlier mistakes (Convention on Biological Diversity, 2014). Natural product-based drug discovery has a past as well as a future contribution to make to malaria. Quinine and artemisinin serve to illustrate the potential of natural products to revolutionize treatment, and continued efforts in biodiversity hotspots hold out the prospect of additional breakthroughs. But problems of resistance, production, and equity must be wisely managed if long-term success is to be realized.

LINKING BURDEN TO DISCOVERY

How Burden Mapping Directs Lead Compound Discovery

Burden mapping is being used to direct malaria drug discovery. By outlining regions of highest incidence, mortality, and drug resistance, researchers can prioritize regions in most need of new medicines (Ogidi et al., 2025a; Snow et al., 2017). For example, the WHO's High Burden to High Impact (HBHI) initiative names 11 countries that are home to two-thirds of the world's malaria burden. Research priorities also align with such countries because they are areas where resistance is spreading and treatment failure would be disastrous (WHO, 2024). Plotting out resistance "hotspots" also informs discovery pipelines. Artemisinin resistance discovered in Southeast Asia and East Africa has targeted screening campaigns on compounds active against resistant parasite strains (Uwimana et al., 2021).

Geospatial mapping also facilitates the determination of parasite diversity. Molecular epidemiology studies in Africa reveal regional variation in Plasmodium falciparum strains, with implications for drug candidate development that is effective against local genetic variants (Amambua-Ngwa et al., 2019). Burden mapping also aids drug discovery target funding. Global Fund and Medicines for Malaria Venture (MMV) are among global donors that allocate funding for discovery programs based on epidemiological data from high-burden areas (MMV, 2023).

Community-Based Ethnobotanical Approaches

Ethnobotanical data have historically provided the foundation of antimalarial drug discovery, and both artemisinin and quinine are sourced from traditional medicine systems (Butler & Newman, 2008). Today, individuals in endemic communities continue to play a significant role in the identification of new leads. Field ethnobotanical surveys document local knowledge of medicinal plants used to treat fevers and malaria-like illnesses. These plants may then be screened for antiplasmodial activity, forming the basis of modern discovery programs (Willcox et al., 2011). For instance, Cryptolepis sanguinolenta was traditionally used to treat malaria in West Africa for centuries. Laboratory studies confirmed that its alkaloids have significant antimalarial activity, demonstrating the value of communal practice (Boye & Ampofo, 2018).

Similarly, in East Africa, *Azadirachta indica* (neem) and Artemisia afra feature conspicuously in herbal medicines, and laboratory research has validated their potential (Chinsembu, 2016). These findings bridge traditional medicine and biomedical science. Public interest also enables biocultural conservation. By recognizing the utility of local knowledge, discovery programs can promote sustainable utilization of biodiversity with adherence to intellectual property rights under the Nagoya Protocol (Convention on Biological Diversity, 2014).

Partnerships Between Endemic-Country Institutions and Global Research Networks

Drug discovery increasingly depends on the collaboration of endemic-country institutions and global research networks. This collaboration ensures that research becomes relevant, equitable, and sustainable. African, Asian, and Latin American institutions are at the forefront of ethnopharmacological research. The Noguchi Memorial Institute for Medical Research in Ghana and the National Institute for Pharmaceutical Research and Development in Nigeria, for example, are leading natural product discovery (Chinsembu, 2016). Collaborations with organizations such as Medicines for Malaria Venture (MMV) provide technical expertise, funding, and international compound library access (MMV, 2023). This collaboration accelerates local plant extracts and chemical derivative screening.

Such networks as the Multilateral Initiative on Malaria (MIM) also increase collaboration by linking African institutions with global research laboratories. This enables training, technology transfer, and co-authorship of cutting-edge malaria work (Njama-Meya et al., 2017). Involvement of local countries in global networks ensures benefit sharing. Unlike earlier extractive models of "biopiracy," today's architectures pay attention to local intellectual property rights and equitable access to resultant medicines (Convention on Biological Diversity, 2014). Collaborations also enhance clinical trial capacity. For example, Tanzanian, Burkinabé, and Malian research sites in Africa are now part of global networks of drug trials, so it is feasible for candidate molecules to be tested in actual-world high-burden contexts (Tinto et al., 2015).

Coupled with drug discovery, burden mapping ensures that research addresses the most important issues in malaria control. Research can focus where it will do the most good since high-burden populations and areas of resistance hotspots are local, by knowing where high-burden areas and resistance hotspots are. Community-led ethnobotany continues to produce valuable leads by being coupled with centuries of customary information. When verified by contemporary science, these remedies can promise new therapies, as quinine and artemisinin once did. Finally, an exchange between endemic-country institutions and global research networks is the foundation of equity and sustainability of drug discovery. By combining local expertise with global resources, these partnerships provide pathways to innovative, accessible, and culturally appropriate solutions to malaria.

OPPORTUNITIES AND FUTURE DIRECTIONS

Advances in Screening Technologies, Synthetic Biology, and Drug Safety

High-throughput screening technologies have transformed the discovery of antimalarial drugs. It is possible to screen thousands of synthetic compounds and natural product extracts for antimalarial activity on automated platforms in a significantly shorter time compared to the past (Harvey et al., 2015). Phenotypic screening approaches allow researchers to directly observe parasite inhibition without prior knowledge of molecular targets. This is particularly valuable for malaria, where parasite biology remains complex and not completely understood (Burrows et al., 2017). Genomics and metabolomics have also enhanced drug discovery. By studying parasite transcriptomes and metabolomes, researchers can identify druggable pathways and screen compounds that disrupt parasite metabolism (Cowell & Winzeler, 2019).

Synthetic biology represents another frontier. Microbes such as yeast and bacteria have been redesigned to make complex natural products, and this has already revolutionized artemisinin supply chains, making production more reliable and scalable (Paddon et al., 2013). Advances in medicinal chemistry also enable the creation of semi-synthetic derivatives of natural products. Artemisinin derivatives and novel endoperoxides have been and are being created to combat emerging resistance (Burrows et al., 2017). Drug safety testing has also improved. Modern toxicology platforms, including organ-on-a-chip technologies, can assess safety profiles early, reducing costly failures in later clinical trials (Ewart et al., 2018).

Integrating Traditional Knowledge with Modern Drug Development

Traditional medicine is still the key foundation for the inspiration of drug discovery for malaria. Ethnopharmacology produces leads that can be verified and improved through modern pharmacological tools (Willcox et al., 2011). *Cryptolepis sanguinolenta*, for example, which has been used in West African medicine for centuries, has yielded alkaloids of possible antimalarial activity (Boye & Ampofo, 2018). Other than plant-based medicine, traditional knowledge about preparation methods and polyherbal blends may provide insight into synergies that are sometimes lost in modern screening (Chinsembu, 2016).

There is a need for collaborative platforms in the integration of indigenous knowledge. Partnerships among national research institutions, local communities, and global drug discovery programs are needed to ensure equitable benefits sharing and scientific validation (Convention on Biological Diversity, 2014). The Nagoya Protocol provides a legal platform for the preservation of community rights as well as bioprospecting for international health needs. This ensures that communities benefit from the commodification of resources and knowledge (CBD, 2014). Asian and African examples have proven that involving local healers in research not only strengthens discovery pipelines but also enhances cultural acceptance of new drugs (Willcox et al., 2011).

Building Regional Research and Development Infrastructure and Capacity

A main opportunity is establishing research capacity in the malaria-endemic nations. A great deal of the pipeline for drug discovery is still in the Global North, with limited local ownership (Njama-Meya et al., 2017). The addition of laboratory infrastructure in Africa, Asia, and Latin America would allow regional scientists to conduct sophisticated screening, pharmacological confirmation, and clinical trials close to the sources of biodiversity (Chinsembu, 2016). Investment in compound libraries and biobanking in endemic nations can facilitate systematic exploration of domestic biodiversity for antimalarial compounds (Harvey et al., 2015).

Training programs are no less critical. Building capacity in medicinal chemistry, pharmacognosy, and clinical pharmacology will make endemic-country scientists first-string leaders of discovery research rather than second-string partners (Njama-Meya et al., 2017). Regional excellence centers are on the horizon. South Africa's Medical Research Council and Nigeria's National Institute for Pharmaceutical Research and Development (NIPRD), for instance, have established strong platforms for validating herbal medicines (Chinsembu, 2016). These can be replicated across other regions. Cross-border collaboration further enhances research sustainability. Regional consortia, such as the African Network for Drugs and Diagnostics Innovation (ANDI), provide shared infrastructure and facilities for discovery (Nwaka et al., 2010).

Policy and Funding Models Supporting South-Led Innovation

Financing has been a persistent constraint to malaria drug discovery. Donor-driven models in the past have, by default, supported short-term solutions over long-term pipelines for discovery (WHO, 2024). New funding arrangements are needed to support South-led discovery. Public-private partnership models, such as those established by the Medicines for Malaria Venture (MMV), demonstrate how risk-sharing can accelerate innovation while making products affordable (MMV, 2023). Funding within endemic countries is also important. Governments should invest in Research and Development (R&D) capacities such that the identification of drugs against malaria becomes a national priority rather than a donor agenda (Nwaka et al., 2010).

South-South collaboration is also able to stimulate innovation. By the sharing of experience and resources, African, Asian, and Latin American nations can collectively drive natural product investigation (Njama-Meya et al., 2017). Intellectual property and access issues will also need to be addressed through policy frameworks. Reasonable license deals have the potential to balance innovation incentives with public health demands, providing new drugs in poor settings (Sachs & Malaney, 2002). International agencies such as the WHO and the African Union can play a coordinating function in aligning national policies with international strategies to avoid duplication and ensure complementarity (WHO, 2024). The future opportunities in malaria drug discovery are based on the merging of technological advancements and local knowledge and infrastructure.

High-throughput screening, synthetic biology, and improved safety testing are opening new avenues for effective and scalable medicine. There are still excellent leads from conventional medicine, and respectful interaction with indigenous communities can enrich drug discovery pipelines while preserving cultural and ethical integrity. Building strong regional R&D infrastructure is key to bringing the center of discovery closer to endemic areas. This will not only empower local researchers but also make sure that research priorities take into consideration local needs. Finally, new funding and policy models must support South-led innovation. Without sustainable funding and equitable policies, exciting scientific advances may not translate into medicines that reach everyone. Through combinations of technological innovation, local knowledge, capacity development in the region, and enabling policy frameworks, the global community can unlock new paths to sustainable malaria elimination.

CONCLUSION

Malaria continues to be one of the biggest 21st-century global health burdens, with sustained morbidity and mortality following decades of control. While tremendous progress was made in the early 2000s through global scale-up of insecticide-treated nets, artemisinin-based combination treatments, and enhanced surveillance, recent times have witnessed a flagging of progress due to drug and insecticide resistance, health system shortcomings, and funding gaps. The disease remains deeply entrenched in sub-Saharan Africa, and it has serious impacts on households, the economies of nations, and human development, which reaffirms its dual character as a health and economic issue. Malaria chemotherapy history is a testament to the pivotal role that has been occupied by drug discovery based on natural products, with quinine and artemisinin standing out as two of the most important advances in medical history. That legacy hints at the continued relevance of biodiversity and traditional knowledge in the discovery of new compounds. At the same time, burden mapping and resistance tracking are critical intelligence for directing discovery to where, within the regions and parasite strains, new treatments are needed most urgently. Synchronizing burden information with discovery pipelines ensures that scientific inquiry remains in tandem with evolving epidemiologic facts.

In the future, there is the possibility of blending technological advancement with locally oriented approaches. Advances in methodology in high-throughput screening, synthetic biology, and new toxicology provide robust methodologies for drug discovery. Combining conventional medicine knowledge with comprehensive clinical testing can yield culturally acceptable, scientifically sound therapies. Establishing effective research and development capabilities within endemic nations will allow local researchers to lead innovation and make discoveries relevant to local requirements and priorities. Finally, long-term success will hinge on balancing scientific potential with policy platforms and sustainable financing. South-led innovation, supported by fair partnerships and benefit-sharing mechanisms, will be the foundation for creating affordable and accessible solutions. Through incorporating burden metrics, discovery strategies, and sustainable delivery, the international community can come together on the ultimate goal of the eradication of malaria as a public health issue in the 21st century.

REFERENCES

Achan, J., Talisuna, A. O., Erhart, A., Yeka, A., Tibenderana, J. K., Baliraine, F. N., Rosenthal, P. J., & D'Alessandro, U. (2011). Quinine, an old anti-malarial drug in a modern world: Role in the treatment of malaria. *Malaria Journal, 10*(1), 144. DOI: 10.1186/1475-2875-10-144 PMID: 21609473

Afakwu-Adimoha, H. C., & Ogidi, O. I., (2025). Health care financing and achieving universal health care in Bayelsa: Changing the narrative through health insurance. *World Journal of Biology Pharmacy and Health Sciences*, *21*(3), 361–373. DOI: 10.30574/wjbphs.2025.21.3.0383

Amambua-Ngwa, A., Tetteh, K. K. A., Manske, M., Gomez-Escobar, N., Stewart, L. B., Deerhake, M. E., & Conway, D. J. (2019). Population genomic scan for candidate signatures of balancing selection to guide antigen characterization in malaria parasites. *PLOS Genetics*, *15*(9), e1008535. PMID: 23133397

Ashley, E. A., Dhorda, M., Fairhurst, R. M., Amaratunga, C., Lim, P., Suon, S., & Dondorp, A. M. (2018). Spread of artemisinin resistance in *Plasmodium falciparum* malaria. *The New England Journal of Medicine*, *371*(5), 411–423. DOI: 10.1056/NEJMoa1314981 PMID: 25075834

Atun, R., & Kazatchkine, M. (2010). The Global Fund's strategic shift: The challenge of integrating HIV, tuberculosis, and malaria programs into health systems. *Health Policy and Planning*, *25*(1), i1–i3. DOI: 10.1093/heapol/czp053 PMID: 19959485

Balikagala, B., Fukuda, N., Ikeda, M., Katuro, O. T., Tachibana, S. I., Yamauchi, M., & Tsuboi, T. (2021). Evidence of artemisinin-resistant malaria in Africa. *The New England Journal of Medicine*, *385*(13), 1163–1171. DOI: 10.1056/NEJMoa2101746 PMID: 34551228

Beat Malaria. (2024). *2024 World Malaria Report: What you need to know*. Retrieved from https://beatmalaria.org

Bhatt, S., Weiss, D. J., Cameron, E., Bisanzio, D., Mappin, B., Dalrymple, U., Battle, K. E., Moyes, C. L., Henry, A., Eckhoff, P. A., Wenger, E. A., Briët, O., Penny, M. A., Smith, T. A., Bennett, A., Yukich, J., Eisele, T. P., Griffin, J. T., Fergus, C. A., & Gething, P. W. (2015). The effect of malaria control on *Plasmodium falciparum* in Africa between 2000 and 2015. *Nature*, *526*(7572), 207–211. DOI: 10.1038/nature15535 PMID: 26375008

Bloom, D. E., Sachs, J. D., Collier, P., & Udry, C. (1998). Geography, demography, and economic growth in Africa. *Brookings Papers on Economic Activity*, *1998*(2), 207–273. DOI: 10.2307/2534695 PMID: 12295931

Boye, G. L., & Ampofo, O. (2018). Cryptolepine hydrochloride: An alkaloid from *Cryptolepis sanguinolenta. Journal of Ethnopharmacology*, *213*, 36–45.

Burrows, J. N., van Huijsduijnen, R. H., Mohrle, J. J., Oeuvray, C., & Wells, T. N. (2017). Designing the next generation of medicines for malaria control and eradication. *Malaria Journal*, *16*(1), 187. DOI: 10.1186/1475-2875-12-187 PMID: 23742293

Butler, M. S., & Newman, D. J. (2008). Mother Nature's gifts to diseases of mankind: The impact of natural products on anti-infective drug discovery. *Annals of the New York Academy of Sciences*, *1213*(1), 136–156.

Caminade, C., Kovats, S., Rocklov, J., Tompkins, A. M., Morse, A. P., Colón-González, F. J., Stenlund, H., Martens, P., & Lloyd, S. J. (2014). Impact of climate change on global malaria distribution. *Proceedings of the National Academy of Sciences of the United States of America*, *111*(9), 3286–3291. DOI: 10.1073/pnas.1302089111 PMID: 24596427

Carrara, V. I., Lwin, K. M., Ashley, E., Price, R. N., & Nosten, F. (2013). Malaria burden and artemisinin resistance in mobile populations on the Thai–Myanmar border. *Malaria Journal*, *12*(1), 1–9.

Centers for Disease Control and Prevention. (2024). *Malaria: Biology*. https://www.cdc.gov/malaria/

Chima, R. I., Goodman, C. A., & Mills, A. (2003). The economic impact of malaria in Africa: A critical review of the evidence. *Health Policy (Amsterdam)*, *63*(1), 17–36. DOI: 10.1016/S0168-8510(02)00036-2 PMID: 12468115

Chinsembu, K. C. (2016). Plants as antimalarial agents in Sub-Saharan Africa. *Acta Tropica*, *152*, 32–48. DOI: 10.1016/j.actatropica.2015.08.009 PMID: 26297798

Chirangi, R. B., Pandey, D. K., Kumar, N., & Mishra, S. (2018). Phytochemicals of traditional medicinal plants with potential antimalarial activity: An updated review. *Journal of Ethnopharmacology*, *225*, 352–381.

Convention on Biological Diversity. (2014). *Nagoya Protocol on Access and Benefit-Sharing*. CBD.

Cowell, A. N., & Winzeler, E. A. (2019). Exploration of the Plasmodium falciparum kinome for targets of established chemotherapeutic agents. *Nature Reviews. Microbiology*, *17*(1), 33–46.

Datoo, M. S., Natama, H. M., Somé, A., Traoré, O., Rouamba, T., Bellamy, D., Yameogo, P., Valia, D., Tegneri, M., Ouedraogo, F., Soma, R., Sawadogo, S., Sorgho, F., Derra, K., Rouamba, E., Orindi, B., Ramos Lopez, F., Flaxman, A., Cappuccini, F., & Tinto, H. (2021). Efficacy of a low-dose candidate malaria vaccine, R21/Matrix-M, with seasonal administration to children in Burkina Faso: A randomized controlled trial. *Lancet, 397*(10287), 1809–1818. DOI: 10.1016/S0140-6736(21)00943-0 PMID: 33964223

Dondorp, A. M., Fairhurst, R. M., Slutsker, L., MacArthur, J. R., Breman, J. G., Guerin, P. J., & Ringwald, P. (2009). The threat of artemisinin-resistant malaria. *The New England Journal of Medicine, 361*(5), 455–457. DOI: 10.1056/NEJMoa0808859 PMID: 19641202

Enenebeaku, C. K., Ogukwe, C. E., Nweke, C. O., Anyado-Nwadike, S. O., Obi, M., Duru, I. A., Enenebeaku, U. E., & Ogidi, O. I. (2022a). Antiplasmodial and *in vitro* antioxidant potentials of crude aqueous and methanol extracts of *Chasmanthera dependens* (Hochst). *Bulletin of the National Research Center, 46*(33), 1–12. DOI: 10.1186/s42269-022-00721-3

Enenebeaku, U. E., Duru, C. E., Okotcha, E. N., Ogidi, O. I., Mgbemena, I. C., Nwigwe, H. C., & Enenebeaku, C. K. (2022b). Phytochemical analysis and antioxidant evaluation of crude extracts from the roots, stem and leaves of *Dictyandra arborescens* (Welw.). *Tropical Journal of Natural Product Research, 6*(1), 62–70. DOI: 10.26538/tjnpr/v6i1.12

Enenebeaku, U. E., Ukwandu, N. C., Mgbemena, I. C., Nwigwe, H. C., Enenebeaku, C. K., Duru, C. E., & Ogidi, O. I. (2021). Oral acute toxicity and antimalarial potentials of aqueous and methanolic extracts of roots, leaves and stem of *Dictyandra arborescens* (Welw.) on *Plasmodium berghei* infected mice. *Bulletin of the National Research Center, 45*(75), 1–12. DOI: 10.1186/s42269-021-00530-0

Ettling, M. B., McFarland, D. A., Schultz, L. J., & Chitsulo, L. (1994). Economic impact of malaria in Malawian households. *Tropical Medicine and Parasitology, 45*(1), 74–79. PMID: 8066390

Ewart, L., Dehne, E. M., Fabre, K., Gibbs, S., Hickman, J., Hornberg, E., & Swanson, B. (2018). Application of microphysiological systems to enhance safety assessment in drug discovery. *Annual Review of Pharmacology and Toxicology, 58*(1), 65–82. DOI: 10.1146/annurev-pharmtox-010617-052722 PMID: 29029591

Feachem, R. G., Chen, I., Akbari, O., Bertozzi-Villa, A., Bhatt, S., Binka, F., & Weiss, D. J. (2019). Malaria eradication within a generation: Ambitious, achievable, and necessary. *Lancet*, *394*(10203), 1056–1112. DOI: 10.1016/S0140-6736(19)31139-0 PMID: 31511196

Gallup, J. L., & Sachs, J. D. (2001). The economic burden of malaria. *The American Journal of Tropical Medicine and Hygiene*, *64*(1–2), 85–96. DOI: 10.4269/ajtmh.2001.64.85 PMID: 11425181

Gavi. (2024). *Rolling out vaccines to beat malaria together: Time to harness the power of immunisation for a malaria-free future*. https://www.gavi.org/news-resources/resources/knowledge-products/rolling-out-vaccines-beat-malaria-together-time-harness-power-immunisation-malaria-free-future

Gleave, K., Lissenden, N., Richardson, M., Choi, L., & Ranson, H. (2018). Piperonyl butoxide (PBO) combined with pyrethroids in insecticide-treated nets to prevent malaria in Africa. *Cochrane Database of Systematic Reviews*, *2018*(11). Advance online publication. DOI: 10.1002/14651858.CD012776.pub2 PMID: 30488945

Global Fund. (2023). *Malaria: Global Fund results report 2023*. Retrieved from https://www.theglobalfund.org

Graziose, R., Lila, M. A., & Raskin, I. (2010). Merging traditional Chinese medicine with modern drug discovery technologies to find novel drugs and functional foods. *Current Drug Discovery Technologies*, *7*(1), 2–12. DOI: 10.2174/157016310791162767 PMID: 20156139

Hailu, A., Lindtjørn, B., Deressa, W., Gari, T., & Loha, E. (2009). Economic burden of malaria and predictors of cost variability to rural households in south-central Ethiopia. *Malaria Journal*, *8*(1), 214.

Haines, A., Sanders, D., Lehmann, U., Rowe, A. K., Lawn, J. E., Jan, S., Walker, D. G., & Bhutta, Z. (2007). Achieving child survival goals: Potential contribution of community health workers. *Lancet*, *369*(9579), 2121–2131. DOI: 10.1016/S0140-6736(07)60325-0 PMID: 17586307

Harvey, A. L., Edrada-Ebel, R., & Quinn, R. J. (2015). The re-emergence of natural products for drug discovery in the genomics era. *Nature Reviews. Drug Discovery*, *14*(2), 111–129. DOI: 10.1038/nrd4510 PMID: 25614221

Hemingway, J., Ranson, H., Magill, A., Kolaczinski, J., Fornadel, C., Gimnig, J., & Gething, P. W. (2016). Averting a malaria disaster: Will insecticide resistance derail malaria control? *Lancet*, *387*(10029), 1785–1788. DOI: 10.1016/S0140-6736(15)00417-1 PMID: 26880124

Holding, P. A., & Snow, R. W. (2001). Impact of *Plasmodium falciparum* malaria on performance and learning: Review of the evidence. *The American Journal of Tropical Medicine and Hygiene*, *64*(1–2), 68–75. DOI: 10.4269/ajtmh.2001.64.68 PMID: 11425179

Keiser, J., Singer, B. H., & Utzinger, J. (2005). Reducing the burden of malaria in different eco-epidemiological settings with environmental management: A systematic review. *The Lancet. Infectious Diseases*, *5*(11), 695–708. DOI: 10.1016/S1473-3099(05)70268-1 PMID: 16253887

Martens, P., & Hall, L. (2000). Malaria on the move: Human population movement and malaria transmission. *Emerging Infectious Diseases*, *6*(2), 103–109. DOI: 10.3201/eid0602.000202 PMID: 10756143

Martins, A., Vieira, H., Gaspar, H., & Santos, S. (2019). Marketed marine natural products in the pharmaceutical and cosmeceutical industries: Tips for success. *Marine Drugs*, *17*(3), 145. PMID: 30832207

Medicines for Malaria Venture. (2023). *Annual report 2023: Advancing the fight against malaria*. MMV.

Njama-Meya, D., Clark, T. D., Nzarubara, B., Staedke, S. G., Kamya, M. R., Dorsey, G., & Rosenthal, P. J. (2017). Treatment of malaria restricted to laboratory-confirmed cases: A prospective cohort study in Ugandan children. *Malaria Journal*, *16*(1), 1–8. PMID: 28049519

Nwaka, S., Ilunga, T. B., Da Silva, J. S., Rial Verde, E., Hackley, D., De Vré, R., & Ridley, R. G. (2010). Developing ANDI: A novel approach to health product R&D in Africa. *Nature Reviews. Drug Discovery*, *9*(6), 437–443. PMID: 20613865

Ogidi, O. I. (2020). A review on the use of herbal remedies and clinical therapeutics for the management of COVID-19 pandemic. *ASIO Journal of Pharmaceutical & Herbal Medicines Research*, *6*(2), 68–77. http://doi.org/doilink/10.2020.85722646

Ogidi, O. I. (2022). Omicron (B.1.1.529): Variant of concern—A mini review. *Biomedical Journal of Scientific & Technical Research*, *41*(5), 33106–33112. DOI: 10.26717/BJSTR.2022.41.006672

Ogidi, O. I., Afakwu-Adimoha, H. C., & Indiamaowei, D. L. (2023). E-health care system in Nigeria: The current status, issues and future prospective. *World Journal of Advanced Healthcare Research*, *7*(4), 75–83.

Ogidi, O. I., Aye, T., & Felagha, I. (2025b). Antiviral therapeutics for emerging viruses. In Aslam, M., Yingngam, B., Javed, T., & Riaz, S. (Eds.), *Global perspectives on antiviral drug development* (pp. 217–260). IGI Global., DOI: 10.4018/979-8-3693-9276-8.ch006

Ogidi, O. I., Berefagha, W. L., & Okara, E. (2021). COVID-19 vaccination: The pros and cons. *World Journal of Biology Pharmacy and Health Sciences*, *7*(1), 15–22. DOI: 10.30574/wjbphs.2021.7.1.0072

Ogidi, O. I., Ebong, C. U., & Ikimi, C. G. (2025c). Lifespan-extending natural compounds. In Chen, J. (Ed.), *Drug discovery and antiaging approaches for human longevity* (pp. 351–390). IGI Global., DOI: 10.4018/979-8-3693-9730-5.ch010

Ogidi, O. I., Ogoun, T. R., & Tobia, P. S. (2025a). Antimalarial activities and lipid profile of ethanolic extract of *Ficus sur* Forssk (described by Peter Forsskål) in *Plasmodium berghei* infected albino rats. *Journal of Ethnopharmacology*, *348*, 119901. DOI: 10.1016/j.jep.2025.119901 PMID: 40306496

Oliveira-Ferreira, J., Lacerda, M. V. G., Brasil, P., Ladislau, J. L. B., Tauil, P. L., & Daniel-Ribeiro, C. T. (2010). Malaria in Brazil: An overview. *Malaria Journal*, *9*(1), 115. DOI: 10.1186/1475-2875-9-115 PMID: 20433744

Oxborough, R. M. (2016). Trends in US President's Malaria Initiative–supported indoor residual spray coverage and insecticide choice in sub-Saharan Africa (2008–2015): Implications for future vector control. *Malaria Journal*, *15*(1), 146. DOI: 10.1186/s12936-016-1201-1 PMID: 26957210

Paddon, C. J., Westfall, P. J., Pitera, D. J., Benjamin, K., Fisher, K., McPhee, D., Leavell, M. D., Tai, A., Main, A., Eng, D., Polichuk, D. R., Teoh, K. H., Reed, D. W., Treynor, T., Lenihan, J., Jiang, H., Fleck, M., Bajad, S., Dang, G., & Newman, J. D. (2013). High-level semi-synthetic production of the potent antimalarial artemisinin. *Nature*, *496*(7446), 528–532. DOI: 10.1038/nature12051 PMID: 23575629

Patouillard, E., Griffin, J., Bhatt, S., Ghani, A. C., Cibulskis, R., & Eckert, E. (2017). Global investment targets for malaria control and elimination between 2016 and 2030. *BMJ Global Health*, *2*(2), e000176. DOI: 10.1136/bmjgh-2016-000176 PMID: 29242750

Payne, D. (1987). Spread of chloroquine resistance in Plasmodium falciparum. *Parasitology Today (Personal Ed.)*, *3*(8), 241–246. DOI: 10.1016/0169-4758(87)90147-5 PMID: 15462966

Price, R. N., Commons, R. J., Battle, K. E., Thriemer, K., & Mendis, K. (2020). Plasmodium vivax in the era of the shrinking P. falciparum map. *Trends in Parasitology, 36*(6), 560–570. DOI: 10.1016/j.pt.2020.03.009 PMID: 32407682

Pulford, J., Hetzel, M. W., Bryant, M., Siba, P. M., & Mueller, I. (2011). Reported reasons for not using a mosquito net when one is available: A review of the published literature. *Malaria Journal, 10*(1), 83. DOI: 10.1186/1475-2875-10-83 PMID: 21477376

Ranson, H., & Lissenden, N. (2016). Insecticide resistance in African *Anopheles* mosquitoes: A worsening situation that needs urgent action to maintain malaria control. *Trends in Parasitology, 32*(3), 187–196. DOI: 10.1016/j.pt.2015.11.010 PMID: 26826784

Roll Back Malaria Partnership. (2020). *The RBM Partnership to End Malaria: Annual Report*. Retrieved from https://endmalaria.org

Rowe, A. K., Rowe, S. Y., Snow, R. W., Korenromp, E. L., Schellenberg, J. R., Stein, C., & Bryce, J. (2009). The burden of malaria mortality among African children in the year 2000. *International Journal of Epidemiology, 38*(3), 791–801. PMID: 19351697

Ryan, S. J., Carlson, C. J., Mordecai, E. A., & Johnson, L. R. (2020). Global expansion and redistribution of Aedes-borne virus transmission risk with climate change. *PLoS Neglected Tropical Diseases, 14*(3), e0007213. DOI: 10.1371/journal.pntd.0007213 PMID: 30921321

Sachs, J., & Malaney, P. (2002). The economic and social burden of malaria. *Nature, 415*(6872), 680–685. DOI: 10.1038/415680a PMID: 11832956

Shepard, D. S., Ettling, M. B., Brinkmann, U., & Sauerborn, R. (2013). The economic cost of malaria in Africa. *Tropical Medicine and Parasitology, 45*(1), 74–79. PMID: 1801147

Sherrard-Smith, E., Hogan, A. B., Hamlet, A., Watson, O. J., Whittaker, C., Winskill, P., & Ghani, A. C. (2022). The potential public health consequences of COVID-19 on malaria in Africa. *Nature Medicine, 26*(9), 1411–1416. DOI: 10.1038/s41591-020-1025-y PMID: 32770167

Sinka, M. E., Pironon, S., Massey, N. C., Longbottom, J., Hemingway, J., Moyes, C. L., & Hay, S. I. (2020). A new malaria vector in Africa: Predicting the expansion range of Anopheles stephensi and identifying the urban populations at risk. *Proceedings of the National Academy of Sciences of the United States of America, 117*(40), 24900–24908. DOI: 10.1073/pnas.2003976117 PMID: 32929020

Siraj, A. S., Santos-Vega, M., Bouma, M. J., Yadeta, D., Ruiz Carrascal, D., & Pascual, M. (2014). Altitudinal changes in malaria incidence in highlands of Ethiopia and Colombia. *Science, 343*(6175), 1154–1158. DOI: 10.1126/science.1244325 PMID: 24604201

Slater, L. B. (2009). *War and disease: Biomedical research on malaria in the twentieth century*. Rutgers University Press.

Snow, R. W., Sartorius, B., & Kyalo, D.. (2021). The prevalence of *Plasmodium falciparum* in sub-Saharan Africa since 1900. *Nature, 601*(7891), 547–553. DOI: 10.1038/s41586-021-04264-3 PMID: 29019978

Snow, R. W., Sartorius, B., Kyalo, D., Maina, J., Amratia, P., Mundia, C. W., Bejon, P., & Noor, A. M. (2017). The prevalence of *Plasmodium falciparum* in sub-Saharan Africa since 1900. *Nature, 550*(7677), 515–518. DOI: 10.1038/nature24059 PMID: 29019978

Tinto, H., Valea, I., Sorgho, H., Rouamba, N., Kaboré, Y., Kazienga, A., & D'Alessandro, U. (2015). Efficacy and safety of the candidate malaria vaccine RTS,S/AS01 administered according to different schedules in African children: A randomised controlled trial. *The Lancet. Infectious Diseases, 15*(12), 1451–1460.

Tu, Y. (2011). The discovery of artemisinin (Qinghaosu) and gifts from Chinese medicine. *Nature Medicine, 17*(10), 1217–1220. DOI: 10.1038/nm.2471 PMID: 21989013

Tusting, L. S., Rek, J., Arinaitwe, E., Staedke, S. G., Kamya, M. R., Cano, J., & Lindsay, S. W. (2017). Why is malaria associated with poverty? Findings from a cohort study in rural Uganda. *Infectious Diseases of Poverty, 5*(1), 78. DOI: 10.1186/s40249-016-0164-3 PMID: 27488674

United Nations. (2015). *Transforming our world: The 2030 Agenda for Sustainable Development*. Retrieved from https://sdgs.un.org

Uwimana, A., Umulisa, N., Venkatesan, M., Svigel, S. S., Zhou, Z., Munyaneza, T., & Udhayakumar, V. (2021). Association of *Plasmodium falciparum* kelch13 R561H genotypes with delayed parasite clearance in Rwanda. *Nature Medicine, 27*(2), 378–381. PMID: 33864801

van Agtmael, M. A., Eggelte, T. A., & van Boxtel, C. J. (1999). Artemisinin drugs in the treatment of malaria: From medicinal herb to registered medication. *Trends in Pharmacological Sciences, 20*(5), 199–205. DOI: 10.1016/S0165-6147(99)01302-4 PMID: 10354615

Wangdi, K., Gatton, M. L., Kelly, G. C., & Clements, A. C. (2021). Cross-border malaria: A major obstacle for malaria elimination. *Advances in Parasitology, 89*, 79–107. DOI: 10.1016/bs.apar.2015.04.002 PMID: 26003036

Weiss, D. J., Bertozzi-Villa, A., Rumisha, S. F., Amratia, P., Arambepola, R., Battle, K. E., & Bhatt, S. (2021). Indirect effects of the COVID-19 pandemic on malaria intervention coverage, morbidity, and mortality in Africa. *Nature Medicine, 27*(3), 703–709. PMID: 32971006

Whitty, C. J., Ansah, E. K., & Reyburn, H. (2021). Malaria control in Africa: Progress but still much to do. *BMJ (Clinical Research Ed.), 375*(2434).

WHO. (2021). *Malaria in the WHO South-East Asia Region 2000–2020*. World Health Organization. https://www.who.int [Access September 15, 2025]

WHO. (2022). *World Malaria Report 2022*. World Health Organization. https://www.who.int [Access September 15, 2025]

WHO. (2023). *WHO's annual malaria report spotlights the growing threat of climate change*. World Health Organization. https://www.who.int[Access September 15, 2025]

WHO. (2024). *World Malaria Report 2024*. World Health Organization. https://www.who.int [Access September 15, 2025]

Willcox, M., Graziose, R., & Bodeker, G. (2011). Traditional herbal medicines for malaria. *BMJ (Clinical Research Ed.), 343*, d7303. PMID: 15539672

World Health Organization. (2015). *Global Technical Strategy for Malaria 2016–2030*. WHO.

World Health Organization. (2025). *Malaria vaccines (RTS,S and R21): Questions and answers*. Retrieved from https://www.who.int/news-room/questions-and-answers/item/q-a-on-rts-s-malaria-vaccine [Access September 15, 2025]

Chapter 2
The Science of Phytochemicals An Introduction to Plant-Based Therapeutics

Aamir Abdullah
https://orcid.org/0000-0002-1046-9422
Annamalai University, India

Abdullah Khan
https://orcid.org/0009-0000-9609-6438
C.G. Bhakta Institute of Biotechnology, Uka Tarsadia University, Surat, India

R. Somasundaram
Annamalai University, Cuddlore, India

Sana Rais
https://orcid.org/0009-0005-3435-9251
Department of Botany, Aligarh Muslim University, Aligarh, India

ABSTRACT

Phytochemicals, the bioactive secondary metabolites produced by plants as part of their defense mechanisms, have gained significant attention for their multifaceted role in plant-based therapeutics. These compounds—mainly alkaloids, flavonoids, and terpenoids—not only ensure plant survival under biotic and abiotic stresses but also provide numerous health-promoting effects in hum, phytochemicals contribute to the nutritional, sensory, and therapeutic value of plant-derived foods, while serving as vital resources in modern drug discovery and development.

DOI: 10.4018/979-8-3373-5821-5.ch002

1. INTRODUCTION TO PHYTOCHEMICALS

1.1 Definition and Significance

Phytochemicals, a term that was derived from the Greek word "*phyto*", means plant. These non-nutritive plant compounds contribute majorly to plant growth and provide defense against pathogens and herbivores. Although they have various pharmacological properties, phytochemicals are not considered an essential nutrient in a human diet and are not required for basic survival (Thakur & Sharma, 2018). Medicinal plants are one of the rich source of bioactive compounds, which play a protective role in human health. These compounds include carbohydrates, flavonoids, steroids, tannins, alkaloids, and terpenoids. The synthesis of such compounds occurs through both primary and secondary metabolic pathways (Jan et al., 2021). Plant-derived metabolites show long-term beneficial effects on health and are widely recognized for their therapeutic potential. Secondary metabolites are therefore considered highly important because they are produced in greater quantities and contribute significantly to the medicinal and tonic properties of plants. Phytochemicals support human health by exhibiting a wide range of biological activities, including antioxidant, anti-inflammatory, antibacterial, antiaging, and anticancer effects. These widely distributed compounds are found in dietary sources like fruits, vegetables, grains, and seeds, and are increasingly recognized for their medicinal properties (Hossain et al., 2025). Phytochemicals are classified into various groups, including polyphenols, terpenes, sulphur-containing compounds, nitrogen-containing compounds, flavonoids, and alkaloids. These compounds arise from primary and secondary plant metabolism and are responsible for the flavour, colour, and protective functions in plants (Afzal et al., 2023).

Phytochemicals are increasingly regarded as natural alternatives to synthetic preservatives owing to their antimicrobial, antioxidant, and anti-enzymatic activities. They protect food quality by inhibiting spoilage and pathogenic organisms through mechanisms such as membrane disruption, metabolic interference, and free radical scavenging. Phenolic compounds, especially flavonoids and tannins, have demonstrated antimicrobial activity by targeting bacterial cell walls and vital proteins, while their strong antioxidant capacity plays a major role in preventing lipid peroxidation, one of the primary factors responsible for rancidity and deterioration of food quality (Pons, 2024; Xu et al., 2024). Additionally, bioactive compounds such as catechins and chlorogenic acid are well recognised to suppress enzymatic browning of fruits and vegetables, thus extending shelf life and maintaining visual quality. For example, rosemary extract, rich in carnosic acid and carnosol, acts as an effective natural antioxidant in maintaining the quality in meat and oil-based products (Andrade et al., 2023).

Phytochemicals contribute substantially to the development of dietary supplements, which are commonly available in the form of capsules, tablets, powders, and liquid extracts. Liquid extracts have the advantage of rapid absorption, whereas in capsules and tablets, dosage can be controlled, and storage is easier, enabling longer use (Kato et al., 2023). Phytochemicals have received growing attention in the food industry as natural alternatives to synthetic preservatives in order to improve food quality and shelf life for a wide variety of products. Green tea extract, for example, has been found to improve the stability and functional attributes of dairy products, including yogurt and cheese (Celik et al., 2023). Similarly, cinnamon oil applied in fruit coatings suppresses microbial growth without degrading nutritional value and sensory quality (Piechowiak & Skóra, 2023). Furthermore, starch-based films containing grape seed extract have shown remarkable antimicrobial and antioxidant activities, strong mechanical properties, UV protection, and water resistance, making them highly effective for extending the freshness of moisture-rich foods (Zheng et al., 2023).

1.2 Historical Context of Plant-Based Therapeutics

Medicinal plants have played a critical role in healthcare across civilizations, with established knowledge preserved and transmitted through generations. Despite cultural and scientific transformations, this wisdom remains fundamental to natural medicine. For millennia, medicinal plants have been employed across cultures as reliable therapeutic agents, with knowledge transmitted through ancestral traditions and healer-to-healer practices. Many civilizations have compiled their own *Materia Medica*, documenting the curative use of plants. Integrating this traditional pharmacopeia with modern medical advancements provides a strong foundation for innovation in contemporary healthcare systems. (Kesarwani and Gupta., 2013). The ancient Indian Vedas document the use of medicinal plants, many of which remain indispensable as spices today, including nutmeg, pepper, and clove. Similarly, past records from the Bible and the Jewish Talmud highlight the utilisation of aromatic plants such as myrtle and incense in therapeutic rituals (Tucakov, 1971; Dimitrova, 1999). Theophrastus (371–287 BC) is regarded as the founder of botanical science through his seminal works *De Causis Plantarum* (Plant Etiology) and *De Historia Plantarum* (Plant History), in which he classified more than 500 medicinal plants known at the time. His writings include references to cinnamon, iris rhizome, false hellebore, mint, pomegranate, cardamom, fragrant hellebore, monkshood, and others. Notably, he prioritized the toxicological properties of certain plants and highlighted the concept of gradual dose adaptation in humans (Nikolovski, 1995). The early 19th century marked a key period in the scientific exploration and application of medicinal plants. During this time, the discovery and successful isolation of key alkaloids such as morphine from opium poppy in 1806, emetine from *Cephaelis ipecacuanha* in 1817, strychnine from *Strychnos* in 1817, quinine from cinchona bark in 1820, and pelletierine from pomegranate in 1878, followed by the identification of glycosides, laid the foundation for modern scientific pharmacy. Advancements in chemical techniques further enabled the isolation of additional bioactive compounds, including tannins, saponins, essential oils, vitamins, and hormones. Phytotherapy remains widely practiced, particularly in regions with limited access to conventional healthcare. While its use declined in industrialized nations in favour of synthetic drugs, the 21st century has seen renewed interest driven by research on the efficacy of plant-based compounds. Nonetheless, variability in potency and potential interactions with medications pose risks, highlighting the need for professional guidance. Overall, phytotherapy demonstrates the integration of traditional knowledge with modern scientific investigation in medicine (Ferreira et al., 2014)

1.3 Scope and Objectives

Phytochemicals are naturally occurring bioactive compounds found in plants, functioning in plant defense, growth, and reproduction, while in humans, they contribute to both the prevention and management of various chronic diseases. Phytochemical research mainly focuses on the identification, isolation, and characterization of these compounds to explain their mechanisms of action and explore their applications in nutrition and medicine (Huang et al., 2016). Antioxidants are bioactive compounds that inhibit or delay molecular oxidation and are classified as natural or synthetic. Common synthetic antioxidants, such as butylated hydroxyanisole (BHA) and hydroxytoluene (BHT), propyl gallate, and tert-butylhydroquinone, have raised safety concerns due to their potential toxicity and carcinogenic effects. Hence, there is growing interest in natural antioxidants, particularly from medicinal plants, which are rich sources of phytochemicals with antioxidant properties. Examples of such plant-derived antioxidants include tamarind, cardamom, lemongrass, and galangal basil, which are commonly used in traditional and ethnic foods (Javanmardi et al., 2003).

Numerous studies have demonstrated the antioxidant properties of various medicinal plants. Ethanolic extracts of *Areca catechu* exhibited higher antioxidant activity compared to *Centella asiatica*, *Punica granatum*, and *Glycyrrhiza glabra* (Ashawat et al., 2007). *Pandanus odoratissimus* and *Acorus calamus* were also reported to possess significant antioxidant activity, with a strong correlation observed between total phenolic content and antioxidant capacity (Zahin et al., 2009). Additionally, *Ocimum sanctum* showed dose-dependent inhibition of lipid peroxidation both *in vitro* and *in vivo*. Fruit consumption has also been linked to a reduction in the risk of many diseases. The antibacterial potential of *Punica granatum* extracts varies with the solvent used, with water extracts inhibiting *Bacillus subtilis* and *Staphylococcus aureus,* while organic solvent extracts were effective against a broader range of pathogens (Gil et al., 2002). Similarly, chloroform extracts of *Rauvolfia tetraphylla* and *Physalis minima* leaves demonstrated strong inhibitory activity against pathogenic bacteria (Shariff et al., 2006).

2. CLASSIFICATION OF PHYTOCHEMICALS

2.1 Overview of Major Classes

Figure 1. Schematic representation of phytochemical types

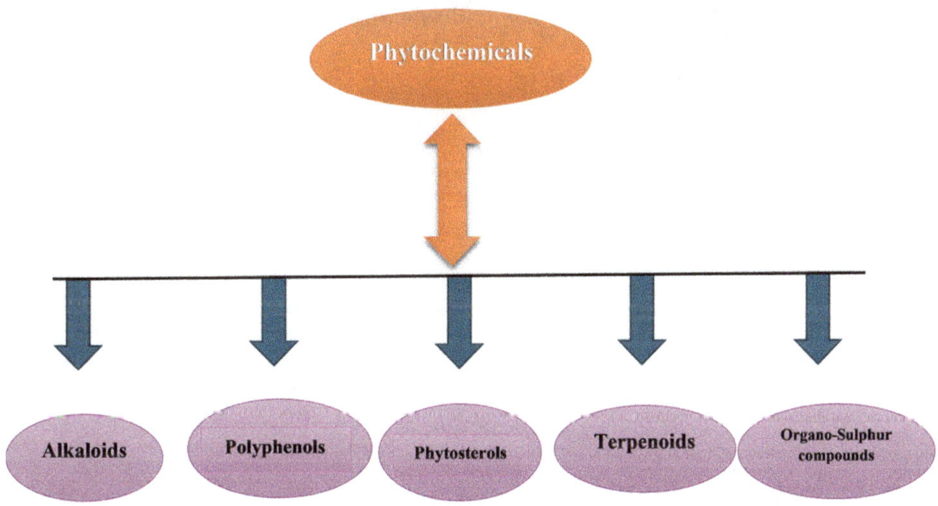

Table 1. Representation of Classes, key Examples, and functions of phytochemicals.

Class	Key Examples	Main Functions
Terpenoids	Carotenoids, essential oils	Pigmentation, aroma, antioxidant activity
Alkaloids	Morphine, caffeine	Defense, neuroactivity, pharmaceuticals
Polyphenols	Flavonoids, tannins	Antioxidant, antimicrobial activity, color
Phytosterols	Beta-sitosterol	Cholesterol absorption inhibition
Organo-sulphur Compounds	Allicin, S-allyl cysteine	Antimicrobial and antioxidant activity

2.2 Chemical Diversity and Biosynthesis

Phytochemicals constitute a structurally diverse group of plant-derived compounds, whose chemo diversity reflects evolutionary processes and ecological adaptations. Their biosynthesis is regulated via multiple metabolic pathways, shaped by genetic factors and influenced by environmental conditions.

Phytochemical diversity comprises of distinct small molecules, including alkaloids, phenolics, terpenoids, glycosides, and saponins. This diversity arises from conserved primary metabolic pathways common to wide range of plant lineages (see figure 2.2), as well as from specialized pathways restricted to particular taxa or ecological niche. Environmental factors such as habitat, climate, and soil conditions together with evolutionary pressures from herbivores and pathogens, have driven the emergence of novel and unique chemical structures across plant groups and ecosystems. Structurally, most phytochemicals can be categorized into four principal biosynthetic classes: alkaloids, phenylpropanoids, polyketides, and terpenoids. (Kumar et al., 2023).

Figure 2. Graphical Representation of Biosynthesis of Phytochemicals

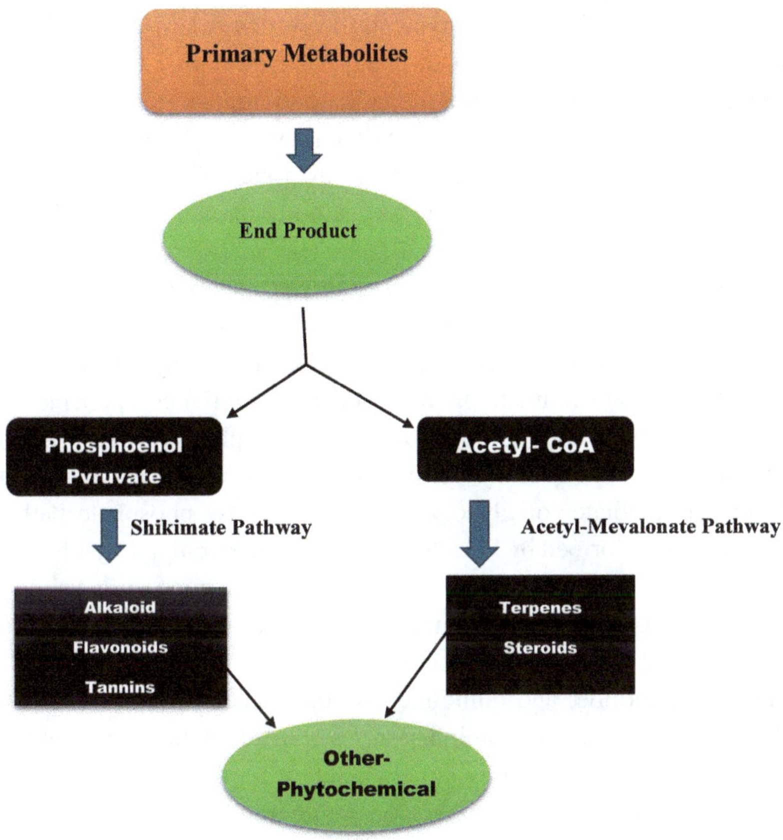

3. ALKALOIDS: CHEMISTRY AND PHARMACOLOGICAL ROLES

3.1 Structural Features and Biosynthesis

Alkaloids are naturally occurring nitrogen-containing compounds found in a wide range of plants, animals, fungi, and microbes, and they are among the most varied and pharmacologically significant categories. They are difficult to classify due to their various biosynthetic origins and structural complexity; however, they are mainly grouped according to their natural origin, chemical structure, and biosynthetic precursors (Gutiérrez-Grijalva et al., 2020). Protoalkaloids (non-heterocyclic), in which nitrogen atom is present in a side chain rather present in the main ring, and in true alkaloids (heterocyclic), nitrogen atom is directly placed into a heterocyclic ring structure. True alkaloids, which also include well-known examples like nicotine (pyridine alkaloid), quinine (quinoline alkaloid), morphine (isoquinoline alkaloid), and atropine (tropane alkaloid), are typically derived from amino acids like ornithine, lysine, tryptophan, and tyrosine (Dey et al., 2020; Gutiérrez-Grijalva et al., 2020). Furthermore, protoalkaloids such as mescaline and similar molecules produced from phenylalanine and tyrosine exhibit strong bioactivity in place of simpler structures (Dey et al., 2020). The third group, known as pseudoalkaloids, is different in its carbon structure and is derived from terpenoids, steroids, and polyketides rather than amino acids (Bhambhani et al., 2021).

Alkaloid biosynthesis is closely linked to key metabolic processes, including those that produce amino acids, nucleosides, and precursors of terpenoid compounds. Aromatic amino acids such as tryptophan, phenylalanine and tyrosine are derived from the shikimate pathway and are essential components for various alkaloids. 3-deoxy-D-arabino-heptulosonate-7-phosphate (DAHP) is formed by the condensation of phosphoenolpyruvate (PEP) and erythrose-4-phosphate (E4P), which are intermediates of glycolysis and the pentose phosphate pathway. This condensation is performed by DAHP synthase. Dehydroquinate synthase, dehydroquinate dehydratase, and shikimate dehydrogenase enzymes work as intermediates in the formation of shikimic acid in a sequential enzymatic reaction. Further from shikimic acid and chorismate, different aromatic amino acids are synthesised such as indole, isoquinoline, and quinoline alkaloids (Gandhi et al., 2023; Batory et al., 2022). Shikimic acid in combination with histidine purine pathway, xanthine alkaloids are also derived through methylation of purine bases (Bhambhani et al., 2021). Alkaloids, including atropine, scopolamine, and cocaine are derived from the ornithine–lysine–nicotinic acid pathway. Arginine and ornithine serve as precursor molecules that undergo decarboxylation, transamination and cyclization processes. Through the glutamine synthetase–glutamate synthase (GS–GOGAT) cycle, glutamate is an essential component in nitrogen metabolism pathways, improving alkaloid formation through nitrogen absorption from soil (Bhambhani et al., 2021; Kohnen-Johannsen & Kayser, 2019).

3.2 Pharmacological Activities

Alkaloids are also well recognised for their pharmacological actions. Indole group present in alkaloids makes its structure interesting for medical uses. Due to various modifications in indole group, it works to treat malaria, depression and cancer. Alkaloids also work against antibacterial, antifungal, antitumor, anticancer, and antimalarial diseases. However, many naturally occurring indolizidine alkaloids, such as Swainsonine, *Rhizoctonia leguminicola* alkaloids, and Slaframine, are extremely poisonous and can cause blood-brain barrier disruptions and neurological abnormalities, which restricts their use in clinical conditions (Omar et al., 2021; Rajput et al., 2022).

Table 2. Different Alkaloids and Their Roles.

Alkaloids	Plant Species	Pharmacological activity	Mechanism of action	Reference
Scopolamine, Hyoscyamine, Atropine	*Datura Stramonium* *Atropa belladonna*	Anticholinergic effect	Inhibiting action on sympathetic nervous system, antibacterial	(Wen et al., 2024)
Scholarisins, Capsaicin	*Alstonia rupestris* *Capsicum annuum*	Antifungal activity	Inhibit fungus *Gibberella pulicaris* and *Cercospora nicotianae,* Inhibit *Candida spp.*	(Periferakis et al., 2023; Uzor, 2020)
Kopsihainins	*Kopsia hainanensis*	antibacterial activities	Inhibit bacteria *Staphylococcus aureus*	(Mohammed et al., 2021)
Berberine, Erchinine	*Berberis Vulgaria, Ervatamia chinensis*	Anti-microbial	Lowers cholesterol through LDL receptor antibacterial and antifungal activities against *Trichophyton rubrum* and *Bacillus subtilis.*	(Huang et al., 2022)
17-nor-excelsinidine and strictamine, Trigonoliimine A, Naucleaoffines	*Alstonia scholaris,* *Trigonostemon lii, Nauclea officinalis*	Antiviral Activity	inhibit herpes simplex virus (HSV) and adenovirus (ADV) anti-HIV-1	(Omar et al., 2021)

continued on following page

Table 2. Continued

Alkaloids	Plant Species	Pharmacological activity	Mechanism of action	Reference
Piperine, Tabersonine, Naucleaorals, Vallesiachotamine, vincristine, vinblastine, Evodiamine	*Piper nigrum,* *Melodinus fusiformis,* *Nauclea orientalis,* *Anthocephalus cadamba,* *Vinca rosea,* *Evodia rutaecarpa*	Anticancer Activity	Lowers the tumor growth and exhibits cell cycle arrest and apoptotic cell death Works on human epidermoid carcinoma against the human lung cancer cell line H1299	(Mohammed et al., 2021; Omar et al., 2021)
Melaxillines, Colchicine, Caffeine	*Melodinus axillaris,* *Colchicum autumnale,* *Coffee arabica*	Anti-inflammatory activity	inhibition of β-glucuronidase secretion Inhibits microtubule polymerization Inhibits the activity of nucleotide phosphodiesterase enzyme	(Omar et al., 2021)
Codeine, Brucine, Umbellatine	*Papaver somniferum,* *Strychnos nux-vomica*	Analgesic Activity	CNS-stimulating action and cardiovascular effects, reduce fever, pneumonia, and laryngitis	(Bhambhani et al., 2021; Letchuman et al., 2025)
Vindoline, vindolidine, Akuammicine	*Catharanthus roseus,* *Picralima nitida*	Antidiabetic Activity	Inhibit protein tyrosine phosphatase 1B, enhanced glucose uptake in adipocytes	(Omar et al., 2021)
Ellipticine and olivacine, Flinderoles	*Aspidosperma vargasii* and *Aspidosperma olivaceum.* *Flindersia acuminate*	Antimalarial activity	against *Plasmodium falciparum*	(Omar et al., 2021)
Quinine	*Cinchona spp.*	Antimalaria, mild antipyretic, and analgesic	causes starvation in parasites by interfering with their capacity to digest and break down haemoglobin.	(Uzor, 2020)
Cocaine	*Erythroxylum coca*	Anaesthetic properties	CNS-stimulating action and cardiovascular effects	(Bhambhani et al., 2021)

3.3 Antimalarial Alkaloids: Quinine and Artemisinin

Malaria is a parasite disease that is exceedingly deadly and has noxious effects in many regions of the world. *Plasmodium falciparum* is the causative agent of malaria, a fatal infectious disease. Artemisinin and its derivatives, such as quinine, chloroquine, amodiaquine, and mefloquine used to treat malaria. The quinine alkaloid, which was isolated from the *Cinchona* tree, was the first effective antimalarial medication (Uzor, 2020).

Quinine is one of the oldest and most potent natural remedies for malaria. Malaria is a serious problem in areas like Africa and Asia. It mainly works by disrupting the hemoglobin digestive system of *Plasmodium* (Mishra et al., 2025). Quinine acts by interfering with *Plasmodium falciparum's* ability to generate hemozoin. Hemoglobin breakdown during the parasite blood stage produces free heme, which crystallizes into hemozoin to detoxify it. Because quinine prevents this process-toxic heme builds up and heme–drug complexes are formed, which eventually kill the parasite. Quinine shows disruption of hemozoin crystallization, and heme iron redistribution within the parasite has been verified by microscopic and spectroscopic analyses. Evidence shows quinine inhibits crystal formation by noncovalently adsorbing to heme, while its exact molecular interactions are still being studied. Quinine is still a big deal for treating malaria. Even with artemisinin resistance picking up more these days (de Villiers & Egan, 2021). Artemisinin was extracted from *Artemisia annua* plant.

Artemisinin and its analogues such as artemether, artether and artesunate, are considered as antimalarial drugs. WHO recommends malaria treated with artemisinin in combination with its analogue with additional medications (ACT) to control. They work quickly and effectively against *Plasmodium* species. Through the endoperoxide bridge, which is reductively activated in the parasite digestive vacuole primarily by ferrous heme produced during hemoglobin catabolism, ART pharmacological activity is mediated. Carbon-centered free radicals are created as a result of this activation, and they alkylate a variety of intracellular targets. With much lower heme alkylation found in ART-resistant strains. Recent studies show that using live parasites have validated free heme as a crucial alkylation target, connecting resistance phenotype to altered heme reactivity. The interruption of the heme detoxification pathway is one of the main effects of this heme interaction. Heme liberated during hemoglobin breakdown is typically trapped by crystallization into inert hemozoin. The degree to which ART directly inhibits hemozoin crystallization is under study, since contradicting data have surfaced under various redox conditions that define ferrous by ferric heme availability. However, ART appears to disrupt this process by creating stable heme drug addicts. However, the capacity of ART to alkylate heme and obstruct detoxification highlights heme metabolism as a key pharmacological target, which explains the molecular underpinnings of developing resistance as well as the strong schizonticidal action of ART (Ribbiso et al., 2021).

3.4 Mechanisms of Action in Malaria

Artemisinin, mainly used as an antimalarial treatment, is a sesquiterpene lactone is the most effective antimalarial drug; it has been rapidly replaced by chloroquine, pyrimethamine, and primaquine because of its moderate toxicity. The structural variations in artemisinin resulted in derivatives that improve the drug's solubility and therapeutic uses. All these treatments help to treat malaria and are highly effective against the *Plasmodium* parasite (Das et al., 2024).

Artemisinin works as it attaches to the heme molecule, rich in iron, which is generated in large numbers when hemoglobin breaks down inside infected red blood cells (RBCs). Such molecules accumulate remarkably onto the cell and activate its endoperoxide linkage. It also activates free radicals, which alkylate and deactivate parasitic proteins, and sometimes kill the parasite. Previous findings suggest that several non-heme targets, including glutathione S-transferase, translationally regulate tumour protein (TCTP), and endoplasmic reticulum calcium ATPase (PfATP6), in addition to heme, are a multifaceted process (Das et al., 2024; Yang et al., 2020).

4. FLAVONOIDS: STRUCTURE, FUNCTION, AND THERAPEUTIC POTENTIAL

4.1 Chemical structure and Subclasses

Flavonoids are one of the largest classes of polyphenolic compounds. Flavonoid structure contains a C6-C3-C6 carbon bond with A and B benzene rings that are attached to a heterocyclic C-ring which has oxygen incorporated in it. Based on A, B, and C rings substitution, various structures of flavonoids are formed (Rahaman & Mondal, 2020). Flavonoids exhibit high antioxidant activity in many plants. They also have many applications in the food industry as preservatives, pigments, and antioxidants, as well as in other industries like beauty and pharmaceuticals (Dias et al., 2021; Rahaman & Mondal, 2020).

Flavonoids are categorized as follows: flavones (e.g., apigenin, rutin), flavonols (e.g., quercetin, kaempferol), flavanols (e.g., epigallocatechin), isoflavonoids (e.g., genistein, daidzein), flavanones (e.g., naringenin, hesperidin), and anthocyanidins (e.g., cyanidin, malvidin), depending on the C-ring's oxidation, saturation, and B-ring linkage (Cao et al., 2022).

Flavonones: have a stereogenic C-2 skeleton with a 2S structure, e.g., naringenin. They are commonly found as 7-O-glycosides and may have a prenyl side chain (Dias et al., 2021).

Anthocyanins: found in angiosperms and provide attractive colour to the plant leaves, fruits, and flowers. They are O-glycosides of anthocyanidins; the most common among them are cyanidin, delphinidin, and pelargonidin (Dias et al., 2021).

Isoflavones: flavonones are changed to isoflavones by dehydrogenation and 2,3-aryl relocation. They contain anti-inflammatory qualities and are mostly found in Leguminosae species (Dias et al., 2021).

Flavones: mostly found as O or C glycosides, in their physically active form. They are also present in the form of C methylated, O-methylated, and isoprenylated (Dias et al., 2021).

4.2 Biological Activities

4.2.1 Antidiabetic effect

Flavonoids are mostly obtained from plants and have antidiabetic properties.

Quercetin, kaempferol, fisetin, naringenin, morin, and rutin are some of the flavonoids that have a hypoglycemic effect (Sok Yen et al., 2021). Additional work of flavonoids is to regulate adipogenesis and preventing the synthesis of aldose reductase, glycogen phosphorylase and glycation end products (AGE). Moreover, flavonoids also influence antidiabetic efficacy by hydroxylation, methoxylation, prenylation and glycosylation processes (Shamsudin et al., 2022).

4.2.2 Anti-inflammatory effect

Flavonoids are well known for their anti-inflammatory effect. Previous findings suggest that twelve different flavonoids help to inhibit the transcription of the cyclooxygenase-2 (COX-2) gene in DLD-1 cells, in a human colon cancer cell line. Some of the well-known flavonoids are quercetin, rhamnetin, genistein, eriodyctiol, luteolin, kaempferol, fisetin, phloretin, epicatechin, epigallocatechin, myricetin, and catechin. Additionally, flavonoids also reduce inflammation inhibiting LOX and COX-2 (Shamsudin et al., 2022).

4.2.3 Antioxidant effect

Flavonoids have strong antioxidant properties through various mechanisms, such as directly scavenging reactive oxygen species (ROS), inhibiting ROS-producing enzymes, chelation of transition metals, and amplification of endogenous antioxidant defenses. Flavonoids can also enhance the production of antioxidant enzymes, such as glutathione peroxidase, superoxide dismutase (SOD), and catalase, which together lessen the oxidative stress and help to prevent prolonged diseases such as diabetes, cardiovascular disease, cancer, and neurological disorders (Dias et al., 2021).

4.2.4 Anticancer effect

Cancer continues to be a major global health concern and a major barrier to the increase in life expectancy. Flavonoids show an anticancer effect through a variety of ways, including cell cycle arrest, angiogenesis reduction, apoptosis induction, and inactivation of carcinogens. Flavonoids works against breast, lung and stomach cancers. Kaempferol shows antiproliferative and apoptotic effects (Li et al., 2023). Similarly, genistein causes G2/M arrest and ROS-mediated apoptosis in prostate, breast, and ovarian cancer. Daidzein induces apoptosis in breast cancer cells, osteosarcoma, reduces ROS, and increases antioxidant defense mechanisms. Furthermore, hesperidin increases apoptosis, inhibits cell cycle progression, and improves antitumor as well as shows hepatoprotective effects (Dias et al., 2021).

4.3 Antimalarial Flavonoids: Mechanisms and Examples

Flavonoids are a large class of polyphenolic compounds generated from plants that have strong antimalarial properties (see Table 3), showing this via a variety of mechanisms. They prevent Plasmodium parasites from developing and multiplying by interfering with important metabolic and enzymatic functions. To prevent the synthesis of non-toxic hemozoin, certain flavonoids such as silymarin and its derivatives interfere with heme detoxification and lead to the accumulation of cytotoxic free heme. Flavonoids not only directly fight parasites but also work in concert to increase the effectiveness of traditional therapies. This also changes the host's immunological response to help in the removal of parasites.

Table 3. Plants with anti-malarial activity.

Plant	Flavonoids and/or their glycosides	Flavonoids class	Therapeutic activities	Reference
Prosopis spp	Quercetin, kaempferol derivatives	Flavonols, Flavones	Traditionally used in malaria treatment	(Sharifi-Rad et al., 2019)
Psiadia dentata, P. arguta	Lutenolin, apigenin glycosides; quercetin derivatives	Flavonols, Flavones	Inhibit growth of *P. falciparum*	(Ullah et al., 2020)
Euphorbia hirta	Quercitrin, myricitrin	Flavonols	In vivo antiplasmodial studies: reduced parasitemia by 44.36%	(Magozwi et al., 2021)
Waltheria indica (*W. americana*)	Epicatechin, kaempferol, quercetin	Flavonols	Antimalarial, toxic to animals in high doses.	(Nirmala & Sridevi, 2021)
Euphorbia cuneata	isoaromadendrin-7-*O*-*β*-d-glucopyranoside (isosinemsin)	Flavanones	In vivo studies in rats: decreased mean arterial blood pressure and heart rate	(Magozwi et al., 2021)
Vitis vinifera	Resveratrol	Flavonoids	*Plasmodium* spp. (malaria)-Highly effective, basis of ACTs	(Hermanto et al., 2024)
Artemisia annua	Acacetin, Artemetin, casticin, eupatorine, Quercetin-3,3'-dimethylether rhamnoglucoside	Flavones	*Plasmodium* spp. (malaria)- Highly effective, basis of ACTs	(J. Sun et al., 2025)
Silybum marianum	Silymarin complex (silybin, silydianin, silychristin)	Flavonolignans	Form silymarin heme complex; block hemozoin formation	(Ullah et al., 2020)
Camellia sinensis	Epigallocatechin-3-gallate	Flavanols	Inhibit parasitic growth	(Lacerda et al., 2025)

4.4 Flavonoids in Disease Prevention

Flavonoids' anti-inflammatory, antioxidant, and cardioprotective properties make them effective preventive agents against chronic diseases. They also reduce the risks of brain, heart, metabolic disorders, and cancer by improving oxidative stress, increasing vascular health, and modulating the key cellular pathways (Zeka et al., 2017). Some flavonoids such as chalcones, anthocyanins and citrus-derived compounds inhibit tumor, cell proliferation, apoptosis and signalling pathway regulation (Rupasinghe, 2020; Samtiya et al., 2021).

Flavonoids also work in reducing the risk of obesity related diseases such as hypertension, diabetes and cardiovascular diseases by inhibiting adipogenesis, increasing lipolysis, activating AMPK signalling and decreasing inflammation in adipose tissue. Nitric oxide and eNOS-mediated vasodilatory actions help in improves blood pressure regulation. Furthermore, flavonoids also works by lowering oxidative damage, promoting autophagy, and slow down the aging process (Rupasinghe, 2020).

Flavonoids also protect the blood-brain barrier and prevent from neurodegenerative disorders by regulating oxidative stress, protein aggregation, mitochondrial malfunction and neuro-inflammation. Extract of epigallocatechin-3-gallate, *Ginkgo biloba,* and quercetin protect dopaminergic neurons, lower oxidative stress, and delay Parkinson's disease-related motor impairment (Li et al., 2023). Frequent ingestion of foods or supplements high in flavonoids has been associated with better long-term health and may help avoid age-related neurological impairment (Zeka et al., 2017).

5. TERPENOIDS: NATURE'S LARGEST CLASS OF SECONDARY METABOLITES

5.1 Biosynthetic Pathways

Terpenoids are synthesized by two distinct pathways, the MVA and the MEP pathways. Also known as the 1-deoxy-D-xylulose-5-phosphate (DXP) mechanism. The MVA pathway, which is present in the cytoplasm of eukaryotes, begins with the condensation of two acetyl-CoA molecules to produce 3-hydroxyl-3-methylglutaryl (HMG-CoA) (Desmet et al., 2021). This intermediate is then reduced by HMG-CoA reductase (HMGR) to produce MVA, which is eventually converted to isopentenyl diphosphate (IPP). IPP isomerizes to dimethylallyl diphosphate (DMAPP) by isopentenyl diphosphate isomerase. Polyisoprene pyrophosphate synthetases use IPP and DMAPP as substrates to form sesquiterpene, triterpene, and steroid precursors (C. Zhang & Hong, 2020).

In addition, the MEP pathway is mostly present in plants and prokaryotes. In the MEP pathway, a sequence of enzymatic processes occurs to mediate the condensation of glyceraldehyde-3-phosphate (G3P) and pyruvate that finally form IPP and DMAPP. This helps in the formation of monoterpenes, diterpenes and tetraterpenes flavonoids in plants (Couillaud et al., 2021).

The three general phases of the MVA and MEP pathways are (i) the same synthesis of prenyl diphosphate precursors, (ii) the creation of the universal C5 intermediates IPP and DMAPP, and (iii) the generation of various terpenoid skeletons followed by structural changes. These two pathways are connected via metabolic crosstalk, even though they are separated into different subcellular locations in eukaryotes. Important, the MEP pathway directly obtains precursors from Calvin cycle intermediates, establishing a close relationship between terpenoid biosynthesis and photosynthesis (Huang et al., 2022).

5.2 Structural Diversity and Bioactivity

Terpenoids is one of the most structurally diverse form of natural chemicals, all are composed of five carbon isoprene unit attach in various ways by the isoprene unit. Depending on the number and arrangement of these units, terpenoids show a wide variety of structural frameworks, ranging from simple linear hydrocarbons to incredibly complex polycyclic molecules.

Hemiterpenes (C5): one isoprene unit is the source of the smallest terpenes, isoprene (C5H8), which plants release to protect themselves from stress (Mosquera et al., 2021).

Monoterpenes (C10): Monoterpenes form from two isoprene units which are present in different forms such as acyclic, monocyclic and bicyclic (Mosquera et al., 2021; Wu ct al., 2023).

Sesquiterpenes (C15): made up of three isoprene units, constitute these structurally varied compounds, which have both food and medical applications (Mosquera et al., 2021; Wu et al., 2023).

Diterpenes (C20): four isoprene units combinedly form diterpenes, which have pharmacological uses such as anti-inflammatory, antibacterial, and anticancer properties. It is present in different forms, such as macrocyclic, cyclic, and linear forms (Mosquera et al., 2021; Wu et al., 2023).

Triterpenes (C30): formed from squalene cyclization, include sterols and pentacyclic units, which are essential for membrane stability and therapeutic uses (Mosquera et al., 2021).

Tetraterpenes (C40): Formed from a long polyene chain with conjugated double bonds. Tetraterpenes give colour to plants, help in the formation of vitamin A and also have antioxidant activity (Mosquera et al., 2021).

5.3 Antimalarial Terpenoids: Artemisinin and Beyond

Artemisinin is commonly used as an antimalarial drug. Beyond it, a variety of terpenoids keep showing promise as effective treatments for drug-resistant *Plasmodium* strains. Pyrimethamine, primaquine, and chloroquine as the most effective antimalarial drugs due to their exceptionally high efficiency and low toxicity. The structural changes in artemisinin resulted in derivatives that improved the drug's solubility and therapeutic uses. Due to their reduced adverse effects and high effectiveness against *Plasmodium* blood stage parasites, these drugs are important to malaria treatment (Das et al., 2024).

Artemisinin works by using iron rich heme molecule, generated during the breakdown of haemoglobin in infected erythrocytes. Due to this breakdown reactive free radicals are form, which help to reduce parasitic proteins and sometimes kill parasites. Artemisinin also targeted some non-heme molecules including glutathione S-transferase, TCTP, and PfATP6, in addition to heme, suggesting a multifactorial process (Das et al., 2024; Yang et al., 2020).

5.4 Therapeutic Application

5.4.1 Antibacterial Action

Terpenoids work as antibacterial agents in a variety of ways, such as membrane rupture, biofilm suppression, and antibiotic effects. Menthol is a monoterpene that inhibits *Candida albicans* biofilm. Artemisinin derivatives inhibit microbes in a dose-dependent manner, and andrographolide suppresses *Pseudomonas aeruginosa* biofilm and increases azithromycin activity against *Staphylococcus aureus* (Yang et al., 2020).

5.4.2 Antimicrobial Action

Terpenoids have significant therapeutic potential in the treatment of inflammation and infections. It inhibits NF-κB, and other compounds such as linalool, D-limonene, and borneol reduce pro-inflammatory cytokines (Del Prado-Audelo et al., 2021). Additionally, either alone or in combination with antibiotics, monoterpene (carvacrol), sesquiterpenes (farnesol), diterpenes (salvipisone), and triterpenes (oleanolic acid) exhibit efficacy against drug-resistant *Mycobacterium tuberculosis* infection (Das et al., 2024).

5.4.3 Antiviral Action

Terpenoids also work as antiviral agents. Two monoterpenoids, such as isoborneol and borneol, inhibit HSV effects. Diterpenes such as andrographolide work against HSV-2, dengue, and chikungunya (moronic acid). It also inhibits HIV, HSV, and SARS-CoV. Pentacyclic triterpenoids such as ursolic, betulinic acid, and oleanolic acid are significant anti-HIV medicines, while derivatives of artemisinin (artesunate) exhibit strong anti-HBV/HCV activities (Das et al., 2024; de Sousa et al., 2023).

5.4.4 Neuroprotection and other applications of Terpenoids

Terpenoids have anti-inflammatory, antioxidant, and anti-apoptotic properties that help in neuroprotection. While limonene protects mitochondria, it inhibits protein aggregation and balances oxidative stress. *Ginkgo biloba* extracts (ginkgolides) decrease cytokines and inhibit COX-2, 5-LOX, and NF-κB, helping to prevent strokes and Parkinson's disease (de Lima et al., 2025).

6. PHYTOCHEMICAL EXTRACTION AND CHARACTERIZATION

6.1 Methods of Extraction

To isolate bioactive substances from plant material, phytochemical extraction techniques are employed

- **Maceration**: plant material is soaked in a solvent for two to seven days. This process is beneficial for thermolabile chemicals such as terpenoids, alkaloids, and phenolics (Abubakar & Haque, 2020; J. Sun et al., 2025).
- **Percolation:** the solvent passes through the plant material continuously. The wet mass is pressed to obtain the remaining extract. Although it requires a lot of solvent and takes a long time to extract, it is effective for essential oils and other phytochemicals (Bitwell et al., 2023).
- **Decoction:** in this process, plant material is boiled in water for 1-2 hours and the extract is collected to quantify flavonoids, tannins, and saponins (Bitwell et al., 2023).
- **Soxhlet Extraction**: dry plant material is repeatedly extracted in a thimble using refluxed solvent. It works well for flavonoids, terpenoids, steroids, and essential oils (J. Sun et al., 2025).
- **Enzyme-assisted extraction (EAE):** enzyme hydrolysis from cell wall through cellulose, hemicellulose and pectinases, bioactive compounds are extracted at a temperature of 33-67^{0}C and maintain pH ~ 4.5 for 20-220 minutes (Bitwell et al., 2023).
- **Supercritical Fluid Extraction (SFE):** supercritical CO_2 is used at above critical temperature (40-80 °C) and pressure (10-35 MPa) to extract compounds (Bitwell et al., 2023).

6.2 Solvent Selection and Green Chemistry

The polarity of the solvent with respect to the targets of the phytochemical determines the choice of solvent for phytochemicals, which are highly effective bioactive compound extracts from plants. The yield and activity of phytochemicals extraction are influenced by temperature, pH, particle size, solvent type, and pretreatments (S. Sun et al., 2025).

6.2.1 Solvent selection:

Polar solvent includes ethanol, water and methanol (Tzanova et al., 2020). Mixed solvents also improve bioactivity and yield. These high-yield and sustainable substitutes are provided by green solvents, such as Deep eutectic solvents (DES) (Natolino et al., 2024).

6.2.2 Time and Temperature:

high heat generally breaks down sensitive compounds, while moderate heat (40-60°C) enhances the extraction of phenolic or flavonoid compounds (Antony & Farid, 2022). Highly heat sensitive compounds are preserved by using supercritical CO_2 (Wang et al., 2021).

6.2.3 pH and Enzyme:

pH plays an important role as acidic pH increases anthocyanin, while alkaline pH enhances alkaloid formation. Cell wall are broken down by using cellulose and pectinases enzymes which improves extraction in plants (S. Sun et al., 2025).

6.2.4 Particle size and pre-treatment:

solvent penetration and yield are enhanced by smaller particles, grinding, freeze-drying, ultrasound, and microwaves (S. Sun et al., 2025).

6.3 Analytical Techniques for Phytochemical Identification

Accurate identification and detailed characterization of phytochemicals are crucial for corroborating their pharmacological properties and guaranteeing reproducibility in the pursuit of antimalarial agents. The isolation, identification, and structural elucidation of bioactive plant compounds requires the application of both classical and modern analytical techniques (Banu & Cathrine, 2015; Mutha et al., 2025).

Chromatographic techniques constitute a foundational element of phytochemical analysis. Specifically, Thin-Layer Chromatography (TLC) distinguishes compounds by exploiting their differential polarities in relation to the mobile phase. Owing to its economic viability and operational simplicity, TLC remains a widely favoured initial screening methodology for plant extracts. High-performance liquid chromatography (HPLC) and ultra-performance liquid chromatography (UPLC) provide higher resolution and sensitivity, enabling both qualitative and quantitative assessment of alkaloids, flavonoids, and terpenoids in complex mixtures. Coupling HPLC with diode array detection (DAD) or mass spectrometry (LC-MS) further increases compound identification by providing molecular mass and fragmentation patterns (T et al., 2024; Vij & Pathania, 2023).

Spectroscopic techniques are indispensable for structural elucidation. UV-Visible spectroscopy is commonly employed for the rapid detection of phenolic compounds, while Fourier Transform Infrared Spectroscopy provides extensive information regarding the functional groups within these compounds (Dev & Mukadam, 2025). Nuclear magnetic resonance spectroscopy remains the gold standard procedure for absolute structural elucidation as it provides detailed insights into molecular connections and stereochemistry (Abu Khalaf et al., 2019). For determining three-dimensional structures of phytochemicals possessing antimalarial properties, X-ray crystallography (XRC) is invaluable. By precisely mapping atomic arrangements, XRC facilitates identification of structural motifs effective against parasites (Amado et al., 2022).

In phytochemical analysis, mass spectrometry-based platforms have demonstrated efficacy. Gas chromatography-mass spectrometry (GC-MS) is a well-known technique for analyzing volatile compounds like essential oils and terpenoids, whereas liquid chromatography-tandem mass spectrometry (LC-MS/MS) stand out in profiling non-volatile and thermolabile metabolites (Frolova et al., 2025). Advances in high-resolution MS (HR-MS) and metabolomics approaches enable untargeted screening of almost the entire phytochemical profiles, thus facilitating the discovery of novel bioactive compounds. Advanced hyphenated techniques, such as LC-NMR, LC-MS, and GC-MS, not only accelerate the phytochemical identification process (Ahmad & Nadeem, 2022) but also improve sensitivity, reproducibility, and reliability, which are necessary for drug discovery programs targeting malaria (Mabuza, 2022.; Mutha et al., 2025).

7. TRANSLATIONAL APPLICATIONS IN MODERN MEDICINE

7.1 Phytochemicals in Drug Discovery

The discovery of antimalarial drugs has relied heavily on phytochemicals, which can act as direct therapeutic agents or scaffolds for synthetic alterations. The evolution of natural substances by which ethnobotanical knowledge contributes to a nationally accepted antimalarial medicine that can subsequently be used on an international scale includes quinine and artemisinin (Barman & Biswas, 2025). Recent advancements in computational biology, metabolomics, and high-throughput screening (HTS) have made the identification of novel phytochemicals with antimalarial effects much easier (Bankole et al., 2016; Mamede & Cristina, 2024; Tarkang et al., 2016). Due to their structural diversity and ability to act against *Plasmodium* strains, plant-derived alkaloids, terpenoids, and flavonoids remain interesting leads (Yu-Ping et al., 2024). Synthetic biology has enabled the use of designed microorganisms for the production of artemisinin precursors on a large scale, reducing dependency on natural plant harvests and ensuring supply stability (Paddon & Keasling, 2014; Seshadri et al., 2025). These examples highlight how phytochemicals have contributed to creative drug discovery pipelines both in the present and in the past.

7.2 Functional Foods and Nutraceuticals

Besides conventional drug development, phytochemicals are increasingly being investigated as functional foods and nutraceuticals that support general health and malaria prevention. High-flavonoid diets have been associated with improved oxidative balance and immunological modulation, which may reduce vulnerability to malaria indirectly (Zhang et al., 2024). It has been shown that polyphenols from medicinal herbs can increase the host's protective mechanism against parasite diseases (Sytar Oksana, 2012). A cost-effective way to supplement pharmacological interventions in endemic regions of the Global South is to incorporate such bioactive compounds into dietary practices. Nutraceutical formulations derived from plants like *Moringa oleifera* (Bezerra et al., 2023) and *Curcuma longa* (Jamil et al., 2023) have shown both nutritional and antimalarial supportive effects, offering systemic approaches to health management (Jamil et al., 2025). Phytochemicals signify the translational potential of food-derived compounds in malaria treatment, effectively connecting nutritional strategies with medicinal approaches.

7.3 Combination Therapies and Synergistic Effects

Perhaps the most promising translational uses of phytochemicals in this respect are their ability to act synergistically with notable antimalarial drugs. ACTs are the most successful example, combining a fast-acting phytochemical derivative with a longer-acting partner drug for enhanced efficacy and delaying resistance (Kangwanrangsan et al., 2025). It was determined that when phytochemicals were combined with standard antimalarial drugs, complementary effects could be produced (Alum, 2024). For example, it has been observed that flavonoids such as quercetin increase the effectiveness of chloroquine, while curcumin has demonstrated the ability to increase the activity of artemisinin (Jamil et al., 2023). Similarly, it has been shown that polyphenolic compounds inhibit efflux pumps in *Plasmodium*, making traditional medications more effective (Duda-Madej et al., 2025). Moreover, enhancing parasite clearance, the development of such synergic combinations presents a calculated approach against resistance (Yu-Ping et al., 2024). Since resistance to drugs remains one of the challenges facing malaria management, combination treatments based on phytochemicals represent a new and sustainable method for future curative strategies.

8. Case Studies: Phytochemicals in Antimalarial Therapy

8.1 Historical and Contemporary Use

Phytochemicals have revolutionized the history of malaria treatment. Quinine, which comes from the bark of *Cinchona* trees, was the first plant-derived substance to reliably alleviate the symptoms of malaria and was the mainstay of treatment for centuries. Its effectiveness prompted more research into alkaloids and set the stage for the creation of synthetic analogues, including chloroquine (Manisha et al., 2025). Beyond these classical examples, other classes of phytochemicals, most notably flavonoids and terpenoids, have also been examined for their antimalarial potential, underlining the continued relevance of plant-based compounds in historical and modern contexts. Other advancements in the late 20th century were represented by the discovery of artemisinin, which offered quick parasite eradication and effectiveness against drug-resistant *Plasmodium falciparum* strains. ACTs are still the gold standard for malaria management (Tu, 2017).

8.2 Mechanisms of Action Against Malarial Parasites

Phytochemicals target both the parasite and host processes in various ways to mediate their antimalarial activity. Quinine and other alkaloids, besides antimalarials like mefloquine and chloroquine, interfere with the detoxification of heme by inhibiting hemozoin synthesis. This leads to a toxic accumulation of free heme inside the parasite, which is associated with poor survival of the parasite (Combrinck et al., 2013). Intraparasitic iron activates artemisinin and its derivatives, which are sesquiterpene lactones, producing ROS that extensively damage parasite proteins and membranes (Hu et al., 2022). It has been demonstrated that flavonoids, like quercetin, enhance oxidative stress in infected red blood cells, interfere with important enzymatic pathways, and inhibit DNA synthesis (Remigante et al., 2022). With molecular docking studies showing high binding affinity with parasite proteases such as falcipain and plasmepsins, terpenoids other than artemisinin, such as cucurbitacin and oleanolic acid, are emerging as potential leads (Ishola et al., 2023). These processes collectively highlight how phytochemicals target vital *Plasmodium* metabolic pathways as a part of an inclusive strategy to counter infection.

8.3 Overcoming Drug Resistance

One of the main challenges in fighting malaria is the increasing resistance of the parasite to frontline drugs. To counteract resistance, structural diversity, and synergistic effects, phytochemicals present special options. For example, by blocking efflux pumps, certain flavonoids function as resistance modulators, regaining the effectiveness of usual antimalarial medications (Duda-Madej et al., 2025). Combination treatments that include both traditional medications and chemicals derived from plants have shown potential in decreasing parasite survival rates and delaying the emergence of resistance (Singh & Sharma, 2019). Furthermore, a dynamic chemical reservoir changing resistance patterns is provided by the ongoing discovery of new terpenoids, alkaloids, and polyphenols from biodiversity hotspots in the Global South. It will be important to prioritize green chemistry for scalable production and incorporate phytochemicals within carefully planned combination regimens to ensure long-term sustainability.

9. FUTURE PERSPECTIVES AND CHALLENGES

9.1 Advances in Phytochemical Research

Recent scientific advancements have expanded research on phytochemicals for the development of antimalarial drugs. Rapid identification of active compounds from complex plant matrices is made possible by modern bioinformatics tools, metabolomics, and HTS technologies (W. Zhang et al., 2023). Predicting phytochemical-parasite interactions by structural biology and computational modeling is becoming more prevalent, which accelerates the development of more effective and tailored analogs (Chihomvu et al., 2024). Additionally, advances in synthetic biology have improved the efficiency and scalability of supply chains by modifying microbes to produce phytochemical drugs (Gunaseelan et al., 2025). These advancements not only improve drug discovery efficiency but also reduce the need for wild plant populations, making phytochemical-based research more accessible and sustainable globally.

9.2 Integration with Conventional Medicine

To effectively treat malaria, phytochemicals must be integrated with conventional medicine. History provides powerful examples in artemisinin and quinine, which demonstrate how natural compounds can become the foundation of modern pharmacology. Current research is exploring these plant-based chemicals not as replacements, but as complementary supplements to standard antimalarial drugs, aiming to boost efficacy while minimizing side effects. Moreover, transforming plant metabolites into safe and reliable medicines requires standardized extraction methods, clinical trials, and detailed pharmacokinetic studies (Ezeanochie et al., 2024). This integration is especially crucial in the Global South, where indigenous medicine remains widespread. Merging this local knowledge with evidence-based clinical practices is key to making phytochemicals a legitimate part of contemporary healthcare.

9.3 Sustainable and Ethical Considerations

As phytochemicals continue to influence the development of antimalarial drugs, sustainability and ethics are emerging as principal concerns. Many medicinal plants come from ecologically delicate areas, and unsustainable harvesting practices can put biodiversity and community maintenance at risk (Hamilton, 2004). In order to solve this problem, green chemistry-based extraction methods must be given top priority, along with conservation initiatives and farming (Alum, 2025). Equally important ethical aspects are ensuring indigenous groups receive proper recognition and profit sharing since their traditional knowledge often informs the choice of plants for study (Patil et al., 2024). Reinforcing intellectual property rights, building community relationships, and encouraging ethical supply chains will be necessary to ensure phytochemical-based treatments not only prove successful but also are socially and environmentally responsible.

10. CONCLUSION

From historically important compounds like quinine and artemisinin to recently discovered flavonoids and terpenoids with promising bioactivities, phytochemicals demonstrate both therapeutic significance and research value: the study of phytochemicals and their antimalarial properties highlight the great potential of plant-derived metabolites in addressing continuing global health issues. Their diverse mechanisms of action, going from interference with parasite metabolism to the improvement of host immunity, underpin their importance as versatile agents in malaria prevention.

This chapter has highlighted not only the pharmacological importance of alkaloids, flavonoids, and terpenoids but also the transitional opportunities offered by phytochemicals in modern medicine. Examples indicate how the biodiversity and long-established knowledge in the Global South have shaped current antimalarial treatments, but advances in phytochemical research, integrated with common medicine, and sustainable practices are needed, considering present-day problems like drug resistance, environmental stress, and restricted access. Besides scientific effort, the research into phytochemicals is a call for responsible innovation that unites traditional knowledge, modern technology, and the needs of global health. By bridging these fields, phytochemicals can continue to be at the forefront of the development of natural antimalarial medications, particularly in the Global South, where the potential of biodiversity and the prevalence of malaria converge.

REFERENCES

Abu Khalaf, R., Alhusban, A. A., Al-Shalabi, E., Al-Sheikh, I., & Sabbah, D. A. (2019). Chapter 10—Isolation and structure elucidation of bioactive polyphenols. In Atta-ur-Rahman (Ed.), *Studies in Natural Products Chemistry* (Vol. 63, pp. 267–337). Elsevier. DOI: 10.1016/B978-0-12-817901-7.00010-1

Abubakar, A. R., & Haque, M. (2020). Preparation of Medicinal Plants: Basic Extraction and Fractionation Procedures for Experimental Purposes. *Journal of Pharmacy & Bioallied Sciences*, *12*(1), 1–10. DOI: 10.4103/jpbs.JPBS_175_19 PMID: 32801594

Afzal, I., Habiba, U., & Yasmeen, H. (2023). Review on therapeutic potential of phytochemicals from medicinal plants. *Journal of Bioresource Management*, *10*(4), 7.

Ahmad, F., & Nadeem, H. (2022). *Mass Spectroscopy as an Analytical Tool to Harness the Production of Secondary Plant Metabolites: The Way Forward for Drug Discovery*. DOI: 10.1007/978-1-0716-2716-7_5

Alum, E. U. (2025). Sustainable harvesting of medicinal plants: Balancing therapeutic benefits with environmental conservation. *Agroecology and Sustainable Food Systems*, *49*(3), 380–385. DOI: 10.1080/21683565.2024.2421948

Amado, P. S. M., Jesus, A. J. L., Paixão, J. A., Fausto, R., & Cristiano, M. L. S. (2022). Unravelling the Structure of Peroxides with Antiparasitic Activity: The Relative Impact of a Trioxolane or a Tetraoxane Pharmacophore on the Overall Molecular Structure. *ChemPlusChem*, *87*(8), e202200207. DOI: 10.1002/cplu.202200207 PMID: 36000152

Andrade, M. A., Barbosa, C. H., Cerqueira, M. A., Azevedo, A. G., Barros, C., Machado, A. V., Coelho, A., Furtado, R., Correia, C. B., Saraiva, M., Vilarinho, F., Silva, A. S., & Ramos, F. (2023). PLA films loaded with green tea and rosemary polyphenolic extracts as an active packaging for almond and beef. *Food Packaging and Shelf Life*, *36*, 101041. DOI: 10.1016/j.fpsl.2023.101041

Antony, A., & Farid, M. (2022). Effect of Temperatures on Polyphenols during Extraction. *Applied Sciences (Basel, Switzerland)*, *12*(4), 2107. DOI: 10.3390/app12042107

Ashawat, M. S., Saraf Shailendra, S. S., & Saraf Swarnlata, S. S. (2007). In vitro antioxidant activity of ethanolic extracts of Centella asiatica, Punica granatum, Glycyrrhiza glabra and Areca catechu.

Bankole, A. E., Adekunle, A. A., Sowemimo, A. A., Umebese, C. E., Abiodun, O., & Gbotosho, G. O. (2016). Phytochemical screening and in vivo antimalarial activity of extracts from three medicinal plants used in malaria treatment in Nigeria. *Parasitology Research, 115*(1), 299–305. DOI: 10.1007/s00436-015-4747-x PMID: 26391173

Banu, K. S., & Cathrine, D. L. (2015). *General Techniques Involved in Phytochemical Analysis*.

Barman, P., & Biswas, A. (2025). *The Contribution of Traditionally Used Medicinal Plants to Modern Medicine: An Update on the Successful Journey of Medicinal Plants of North East Africa*. Bentham Science Publishers. https://www.benthamdirect.com/content/books/9789815313178.chapter-6

Bezerra, J. J. L., Pinheiro, A. A. V., & Dourado, D. (2023). *Antimalarial potential of* Moringa oleifera *Lam. (Moringaceae): A review of the ethnomedicinal, pharmacological, toxicological, and phytochemical evidence*. https://doi.org/DOI: 10.1590/1678-9199-JVATITD-2022-0079

Bhambhani, S., Kondhare, K. R., & Giri, A. P. (2021). Diversity in Chemical Structures and Biological Properties of Plant Alkaloids. *Molecules (Basel, Switzerland), 26*(11), 3374. DOI: 10.3390/molecules26113374 PMID: 34204857

Bitwell, C., Indra, S. S., Luke, C., & Kakoma, M. K. (2023). A review of modern and conventional extraction techniques and their applications for extracting phytochemicals from plants. *Scientific African, 19*, e01585. DOI: 10.1016/j.sciaf.2023.e01585

Celik, O. F., Kilicaslan, M., Akcaoglu, S., & Ozturk, Y. (2023). Improving the antioxidant activity of yogurt through black and green tea supplementation. *International Journal of Food Science & Technology, 58*(11), 6121–6130. DOI: 10.1111/ijfs.16722

Chihomvu, P., Ganesan, A., Gibbons, S., Woollard, K., & Hayes, M. A. (2024). Phytochemicals in Drug Discovery—A Confluence of Tradition and Innovation. *International Journal of Molecular Sciences, 25*(16), 8792. DOI: 10.3390/ijms25168792 PMID: 39201478

Combrinck, J. M., Mabotha, T. E., Ncokazi, K. K., Ambele, M. A., Taylor, D., Smith, P. J., Hoppe, H. C., & Egan, T. J. (2013). Insights into the Role of Heme in the Mechanism of Action of Antimalarials. *ACS Chemical Biology, 8*(1), 133–137. DOI: 10.1021/cb300454t PMID: 23043646

Couillaud, J., Leydet, L., Duquesne, K., & Iacazio, G. (2021). The Terpene Mini-Path, a New Promising Alternative for Terpenoids Bio-Production. *Genes, 12*(12), 1974. DOI: 10.3390/genes12121974 PMID: 34946923

Das, G., Shin, H.-S., & Patra, J. K. (2024). The Antiviral and Antimalarial Prodrug Artemisinin from the Artemisia Species: A Review. *Current Issues in Molecular Biology*, *46*(11), 12099–12118. DOI: 10.3390/cimb46110718 PMID: 39590312

de Lima, E. P., Laurindo, L. F., Catharin, V. C. S., Direito, R., Tanaka, M., Jasmin Santos German, I., Lamas, C. B., Guiguer, E. L., Araújo, A. C., Fiorini, A. M. R., & Barbalho, S. M. (2025). Polyphenols, Alkaloids, and Terpenoids Against Neurodegeneration: Evaluating the Neuroprotective Effects of Phytocompounds Through a Comprehensive Review of the Current Evidence. *Metabolites*, *15*(2), 124. DOI: 10.3390/metabo15020124 PMID: 39997749

de Sousa, D. P., Damasceno, R. O. S., Amorati, R., Elshabrawy, H. A., de Castro, R. D., Bezerra, D. P., Nunes, V. R. V., Gomes, R. C., & Lima, T. C. (2023). Essential Oils: Chemistry and Pharmacological Activities. *Biomolecules*, *13*(7), 1144. DOI: 10.3390/biom13071144 PMID: 37509180

de Villiers, K. A., & Egan, T. J. (2021). Heme Detoxification in the Malaria Parasite: A Target for Antimalarial Drug Development. *Accounts of Chemical Research*, *54*(11), 2649–2659. DOI: 10.1021/acs.accounts.1c00154 PMID: 33982570

Del Prado-Audelo, M. L., Cortés, H., Caballero-Florán, I. H., González-Torres, M., Escutia-Guadarrama, L., Bernal-Chávez, S. A., Giraldo-Gomez, D. M., Magaña, J. J., & Leyva-Gómez, G. (2021). Therapeutic Applications of Terpenes on Inflammatory Diseases. *Frontiers in Pharmacology*, *12*, 704197. Advance online publication. DOI: 10.3389/fphar.2021.704197 PMID: 34483907

Dev, M., & Mukadam, M. (2025). *Functional group profiling of medicinal plants using FTIR spectroscopy*. World Journal of Biology Pharmacy and Health Sciences., DOI: 10.30574/wjbphs.2025.21.1.0039

Dey, P., Kundu, A., Kumar, A., Gupta, M., Lee, B. M., Bhakta, T., Dash, S., & Kim, H. S. (2020). Analysis of alkaloids (indole alkaloids, isoquinoline alkaloids, tropane alkaloids). *Recent Advances in Natural Products Analysis*, 505–567. DOI: 10.1016/B978-0-12-816455-6.00015-9

Dias, M. C., Pinto, D. C. G. A., & Silva, A. M. S. (2021). Plant Flavonoids: Chemical Characteristics and Biological Activity. *Molecules (Basel, Switzerland)*, *26*(17), 5377. DOI: 10.3390/molecules26175377 PMID: 34500810

Dimitrova, Z. (1999). The history of pharmacy. *Sofija: St Clement of Ohrid*, 13-26.

Duda-Madej, A., Viscardi, S., Niezgódka, P., Szewczyk, W., & Wińska, K. (2025). The Impact of Plant-Derived Polyphenols on Combating Efflux-Mediated Antibiotic Resistance. *International Journal of Molecular Sciences*, *26*(9), 4030. DOI: 10.3390/ijms26094030 PMID: 40362268

Ferreira, T. S., Moreira, C. Z., Cária, N. Z., Victoriano, G., Silva, W. F.Jr, & Magalhães, J. C. (2014). Phytotherapy: An introduction to its history, use and application. *Revista Brasileira de Plantas Medicinais*, *16*(2), 290–298. DOI: 10.1590/S1516-05722014000200019

Frolova, N., Orlova, A., Popova, V., Bilova, T., & Frolov, A. (2025). *GC-MS-based metabolomics–Part 1 Gas chromatography-mass spectrometry (GC-MS) and its place in the plant metabolomics toolbox*. Chemistry. DOI: 10.26434/chemrxiv-2025-5kgvt

Gil, M. I., Tomás-Barberán, F. A., Hess-Pierce, B., & Kader, A. A. (2002). Antioxidant capacities, phenolic compounds, carotenoids, and vitamin C contents of nectarine, peach, and plum cultivars from California. *Journal of Agricultural and Food Chemistry*, *50*(17), 4976–4982. DOI: 10.1021/jf020136b PMID: 12166993

Gunaseelan, R. J., Raj, A., Nagarajan, P., Perumal, S., Kumar, J., & Patil, S. J. (2025). Biotechnological Phytochemical Synthesis: Innovations, Challenges, Advantages, Implications. In *Biotechnology and Phytochemical Prospects in Drug Discovery* (pp. 83–101). Springer., DOI: 10.1007/978-981-96-2790-5_3

Gutiérrez-Grijalva, E. P., López-Martínez, L. X., Contreras-Angulo, L. A., Elizalde-Romero, C. A., & Heredia, J. B. (2020). Plant Alkaloids: Structures and Bioactive Properties. In Swamy, M. K. (Ed.), *Plant-derived Bioactives* (pp. 85–117). Springer Singapore., DOI: 10.1007/978-981-15-2361-8_5

Hamilton, A. C. (2004). Medicinal plants, conservation and livelihoods. *Biodiversity and Conservation*, *13*(8), 1477–1517. DOI: 10.1023/B:BIOC.0000021333.23413.42

Hermanto, F., Haq, F. A., & Khasanah, R. (2024). The effect of resveratrol on the relationship of antioxidant activity and beta-hematin inhibition as an antimalarial action target. *Journal of Advanced Pharmaceutical Technology & Research*, *15*(4), 359–363. DOI: 10.4103/JAPTR.JAPTR_144_24

Hossain, M. S., Wazed, M. A., Asha, S., Amin, M. R., & Shimul, I. M. (2025). Dietary phytochemicals in health and disease: Mechanisms, clinical evidence, and applications a comprehensive review. *Food Science & Nutrition*, *13*(3), e70101. DOI: 10.1002/fsn3.70101 PMID: 40115248

Hu, Y., Guo, N., Yang, T., Yan, J., Wang, W., & Li, X. (2022). The Potential Mechanisms by which Artemisinin and Its Derivatives Induce Ferroptosis in the Treatment of Cancer. *Oxidative Medicine and Cellular Longevity, 2022*(1), 1458143. DOI: 10.1155/2022/1458143 PMID: 35028002

Huang, W., Wang, Y., Tian, W., Cui, X., Tu, P., Li, J., Shi, S., & Liu, X. (2022). Biosynthesis Investigations of Terpenoid, Alkaloid, and Flavonoid Antimicrobial Agents Derived from Medicinal Plants. *Antibiotics (Basel, Switzerland), 11*(10), 1380. DOI: 10.3390/antibiotics11101380 PMID: 36290037

Huang, Y., Xiao, D., Burton-Freeman, B. M., & Edirisinghe, I. (2016). Chemical changes of bioactive phytochemicals during thermal processing

Ishola, A. A., Adewole, K. E., Adebayo, J. O., & Balogun, E. A. (2023). Potentials of Terpenoids as Inhibitors of Multiple Plasmodium falciparum Protein Drug Targets. *Acta Parasitologica, 68*(4), 793–806. DOI: 10.1007/s11686-023-00711-z PMID: 37603126

Jamil, S. N. H., Ali, A. H., Feroz, S. R., Lam, S. D., Agustar, H. K., Mohd Abd Razak, M. R., & Latip, J. (2023). Curcumin and Its Derivatives as Potential Antimalarial and Anti-Inflammatory Agents: A Review on Structure Activity Relationship and Mechanism of Action. *Pharmaceuticals (Basel, Switzerland), 16*(4), 609. DOI: 10.3390/ph16040609 PMID: 37111366

Jamil, S. N. H., Bakar, K. A., Ali, A. H., Marzuki, N. F. N., Shahid, F., Mahmud, F., Feroz, S. R., Lam, S. D., Oka, N., Zakaria, Y., Muhajir, M. I., Maharani, R., Supratman, U., & Latip, J. (2025). *Promising bioactivity of curcumin derivatives against malaria: In silico, in vitro and ITC studies. Research Square*. DOI: 10.21203/rs.3.rs-7148737/v1

Jan, R., Asaf, S., Numan, M., Lubna, , & Kim, K.-M. (2021). Plant secondary metabolite biosynthesis and transcriptional regulation in response to biotic and abiotic stress conditions. *Agronomy (Basel), 11*(5), 968. DOI: 10.3390/agronomy11050968

Javanmardi, J., Stushnoff, C., Locke, E., & Vivanco, J. M. (2003). Antioxidant activity and total phenolic content of Iranian Ocimum accessions. *Food Chemistry, 83*(4), 547–550. DOI: 10.1016/S0308-8146(03)00151-1

Kangwanrangsan, N., Niramolyanun, G., Praikongkatham, C., Chantree, P., Martviset, P., & Pankao, V. (2025). Growth Inhibition and Additive Effect to Antimalarial Drugs of Brucea javanica Extracts on Asexual Blood-Stage Plasmodium falciparum. *Pathogens (Basel, Switzerland), 14*(7), 646. DOI: 10.3390/pathogens14070646 PMID: 40732696

Kato, L. S., Lelis, C. A., da Silva, B. D., Galvan, D., & Conte-Junior, C. A. (2023). Micro-and nanoencapsulation of natural phytochemicals: Challenges and recent perspectives for the food and nutraceuticals industry applications. *Advances in Food and Nutrition Research*, *104*, 77–137. DOI: 10.1016/bs.afnr.2022.10.003 PMID: 37236735

Kesarwani, K., & Gupta, R. (2013). Bioavailability enhancers of herbal origin: An overview. *Asian Pacific Journal of Tropical Biomedicine*, *3*(4), 253–266. DOI: 10.1016/S2221-1691(13)60060-X PMID: 23620848

Kohnen-Johannsen, K. L., & Kayser, O. (2019). Tropane Alkaloids: Chemistry, Pharmacology, Biosynthesis and Production. *Molecules (Basel, Switzerland)*, *24*(4), 796. DOI: 10.3390/molecules24040796 PMID: 30813289

Kumar, A., P, N., Kumar, M., Jose, A., Tomer, V., Oz, E., Proestos, C., Zeng, M., Elobeid, T., K, S., & Oz, F. (2023). Major phytochemicals: Recent advances in health benefits and extraction method. *Molecules (Basel, Switzerland)*, *28*(2), 887. DOI: 10.3390/molecules28020887 PMID: 36677944

Lacerda, U. V., da Costa, C. V. P., Cardoso, R. R., D'Almeida, C. T. dos S., do Carmo, M. A. V., Lima, A. dos S., Cruz, L. da S., de Souza, A. B., Fernandes, P. O., Maltarollo, V. G., Ferreira, M. S. L., Azevedo, L., Eller, M. R., Corich, V., Giacomini, A., & de Barros, F. A. R. (2025). Antioxidant, Antiproliferative, Antibacterial, and Antimalarial Effects of Phenolic-Rich Green Tea Kombucha. *Beverages*, *11*(1), 7. DOI: 10.3390/beverages11010007

Letchuman, S., Madhuranga, H. D. T., Madhurangi, B. L. N. K., Premarathna, A. D., & Saravanan, M. (2025). Alkaloids unveiled: A comprehensive analysis of novel therapeutic properties, mechanisms, and plant-based innovations. *Intelligent Pharmacy*, *3*(4), 268–276. DOI: 10.1016/j.ipha.2024.09.007

Li, M., Qian, M., Jiang, Q., Tan, B., Yin, Y., & Han, X. (2023). Evidence of Flavonoids on Disease Prevention. *Antioxidants*, *12*(2), 527. DOI: 10.3390/antiox12020527 PMID: 36830086

Mabuza, M. J. (2022). *Antiplasmodial properties of extracts from Pappea capensis Eckl. & Zeyh.* Sapindaceae.

Magozwi, D. K., Dinala, M., Mokwana, N., Siwe-Noundou, X., Krause, R. W. M., Sonopo, M., McGaw, L. J., Augustyn, W. A., & Tembu, V. J. (2021). Flavonoids from the Genus Euphorbia: Isolation, Structure, Pharmacological Activities and Structure–Activity Relationships. *Pharmaceuticals (Basel, Switzerland)*, *14*(5), 428. DOI: 10.3390/ph14050428 PMID: 34063311

Mamede, C. C., & Cristina, L. (2024). *Metabolomic Investigation of Natural Anti-plasmodial Agents*. https://orbi.uliege.be/handle/2268/311229

Manisha, M., Babu, R., Begam, A. M., Shakya Chahal, K., & Ashok Harale, A. (2025). Medicinal Plants and Traditional Uses and Modern Applications. *Journal of Neonatal Surgery*, *14*(3), 162–175. DOI: 10.52783/jns.v14.2210

Mishra, R., Xavier, J. da C., Kumar, N., Krishna, G., Dhakad, P. K., Santos, H. S., dos, , Bandeira, P. N., Rodrigues, T. H. S., Gondim, D. R., Ribeiro, W. H. F., Silva, D. S., da, , Teixeira, A. M. R., Pereira, W. F., & Marinho, E. S. (2025). Exploring Quinoline Derivatives: Their Antimalarial Efficacy and Structural Features. *Medicinal Chemistry (Shariqah, United Arab Emirates)*, *21*(2), 96–121. DOI: 10.2174/0115734064318361240827072124 PMID: 40007183

Mohammed, A. E., Abdul-Hameed, Z. H., Alotaibi, M. O., Bawakid, N. O., Sobahi, T. R., Abdel-Lateff, A., & Alarif, W. M. (2021). Chemical Diversity and Bioactivities of Monoterpene Indole Alkaloids (MIAs) from Six Apocynaceae Genera. *Molecules (Basel, Switzerland)*, *26*(2), 488. DOI: 10.3390/molecules26020488 PMID: 33477682

Mosquera, M. E. G., Jiménez, G., Tabernero, V., Vinueza-Vaca, J., García-Estrada, C., Kosalková, K., Sola-Landa, A., Monje, B., Acosta, C., Alonso, R., & Valera, M. Á. (2021). Terpenes and Terpenoids: Building Blocks to Produce Biopolymers. *Sustainable Chemistry*, *2*(3), 467–492. DOI: 10.3390/suschem2030026

Mutha, R. E., Kalaskar, M., & Khan, Z. G. (2025). *Modern Analytical Techniques for Quality Control and Chemical Identification of Phytochemicals*. Retrieved September 28, 2025, from https://onlinelibrary.wiley.com/doi/10.1002/9781394203680.ch09

Natolino, A., Passaghe, P., Brugnera, G., & Comuzzo, P. (2024). Intensification of grape marc (*Vitis vinifera*) exploitation by subcritical water-ethanol extraction: Effect on polyphenol bioactivities and kinetic modelling. *Journal of Food Engineering*, *381*, 112185. DOI: 10.1016/j.jfoodeng.2024.112185

Nikolovski, B. (1995). Essays on the history of health culture in Macedonia. *Skopje: Macedonian pharmaceutical association*, 17-27.

Nirmala, C., & Sridevi, M. (2021). Ethnobotanical, phytochemistry, and pharmacological property of Waltheria Indica Linn. *Future Journal of Pharmaceutical Sciences*, *7*(1), 14. DOI: 10.1186/s43094-020-00174-3

Oksana, S. (2012). Plant phenolic compounds for food, pharmaceutical and cosmetics production. *Journal of Medicinal Plants Research*, *6*(13). Advance online publication. DOI: 10.5897/JMPR11.1695

Omar, F., Tareq, A. M., Alqahtani, A. M., Dhama, K., Sayeed, M. A., Emran, T. B., & Simal-Gandara, J. (2021). Plant-Based Indole Alkaloids: A Comprehensive Overview from a Pharmacological Perspective. *Molecules (Basel, Switzerland), 26*(8), 2297. DOI: 10.3390/molecules26082297 PMID: 33921093

Paddon, C. J., & Keasling, J. D. (2014). Semi-synthetic artemisinin: A model for the use of synthetic biology in pharmaceutical development. *Nature Reviews. Microbiology, 12*(5), 355–367. DOI: 10.1038/nrmicro3240 PMID: 24686413

Patil, P. R, A. R., Sivakumar, B., Bora, N. R., V, V., D, S. S., A, M. V., Rajaram, R., Prathyusha, K., Datta, P. L., & Nath, I. (2024). *A Comprehensive Review on Sustainable Cultivation Practices of Medicinal Plants | International Journal of Plant & Soil Science*. Retrieved September 28, 2025, from https://journalijpss.com/index.php/IJPSS/article/view/5002

Periferakis, A.-T., Periferakis, A., Periferakis, K., Caruntu, A., Badarau, I. A., Savulescu-Fiedler, I., Scheau, C., & Caruntu, C. (2023). Antimicrobial Properties of Capsaicin: Available Data and Future Research Perspectives. *Nutrients, 15*(19), 4097. DOI: 10.3390/nu15194097 PMID: 37836381

Piechowiak, T., & Skóra, B. (2023). Edible coating enriched with cinnamon oil reduces the oxidative stress and improves the quality of strawberry fruit stored at room temperature. *Journal of the Science of Food and Agriculture, 103*(5), 2389–2400. DOI: 10.1002/jsfa.12463 PMID: 36683377

Pons, D. G. (2024). Roles of phytochemicals in cancer prevention and therapeutics. *International Journal of Molecular Sciences, 25*(10), 5450. DOI: 10.3390/ijms25105450 PMID: 38791488

Rahaman, S. T., & Mondal, S. (2020). Flavonoids: A vital resource in healthcare and medicine. *Pharmacy & Pharmacology International Journal, 8*(2), 91–104. DOI: 10.15406/ppij.2020.08.00285

Remigante, A., Spinelli, S., Straface, E., Gambardella, L., Caruso, D., Falliti, G., Dossena, S., Marino, A., & Morabito, R. (2022). Antioxidant Activity of Quercetin in a H2O2-Induced Oxidative Stress Model in Red Blood Cells: Functional Role of Band 3 Protein. *International Journal of Molecular Sciences, 23*(19), 10991. DOI: 10.3390/ijms231910991 PMID: 36232293

Ribbiso, K. A., Heller, L. E., Taye, A., Julian, E., Willems, A. V., & Roepe, P. D. (2021). Artemisinin-Based Drugs Target the Plasmodium falciparum Heme Detoxification Pathway. *Antimicrobial Agents and Chemotherapy, 65*(4), . https://doi.org/DOI: 10.1128/AAC.02137-20

Rupasinghe, H. P. V. (2020). Special Issue "Flavonoids and Their Disease Prevention and Treatment Potential": Recent Advances and Future Perspectives. *Molecules (Basel, Switzerland), 25*(20), 4746. DOI: 10.3390/molecules25204746 PMID: 33081132

Samtiya, M., Aluko, R. E., Dhewa, T., & Moreno-Rojas, J. M. (2021). Potential Health Benefits of Plant Food-Derived Bioactive Components: An Overview. *Foods, 10*(4), 839. DOI: 10.3390/foods10040839 PMID: 33921351

Seshadri, K., Abad, A. N. D., Nagasawa, K. K., Yost, K. M., Johnson, C. W., Dror, M. J., & Tang, Y. (2025). Synthetic Biology in Natural Product Biosynthesis. *Chemical Reviews, 125*(7), 3814–3931. DOI: 10.1021/acs.chemrev.4c00567 PMID: 40116601

Shamsudin, N. F., Ahmed, Q. U., Mahmood, S., Shah, S. A. A., Sarian, M. N., Khattak, M. M. A. K., Khatib, A., Sabere, A. S. M., Yusoff, Y. M., & Latip, J. (2022). Flavonoids as Antidiabetic and Anti-Inflammatory Agents: A Review on Structural Activity Relationship-Based Studies and Meta-Analysis. *International Journal of Molecular Sciences, 23*(20), 12605. DOI: 10.3390/ijms232012605 PMID: 36293459

Shariff, N., Sudarshana, M. S., Umesha, S., & Hariprasad, P. (2006). Antimicrobial activity of Rauvolfia tetraphylla and Physalis minima leaf and callus extracts. *African Journal of Biotechnology, 5*(10).

Sharifi-Rad, J., Kobarfard, F., Ata, A., Ayatollahi, S. A., Khosravi-Dehaghi, N., Jugran, A. K., Tomas, M., Capanoglu, E., Matthews, K. R., Popović-Djordjević, J., Kostić, A., Kamiloglu, S., Sharopov, F., Choudhary, M. I., & Martins, N. (2019). Prosopis Plant Chemical Composition and Pharmacological Attributes: Targeting Clinical Studies from Preclinical Evidence. *Biomolecules, 9*(12), 777. DOI: 10.3390/biom9120777 PMID: 31775378

Singh, R., & Sharma, B. (2019). *Therapeutic Potential of Plant Based Natural Compounds for Malaria—Recent Advances and Future Perspective.*

Sok Yen, F., & Qin, S. (2021). C., Tan Shi Xuan, S., Jia Ying, P., Yi Le, H., Darmarajan, T., Gunasekaran, B., & Salvamani, S. (2021). Hypoglycemic Effects of Plant Flavonoids: A Review. *Evidence-Based Complementary and Alternative Medicine : eCAM, 2057333*(1), 1–12. DOI: 10.1155/2021/2057333 PMID: 34925525

Sun, J., Xufeng, J., Qiu, Z., Gao, Q., Zhu, Z., He, J., Gao, S., & Sui, X. (2025). Artemisiae Annuae Herba: From anti-malarial legacy to emerging anti-cancer potential. *Theranostics, 15*(15), 7346–7377. DOI: 10.7150/thno.115414 PMID: 40756346

Sun, S., Yu, Y., Jo, Y., Han, J. H., Xue, Y., Cho, M., Bae, S.-J., Ryu, D., Park, W., Ha, K.-T., & Zhuang, S. (2025). Impact of extraction techniques on phytochemical composition and bioactivity of natural product mixtures. *Frontiers in Pharmacology, 16*, 1615338. Advance online publication. DOI: 10.3389/fphar.2025.1615338 PMID: 40808686

Tarkang, P. A., Appiah-Opong, R., Ofori, M. F., Ayong, L. S., & Nyarko, A. K. (2016). Application of multi-target phytotherapeutic concept in malaria drug discovery: A systems biology approach in biomarker identification. *Biomarker Research, 4*(1), 25. DOI: 10.1186/s40364-016-0077-0 PMID: 27999673

Thakur, A., & Sharma, R. (2018). Health promoting phytochemicals in vegetables: A mini review. *International Journal of Food and Fermentation Technology, 8*(2), 107–117. DOI: 10.30954/2277-9396.02.2018.1

Tu, Y. (2017). *From Artemisia annua L. to Artemisinins: The Discovery and Development of Artemisinins and Antimalarial Agents*. Academic Press.

Tucakov, J. (1971). Healing with plants–phytotherapy. *Beograd. Culture (Québec), 180*, 90.

Tzanova, M., Atanasov, V., Yaneva, Z., Ivanova, D., & Dinev, T. (2020). Selectivity of Current Extraction Techniques for Flavonoids from Plant Materials. *Processes (Basel, Switzerland), 8*(10), 1222. DOI: 10.3390/pr8101222

Ullah, A., Munir, S., Badshah, S. L., Khan, N., Ghani, L., Poulson, B. G., Emwas, A.-H., & Jaremko, M. (2020). Important Flavonoids and Their Role as a Therapeutic Agent. *Molecules (Basel, Switzerland), 25*(22), 5243. DOI: 10.3390/molecules25225243 PMID: 33187049

Uzor, P. F. (2020). Alkaloids from Plants with Antimalarial Activity: A Review of Recent Studies. *Evidence-Based Complementary and Alternative Medicine : eCAM, 2020*(1), 8749083. DOI: 10.1155/2020/8749083 PMID: 32104196

Vij, I., & Pathania, A. (2023). An Overview- Advances in Chromatographic Techniques in Phytochemistry. *E3S Web of Conferences, 391*, 01038. Retrieved September 28, 2025, from https://www.e3s-conferences.org/articles/e3sconf/abs/2023/28/e3sconf_icmed-icmpc2023_01038/e3sconf_icmed-icmpc2023_01038.html

Wang, W., Rao, L., Wu, X., Wang, Y., Zhao, L., & Liao, X. (2021). Supercritical Carbon Dioxide Applications in Food Processing. *Food Engineering Reviews, 13*(3), 570–591. DOI: 10.1007/s12393-020-09270-9

Wen, M., Zeng, J., Qiu, F., Zhang, F., & Liao, Z. (2024). De Novo Synthesis of Anticholinergic Hyoscyamine and Scopolamine in Nicotiana benthamiana Based on Elucidating Tropane Alkaloid Biosynthetic Pathway of Anisodus luridus. *Agronomy (Basel), 14*(11), 2460. DOI: 10.3390/agronomy14112460

Wu, J., Lv, S., Zhao, L., Gao, T., Yu, C., Hu, J., & Ma, F. (2023). Advances in the study of the function and mechanism of the action of flavonoids in plants under environmental stresses. *Planta, 257*(6), 108. DOI: 10.1007/s00425-023-04136-w PMID: 37133783

Xu, K., Qu, L., Li, H., Ren, X., Yan, N., & Fu, X. (2024). Functional properties of dietary quercetin in cardiovascular health and disease. *Food Frontiers, 5*(5), 1951–1967. DOI: 10.1002/fft2.434

Yang, W., Chen, X., Li, Y., Guo, S., Wang, Z., & Yu, X. (2020). Advances in Pharmacological Activities of Terpenoids. *Natural Product Communications, 15*(3), 1934578X20903555. DOI: 10.1177/1934578X20903555

Yu-Ping, L., Mendonça, D., Sheng-Khai, L., Phan-Sing, Y. A., Chimplee, S., Chuprom, J., Boonhok, R., Mahboob, T., Oliveira, S. M., Rajagopal, M., Pereira, M. L., Girol, A. P., & Nissapatorn, V. (2024). Malaria – the importance of phytochemicals as sources of alternative medicines. *Indian Journal of Natural Products and Resources (IJNPR) [Formerly Natural Product Radiance (NPR)], 15*(2), 274–285. DOI: 10.56042/ijnpr.v15i2.11493

Zahin, M., Aqil, F., & Ahmad, I. (2009). The in vitro antioxidant activity and total phenolic content of four Indian medicinal plants. *International Journal of Pharmacy and Pharmaceutical Sciences, 1*(1), 88–95.

Zeka, K., Ruparelia, K., Arroo, R. R. J., Budriesi, R., & Micucci, M. (2017). Flavonoids and Their Metabolites: Prevention in Cardiovascular Diseases and Diabetes. *Diseases (Basel, Switzerland), 5*(3), 19. DOI: 10.3390/diseases5030019 PMID: 32962323

Zhang, C., & Hong, K. (2020). Production of Terpenoids by Synthetic Biology Approaches. *Frontiers in Bioengineering and Biotechnology, 8*, 347. Advance online publication. DOI: 10.3389/fbioe.2020.00347 PMID: 32391346

Zhang, W., Zeng, Y., Jiao, M., Ye, C., Li, Y., Liu, C., & Wang, J. (2023). Integration of high-throughput omics technologies in medicinal plant research: The new era of natural drug discovery. *Frontiers in Plant Science, 14*, 1073848. DOI: 10.3389/fpls.2023.1073848 PMID: 36743502

Zhang, Y. L., Sun, S. J., & Zeng, L. (2024). *Biological effects and mechanisms of dietary chalcones: Latest research progress, future research strategies, and challenges*. DOI: 10.1039/D4FO03618B

Zheng, M., Zhu, Y., Zhuang, Y., Tan, K. B., & Chen, J. (2023). Effects of grape seed extract on the properties of pullulan polysaccharide/xanthan gum active films for apple preservation. *International Journal of Biological Macromolecules*, *241*, 124617. DOI: 10.1016/j.ijbiomac.2023.124617 PMID: 37119919

Chapter 3

Amazon Ethnomedicine and Malaria Control in Latin America, Field Based Plant Surveys and Partnership With Indigenous Communities

Aman Suresh Tharayil
https://orcid.org/0009-0000-5377-7428
Dr MGR Educational and Research Institute, Chennai, India

Sreya Kosanam
https://orcid.org/0000-0002-0645-5677
Dr. MGR Educational and Research Institute, Chennai, India

Praveen Javali R.
https://orcid.org/0009-0001-3737-5813
Sri Raghavendra College of Pharmacy, Chitradurga, India

Adinarayana Andy
https://orcid.org/0000-0002-5163-1094
Weatherwax Family Pharmacies Inc, Spring Arbor, USA

K. J. Nithin Sujay
https://orcid.org/0009-0007-4689-7940
St. Mary's College of Pharmacy, India

Darshan Huraliganganahalli Balaramegowda
https://orcid.org/0009-0001-3001-3254
University of East Anglia, Norwich, UK

A. M. T. Gurubasavaraj
https://orcid.org/0009-0008-9256-2436
YSS College of Pharmacy, Kudligi, India

Dhanalakshmi Perumal
Faculty of Pharmacy, Dr. MGR Educational and Research Institute, Chennai, India

DOI: 10.4018/979-8-3373-5821-5.ch003

Vikas Huraliganganahalli Balaramegowda
https://orcid.org/0009-0003-0154-5168
Swansea Medical School, Swansea, UK

P.A. Sreeja
https://orcid.org/0009-0000-9297-0757
Dr. MGR Educational and Research Institute, Chennai, India

Aiswarya Nair
Institute of Microbiology, India

ABSTRACT

Malaria persists across the Amazon basin as ecological conditions, deforestation, mobility, and health system gaps sustain transmission in indigenous and riverine communities. This chapter examines ethnomedicine as a complementary pathway for malaria control in Latin America, positioning traditional knowledge within epidemiological, ecological, and political realities. It details participatory, field-based plant surveys semi-structured interviews, guided walks, herbarium validation, and access-and-benefit-sharing to document medicinal plants and link community pharmacopeias to phytochemical profiling and in vitro antiplasmodial testing. Case studies show therapeutic promise, toxicity cautions, and polyherbal synergy. The chapter advances intercultural health models linking traditional healers, community health agents, rapid diagnostics, and conservation-linked medicinal gardens, and proposes policy paths for recognition of indigenous health systems, sustainable harvesting, equitable benefit-sharing, and governance aligning biodiversity stewardship with resilient malaria control.

INTRODUCTION

Globally, malaria continues to be the most persistent vector-borne disease in Latin America, albeit at a decreasing rate. Still, Brazil's Amazon region accounts for hundreds of thousands of malaria cases annually (Ferreira et al., 2022). While malaria is virtually absent in cities, rural and forested regions continue to experience significant transmission.

The Amazon is more than 6 million square kilometers in more than 9 countries. It creates perfect ecological settings for malaria. Periodic flooding, a dense system of rivers and streams, and humid forests for most of the year give *Anopheles darlingi* and other malaria mosquito vectors myriad breeding sites. Human activities increase the risk even more. Isolated riverside communities, temporary mining camps, and shifting agricultural boundaries place large numbers of people in direct contact with malaria mosquito habitats (Amaral et al., 2024). Indigenous people live in communities that are distanced from the health system, which contributes to increased malaria infection and increased delays in treatment. As a result of poverty, inadequate infrastructure, and political silences, these communities are extremely vulnerable. Many of them rely on local knowledge systems and traditional healing practices as a primary response to illness (Hogan et al., 2024).

During the 1940s and 1950s, campaigns aimed at eradicating malaria focused on the widespread ill effects of DDT, which, at the time, was more economically DDT. DDT was used to spray down and kill large mosquito populations, with some success. But, with the negative ecological long-term effects and the eventual defiance of "super" mosquitoes, the health concerns, and the lack of sustainability the DDT campaigns had to be stopped. The same marginal success was observed with the pharmaceuticals, namely chloroquine, artemisinin and combination therapies (Colonia et al, 2024). The lack of success was observed with the uneven distribution of the products, particularly in remote areas. Efforts to contain and control malaria on the Amazon's cartographic spread of communities illustrate the absence of health initiatives which considered local and dispersed realities. Specifically, health campaigns inspired and organized in the Amazon focused on the urban spaces, agricultural frontiers, and dispersed riverine communities with limited success because of the seasonal and territorial movements of miners and loggers (De Salazar et al 2025). To this day, malaria continues to showcase the limited success of centrally planned, uniform, and generalized strategies on focused and defined regions of the world, and in this case, the Amazon (Arisco et al, 2024). The Amazon continues to struggle with the prevailing global and local strategies focused on uprating the region's infrastructure.

The ongoing presence of malaria in the Amazon region highlights the importance of adopting different strategies. Ethnomedicine can be both a pragmatic resource and a philosophical shift on a broader level. Traditional healers and community knowledge about malaria provide immediate access to treatment, especially in settings where biomedical health care is remote or unavailable. Many Amazonian peoples have been using plant-based treatments for fever, chills, and other malaria-like symptoms for centuries (Lindberg et al., 2023). Although not all of these remedies may be effective at reducing malaria, several have been shown through laboratory testing to have substantial antimalarial properties.

Breakthroughs in the treatment of malaria have, in the past, been developed using ethnomedical practices. Quinidne and artemisinin were developed based on ethnomedical practices using Cinchona and Artemisia annua, and each subsequently changed the course of global medicine. In the Amazon, one of the biologically richest regions of the world, the potential for ethnomedical practices to facilitate discovery is still significant. (Ferreira et al., 2022). Ethnomedicine seeks to provide a far more comprehensive and holistic perspective on illness and health, where the body, the land, the spirit, and the community must all be in a balanced state. This is a reminder to us all that treating disease is not only about biology but also about relationships and meaning.

The chapter has five objectives

1. To document the epidemiological and social dimensions of malaria in Amazonia.
2. To describe field-based methods for ethnobotanical plant surveys and knowledge documentation.
3. To present case studies of medicinal plants with demonstrated or potential antimalarial activity.
4. To examine partnerships between indigenous communities and researchers, including successes and ethical challenges.
5. To discuss the broader implications for policy, sustainability, and the integration of traditional medicine into national health strategies.

The scope extends beyond pharmacology. It emphasizes community empowerment, ecological stewardship, and cultural respect, positioning ethnomedicine as both a practical and symbolic tool for rethinking malaria control in the 21st century.

Malaria in Latin America: Epidemiological and Socio-Environmental Landscape

Malaria shows uneven distribution in Latin America, clustering in certain ecological and socio-economic areas. The Amazon basin is responsible for over 90% of the region's cases (Wetzler et al., 2022). Brazil has the highest numbers of infections, particularly in Amazonas, Acre, and Rondônia, states that are considered hotspots (Arisco et al., 2024). Peru, Colombia, and Venezuela also have significant cases, though with different levels of transmission intensity.

In Venezuela, the political and economic crisis and illegal mining operations have triggered a migratory influx into Bolívar state, worsening the malaria case crisis in the endemic region (Fletcher et al., 2022). Colombia has improved in reducing overall malaria incidence during the last decades, but still has significant outbreaks in riverine and Afro-descendant communities (Wetzler et al., 2022). In Peru, the Loreto region, in the heart of the Amazon, has malaria seasonal surges during flooding times and increased riverine mobility (Colonia et al., 2024).

Ecuador, Suriname and Guyana have lower totals of malaria cases, but still have persistent foci of transmission in endemic regions. These areas are often in isolated or marginalised indigenous and migrant communities. This phenomenon clearly illustrates that malaria is more than a continental problem: it is a problem defined by geography, politics, and economic marginalisation.

The amazon is ideal location for malaria carrying mosquitoes, especially, *Anopheles darlingi.* The ecological system in amazon, such as rivers, lakes and seasonally flooded forests make more convenient environment for mosquito growth and survival (Garcia et al., 2025). Along with ecology, high humid climate makes more cozy for breeding and increases human exposure (Colonia et al., 2024; Arisco et al., 2024).

People residing in amazon region are at high risk of malaria. Usually, humans working for infrastructure projects, are forced to work in forest regions making them more prone to malaria. Migrant laborers frequently move between high-transmission areas and urban centers, allowing the parasite to circulate across wider regions (Wetzler et al., 2022). In essence, malaria in the Amazon is not an isolated phenomenon; it is deeply embedded in the region's social and ecological dynamics. This makes people to reduced access to healthcare, increasing morbidity (Wetzler et al., 2022).

Some communities such as riverine caboclo, descendants of indigenous, African and European people, are more at risk for malaria. Because these people depend on agriculture, fishing, making them more in contact with mosquito growing areas. As previously mentioned, limited healthcare, leads to reinfection (Fletcher et al., 2022). Migrant laborers working on agricultural frontiers experience comparable vulnerabilities, especially in areas of rapid forest clearance. Women, pregnant women and children in this region are at greater risk of severe malaria and more fatal to children. These overlapping social, economic, and biological vulnerabilities reveal why malaria persists despite sustained government control efforts.

Deforestation is one of the common reasons which contribute to increase mosquito population. Research from Brazil and Peru, explains about the link between forest loss and increasing malaria cases (Colonia et al., 2024; Arisco et al., 2024; Garcia et al., 2025). Climate change not only compounds for humid temperature but also can lengthen malarial reproductive cycle, and intensifies with seasonal peaks. Extreme floods can damage existing healthcare facilities in forest and increases risk of malaria making it more vulnerable (Garcia et al., 2025).

Sometimes, dams, reservoirs, isolated communities to greater human traffic, accelerating parasite flow with stagnant water makes ideal place for anopheles to grow more. These environmental changes highlight how Amazon is entangled with landscape changes and development. It cannot be separated from debates about conservation, climate resilience, and who bears the burden of frontier expansion.

Ethnomedicine against Malaria:

Ethnomedicine means body of healing and practices within cultural traditions. It is about not only use of medicinal plants but also ritual practices, cosmologies, and community-based understanding of illness (Alum, 2024). Ethnomedicine is inseparable from the traditional ecological knowledge (TEK). Healing involves maintaining harmony between individuals, communities and their environment (Lindberg et al., 2023; Alum, 2024).

Usually researchers focus on identifying active chemical compounds and local healers often focus on spiritual origin of illness, taboos around harvesting, or ritual preparation of remedies. Understanding ethnomedicine therefore requires moving beyond pharmacology to appreciate a holistic worldview where health, ecology, and spirituality are intertwined (Alum, 2024; Lindberg et al., 2023).

In Amazon basin, people consider disease is not only related to biological event but also a disturbance in spiritual relations. People also assume, illness arise from broken taboos, sorcery, or imbalance with the natural world. Common fever and chills are often attributed to spirits of rivers and forest. Treatments are therefore designed not just to eliminate symptoms but to realign patients with cosmic and ecological orders (Alum, 2024). These people mainly depend on healers known as shamans, pajés, or curanderos depending on the cultural group. Healers prescribe plant-based infusions, but accompanied by chants, smoke, or rituals designed to remove harmful influences. Healing is often a communal affair, with family or community members participating in ceremonies (Lindberg et al., 2023; Alum, 2024). Rituals reinforce community cohesion. Importantly, ethnomedical practices are dynamic rather than static. Communities adapt remedies, integrate new plants, and borrow from neighbors, producing a constantly evolving pharmacopeia (Alum, 2024). Medicinal plants are important part of Amazonian ethnomedicine. For malaria, Amazonian people prefer decoctions, infusions, or baths from bark, leaves and roots (de Páscoa Júnior et al., 2021; Milliken et al., 2021).

Some plants are used directly for antimalarial purposes, while others used for symptoms such as fever, chills, or weakness. Bitter-tasting plants commonly prescribed for fever, reflecting an empirical recognition of their pharmacological potential. For some diseases, combinations of plants are used in polyherbal preparations to increase efficacy and to manage side effects (Milliken et al., 2021; Ribeiro et al., 2023). Collection of plant and preparation of medicine will be based on the ritual context. These details highlight how plant use is embedded in cultural logics that go beyond chemistry (Alum, 2024).

Amazonian people believe that wearing roots as amulets burned to ward off harmful spirits, or consumed as tonics to strengthen the body. Whether or not these practices affect parasite loads, they shape community resilience and provide frameworks of meaning in the face of disease (Lindberg et al., 2023; Alum, 2024). The global history of malaria control is deeply tied to indigenous knowledge. For instance, a bark derived from the *Cinchona* genus, was used by Andean communities before European colonization. Most popular marketed drug for malaria, artemisinin though derived from a plant outside the Amazon but best example of ethnomedical insight transforming global medicine (Ribeiro et al., 2023; Alum, 2024).

Within the Amazon itself, numerous plants are under study for antimalarial properties. *Quassia amara* is one such example, having attracted interest for its bitter compounds. While few Amazonian plants have yet been developed into mainstream drugs, the potential remains significant (Milliken et al., 2021; de Páscoa Júnior et al., 2021). However, these contributions raise ethical challenges. The extraction of indigenous knowledge without recognition, is often labeled "biopiracy" (Alum, 2024; "Biopiracy: the largely lawless plundering," 2020). Moving forward, equitable partnerships must ensure indigenous communities are equal stakeholders in benefits derived from their knowledge (Alum, 2024; Lindberg et al., 2023).

Field-Based Plant Surveys Approaches and Methodologies:

In Amazonia, careful methods are required of field-based plant studies. Ethnobotanical studies start with the community rather than random sampling of the vegetation as in conventional ecological studies. Methods such as focus groups to evaluate knowledge, guided walks with communities to collect plant samples, and semi-structured interviews with healers, are traditional methods employed by researchers (Horackova et al., 2023).

When developing a survey, it is important to find a balance between scientific rigor and cultural consideration. Rather than just using rigid questionnaires, ethnobotanists typically allow the healer to talk about their experiences with illness and treatment, thus obtaining better contextual information. Key informants might be chosen based on cultural recognition of who are known or respected experts in a community shamans, midwives, elder women, or other older healers. Likewise, surveys often go beyond experts to recognize what is happening in daily practices among households (Davis et al., 2021).

When conducting surveys, seasonality is also a factor, as some plants may only be available during rainy seasons or certain lunar cycles. This is essential for long-term involvement longer than a few months. Triangulation for example, confirmation of plant identity and/or use by multiple informants, can help avoid over-reliance on just one voice (Bussmann & Sharon, 2022).

Power relations are another significant consideration. As a result of long histories of exploitation and bioprospecting, the community will likely be suspicious of outsiders. Creating this trust takes time, requires transparency about the purpose of the research, joint decision-making, and assurances that the knowledge and specimens will not be exploited (Alum, 2024). After identification has occurred during the field walk, specimens are gathered for scientific documentation. Typically, leaves, flowers, and, at times, bark are pressed between newspaper, dried, and labeled for storage in the herbarium. In each instance, metadata is recorded, including local name, a description of the habitat, plant part used, preparation, and cultural information provided by informants (Horackova et al., 2023).

Taxonomy must be accurately recorded. Many Amazonian species are morphologically similar, making field identification challenging; misidentifications can provide erroneous information to pharmacological research or reduce trust with local communities. Working with local botanists and herbaria is a good option for classification, which is confirmed by cross-referencing the specimens to existing collections in regional or international institutions (Bussmann & Sharon, 2022).

Modern digital technologies (e.g., high-resolution images, GPS coordinates, and DNA barcoding) have taken over some functions of the traditional herbarium model, although the humidity and isolation of the Amazon will prove logistical challenges (Horackova et al., 2023). Herbarium collections do not just hold scientific value; they also hold cultural value as they create connections between indigenous names, their ecological context, and potential biomedical benefits (Davis et al., 2021).

At the heart of ethnobotanical surveys is ethics; generations of bioprospecting have made Amazonian communities skeptical of researchers. Informed consent cannot be seen as a one-off bureaucratic exercise but must be seen as an ongoing back and forth of dialogue to negotiate and talk about. Communities must understand what research is, what is done with the things that are learned, and how they might benefit (Alum, 2024).

Reciprocity is key. Researchers may wish to take the opportunity to contribute to local activities such as community gardens, workshops, or occasion a donation to health service. At the very least, results should be fed back as, at a minimum, locally relevant forms, such as booklets in indigenous languages, illustrated guides, or manuals for applied use (Horackova et al., 2023). Intellectual Property (IP) can be contentious. While frameworks such as the Nagoya Protocol exist to make sure that there is a just access and sharing of benefits, there may still be uneven enforcement in Amazonian regions that are removed. Without safeguards, traditional knowledge may be commercialized by pharmaceutical companies without remuneration for the communities of source (Alum, 2024).

Ethnobotanical studies are often used as a first step toward pharmacological validation. After the plants many then be tested for anti-malarial activity in the lab following ethanol extract preparation and conducting in vitro assays to screen against Plasmodium falciparum. Having identified a promising candidate the next stage would be animal models of antimalarial activity, which reopens or leads to ethical debate. (Ribeiro et al., 2023).

Phytochemical analysis is intended to separate the bioactive compounds. Many plants from the Amazon have members containing alkaloids, flavonoids, terpenes, and quassinoids that may possess anti-malarial activity (Ribeiro et al., 2023). Potentially, certain quassinoids have been derived from Quassia amara (e.g., simalikalactone

E) and shown antiparasitic activity (Cachet et al., 2099; Berlowitz et al., 2021). Still, efficacy is not guaranteed some traditional remedies may act mainly to relieve symptoms rather than eliminate parasites (Davis et al., 2021).

It is crucial to approach combining field and laboratory studies with care. Scientists must be cautious not to fall into the "biopiracy trap," which means taking active ingredients while stripping active ingredients from their cultural or ecological contexts. In an ideal world, research programs would be co-designed with people, including clear agreements on ownership, benefit-sharing, and publication (Alum, 2024).

The methodological challenge is trying to balance two worlds, the holistic, community-based logic and approaches of ethnomedicine and the reductionist, compound-based frameworks of biomedicine. If integration works as hoped, it could result both in new drugs, and in collaborative models for ethical and culturally respectful research (Horackova et al., 2023; Bussmann & Sharon, 2022).

CASE STUDIES

Cinchona spp. The Classic Antimalarial Tree

Cinchona's journey, an ethnomedical story from the Andean-Amazonian transition zones, is likely the most recognized ethnomedical contribution to malaria prevention. Indigenous Quechua and other Andean populations utilized its bitter bark to alleviate fevers long before European colonization (Ceravolo et al., 2021). Jesuit missionaries brought the bark to Europe in the 17th century, referring to it as "Jesuit's powder" (Dewees, J., 2023). Quinine was extracted from the bark in the 19th century, representing the first successful antimalarial to be used globally (Khosropour et al., 2024). After its extraction, while quinine enabled European colonial expansion into Africa and Asia, it also initiated a long-standing history of extracting profit from Indigenous knowledge with neither recognition nor benefit-sharing (Middleton, T., 2024). As synthetic medications and resistance to medications have developed, quinine has become less important, but the legacy of Cinchona persists. Modern treatments such as chloroquine have been designed to model off of the alkaloid structure of quinine (Nosten, F et al., 2022). The story of Cinchona is illustrative of not only the extent of ethnomedicine to reshape global health, but the ethical nuances of such an endeavor.

Quassia amara (Bitterwood Remedies):

Quassia amara, or "pau amargo" or simply "amargo" in local terminology, is a small tree that is broadly distributed throughout the Amazon. Its bark and wood are used by indigenous and riparian populations as infusions due to their intensely bitter taste, which is purportedly useful for fever and gastrointestinal issues (Gomes, A et al., 2021). In laboratory studies, quassinoids, a class of compounds that are highly significant in relation to their biological activity such as antimalarial activity, extracted from Q. amara were capable of inhibiting Plasmodium falciparum in vitro (Nosten, F et al., 2022). However, toxicity is a concern, especially at high doses that can lead to liver damage. As stated, due to the bitter taste, in communities the plant is rarely used alone as healers combine it with other herbs to mitigate its bitter taste or balance thermal properties associated with "hot" versus "cold" in terms of their effects (Siqueira-Neto et al., 2023).

Aspidosperma spp. (Snakewood and Its Alkaloids):

The Aspidosperma genus belongs to the Apocynaceae family, and species in this genus are used throughout the Amazon in the treatment of fevers and malarial illnesses. Locally termed "carapanaúba" or "snakewood," the tree is prepared through the decoction of its bark in rural and indigenous households. Phytochemical studies have documented the presence of alkaloids, including aspidospermine and quebrachine, that have demonstrated antimalarial activity. Historically, they were used in situations where quinine was unavailable, although aspidospermine was reportedly less effective than quinine. The bark is traditionally prepared as a decoction and consumed for several days; it is said to be strong with purgative properties and is reserved for extreme or severe cases (Ceravolo et al., 2024).

Polyherbal Remedies and Synergistic Approaches:

In contrast to Western science, which often searches for a single "active ingredient," many Amazon Remedies are polyherbal, or mixtures of several plants. Healers emphasize synergy, or that the plants work together for salutary effects. For instance, a remedy for fever might combine a bitter plant to suppress parasites, a cooling herb to cool down the fever, and perhaps another plant to ward off danger from the spirit world. Pharmacological research suggests that polyherbal preparations may reduce toxic effects or improve their effects via additive or synergistic interactions. There is evidence in the literature that mixtures can produce greater effects than a decoction of just one plant (de Swiet et al., 2023). Taking these practices into account demonstrates empirical sophistication and the need not to categorize traditional indigenous pharmacologies as 'superstitions.'

CHALLENGES OF EFFICACY, TOXICITY, AND VALIDATION

Not every traditional remedy works according to biomedicine. While some may relieve symptoms, they may not eliminate the parasite, which poses the risk of still allowing the infection to persist; and others may be toxic at high doses. For example, strong alkaloids from the genus Aspidosperma have shown in animal studies to be associated with sedation, respiratory effects, and other signs of toxicity (Lins et al., 2021). This means there is a tension in how to assess the medicines without denying their cultural relevance. Clinical trials are expensive and rarely suitable for traditional contexts; and at the same time, untested remedies with overconfidence in their effects could be threatening to the patient. The communities themselves know this, and identify plant uses as "light" for everyday use, and "strong" requiring expert administration. Therefore, efforts at validation must be cautious, open, and participative. Instead of taking compounds and solely looking for testing pharmacological tests research can work with the communities to co-design of safely and efficacy evaluations, in culturally relevant formats. This method respects both shared standards of biomedicine and indigenous autonomy (Nascimento Brandão et al., 2020).

Indigenous Partnerships in Malaria Control

Relationships between researchers, government, and indigenous communities have changed over the years. Historically, most interactions were exploitative. Researchers encountered indigenous communities, and without proper consult, took plant samples, recorded indigenous knowledge of plant-based remedies, or documented practices, with little benefit to the community or healer (Heinrich, 2020). This generalized method contributed to the continue skepticism and mistrust of researchers.

In the past few decades, collaborative, or participatory, relationships have been developed. In this model, the community does not serve only as informants, to be used by the researcher, but co-researchers. healers and community leaders determine research agendas, priorities, and dissemination of findings. A affirmation of ethics is an essential component for relationships that build reciprocity in ethical research. The scientist gains an additional layer of understanding about the broader context, and community members gain training, benefits, resources, or acknowledgement of their indigenous practices, for example.

Co-management of health programs is yet another model. In this model, indigenous organizations partner with a ministry of health, or non-governmental organization, to administer their own culturally appropriate methods of malaria prevention and treatment. Within these roles, community health workers, often trained in a combination of biomedicine and ethnomedicine and often bilingual, play roles to bridge the two systems.

These shifts in the emphasis in research methods and types of relationships can also be viewed through broader shifts in governance and ethics. Globally, agreements, such as the Nagoya Protocols, have increased awareness of expectations of fair and equitable sharing of benefits in the utilization of indigenous knowledge and thereby protocols. Those legal mechanisms are not sufficient to ensuring equity (Heinrich, 2020; Colella, 2023). Equity implies an element of mutual respect and trust, or lack of mistrust, that is built around indigenous governance and where the community is entitled to the knowledge and not the researcher.

Various initiatives in Latin America demonstrate how partnerships can support malaria control.

- Brazil: In the Upper Rio Negro region, indigenous federations collaborated with researchers to collect and document medicinal plants used to treat fever and infections. Programs of training and support for young Indigenous researchers, as well as for Indigenous health agents who delivered biomedical (e.g. rapid diagnostic tests) and traditional healing methods, built trust in terms of what they both offered for malaria control.
- Peru: In Loreto, NGOs have worked collaboratively with riverine communities to incorporate plant-based remedies into malaria communication and awareness campaigns. Workshops presented opportunities for biomedical care providers and healers to bring their expertise to dialogue with one another and refine these strategies for local malaria prevention (e.g. reframing the use of mosquito nets in local cosmologies) and increase uptake of malaria interventions among the community.
- Colombia: In the Amazonian Vaupés region, collaboratively-developed community medicinal gardens exist in conjunction with traditional medicine and as community pharmacies. These gardens are not to replace pharmaceutical options but are locally-oriented options with medicinal plants, where biomedical care is distant and communities lack access to formal health posts.
- Venezuela: Due to the collapse of the public health systems, many Indigenous communities are relying upon traditional pharmacopeia. Some NGOs are seeking to support communities by documenting traditional remedies and share illustrated guides in their languages. These partnerships may seem small but exemplify resiliency in contexts of weak governance.

These examples reveal the diversity of partnerships some research-oriented, some service-oriented, some conservation-driven. All show that malaria control can be strengthened when communities are treated as partners, not passive beneficiaries.

Partnerships with indigenous communities offer multiple benefits for malaria control:

1. Trust and legitimacy: When programs are respectful of traditional medicine, they are more likely to achieve acceptance. If biomedical interventions are positively endorsed by healers, acceptance rates will surge.
2. Integration of knowledge: Ethnomedical understanding of mosquito behavior, seasonal cycles of illness, or plant-based options for prevention can strengthen epidemiological models.
3. Capacity building: By involving indigenous health care workers and training them in biomedical practices and traditional systems, these approaches build local autonomy, decrease reliance on outside actors, and produce community health care experts.
4. Conservation and sustainability: Projects that create medicinal plant gardens or protected harvesting areas support biodiversity, which should also sustain malaria research and treatment options that can scale over time.
5. Cultural revitalization: Projects that engage partnerships further acknowledge and build capacity for traditional practices in communities and address historical marginalization of indigenous practices, fostering development of community pride, resilience, and cohesion.

Nonetheless, the partnerships are not always free of concerns. The initial power imbalance may exist, allowing scientists to navigate decision-making in projects and limiting communities' understanding of the process or outcome. Alternatively, governments may impose agendas in relationships with little sensibility or consideration from the communities involved. In some communities, there are worries of biopiracy in which knowledge could be utilized and commodified without compensation to the community (Heinrich, 2020).

Clashes between knowledge systems may create further barriers to collaboration. Biomedical staff may view traditional practices as unscientific or unreliable; traditional healers may view biomedical treatments as culturally unsuitable or unsafe for spiritual reasons. Such tensions need to attended adequately to have the potential to encourage mistrust. Logistical challenges are real. Distance, unncertainty about funding, and perhaps governing instability may make it difficult to get intended programs off the ground, let alone to a high standard. Popping, sustainability is tenuous, and after external funding ceases, community members may not know what next or may not feel encouraged to keep going.

Ultimately, the revitalization of traditional practices will generate their own tensions internally. Younger generations may be less interested in maintaining traditional practices, or communities may differ in their levels of comfort about what knowledge to pass on to others. Partnerships will need to carefully consider these and other tensions altogether, but with nuance and in a way that demonstrates respect for community variety and commitment to governance.

Challenges and Ethical Dilemmas

One of the most significant issues in Amazonian ethnomedicine is the threat of biopiracy: the unauthorized use of traditional knowledge and genetic resources without just recognition and sharing of benefits. The history of malaria control is bound up in this dilemma, as quinine from Cinchona bark became a global commodity with little recognition of Andean peoples, and later, fields in Asia removed local monopolies (Gebara et al., 2023).

Today, Amazonian communities are still suspicious of outsiders collecting plants or documenting remedies. Pharmaceutical companies and researchers affiliated with universities can be viewed with suspicion because these patterns of appropriation have occurred in the past. Global agreements, like the Convention on Biological Diversity (CBD), and or the Nagoya Protocol attempt to ensure access and benefit sharing; however, the enforcement of these legal agreements is less reliable in the context of remote forests (Bency Baby et al., 2022).

This creates a dilemma: without working with outsiders, many remedies may go undocumented and the potential to benefit is lost, and with their assistance, knowledge may be commodified, or they could violate their trust. The goal is to build frameworks in which Indigenous people have ownership and agency over who is accessing their knowledge and can share any benefits, whether they are monetary, cultural, and or infrastructural (Berlowitz et al., 2025).

Reconciling Traditional Knowledge with Biomedical Frameworks

Another issue comes in assessing traditional remedies. The expectations of biomedical science include standardized trials, reproducible doses, and quantification of outcomes, whereas ethnomedicine from a community perspective often focuses on personalized treatment, the context of the ritual, and the balance experienced by the patient. These two systems of thought do not always mesh (Ogorzewska 2022; Pesantes et al., 2024). For instance, a healer may explain that a plant works depending on who harvested it, which moon cycle the harvest occurred, and what words were said in the ritual. These things are not measurable through biomedical protocols and while dismissing them may risk alienation in the community, it may also neglect the possibility of toxicity or lack of efficacy (Berlowitz et al. 2025). The vocation is not so much to collapse one system of thought into the other system of thought, but to create a space where respectful dialogue can occur. Attempts to do this in Brazil and Peru are called "intercultural health" initiatives where biomedical clinics build into the services of traditional healers, but these initiatives also remain fragile initiatives and sometimes underfunded (Ogorzewska 2022; Pesantes et al, 2024).

Political Marginalization of Indigenous Communities

Politics and health challenges in the Amazon go hand in hand. Indigenous communities often do not have formal land rights, Health services are historically underfunded, and they are often not part of the decision-making process. Urban capitals design interventions for Malaria that rarely consider the realities on the ground in isolated and remote villages (Ramos, 2022).

Even if an indigenous health system is recognized by a government, it matters very little if there is without incorporation or systems of inclusion. The system of traditional medicine is recognized as a system of supplemental knowledge, not an equal system. This continues cycles of inequity (Berlowitz et al., 2025). Partnerships with NGOs or academic organizations can help fill gaps in capacity and generally support indigenous health systems, but it requires systemic change, including indigenous voices in health governance systems altogether to support long-term change in future health services more generally (Barreto et al., 2025).

Marginalization intersects with the politics of the environment. Deforestation, mining, or some infrastructure projects have an effect on raising the risk of Malaria, and do not allow for Indigenous communities to be part of the decision-making process. In this way, control for Malaria is not separate from control over land, self-determination, and sustainable practices for cultural survival (Barreto et al., 2025).

Logistical and Practical Constraints

The Amazon's natural environment presents significant challenges for malaria control. In this setting, communities could be days away from a health clinic only accessible by a river or a small plane. Implementation of the cold-chain for medicines, distribution of bed nets, or planning and conducting clinical trials will require resources well-beyond the reach of most health programs. For researchers themselves, fieldwork presents obstacles as well we have humidity ruining specimens, unreliable methods of transport and negotiating time away from communities or twice the distance in a longer duration. These logistical hurdles mean that even the best partnerships or the most promising cure for malaria may not work practically (Ramos 2022).

Sustainability of Plant Harvesting and Conservation Concerns

Lastly, we must address the environmental quandary - many plants that yield antimalarials are taken from natural populations. More supply in any context - local and global - leads to higher harvest levels than could be imposed to the detriment of biodiversity or community access. For illustration, cinchona trees approached extinction in some regions during the colonial quinine trade (Kimura et al., 2023). Sustainability means investing in cultivation through community gardens, reforestation, and regulated harvesting - but these approaches do require funding and training, as well as more presume conservation would allow to occur. Absent of these methods, there is potential that ethnomedicine could further compromise the ecosystems from which human medicine is derived (Silva et al., 2025).

Figure 1. Integrating Ethnomedicine and Indigenous Partnerships in Malaria Control in the Amazon

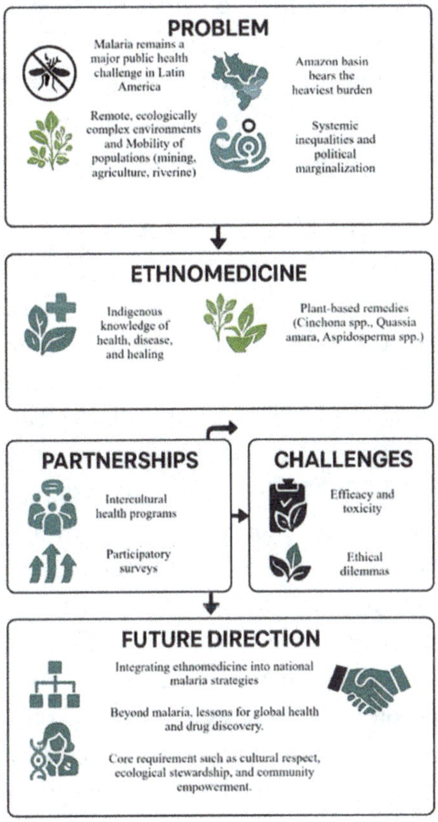

Integrating Ethnomedicine into Malaria Control Policy

Programs of national malaria control throughout Latin America have historically focused attention on biomedical interventions, specifically insecticides for vector control, distribution of treated mosquito nets, and pharmaceutical interventions such as chloroquine or artemisinin combination therapies (ACTs). Although effective in urban and peri-urban contexts, such approaches are challenging to maintain in remote Amazonian locales (Barreto et al. 2025).

Ethnomedicines represent alternative and complementary opportunities. Recognizing indigenous remedies as legitimate, even if not fully validated, increases treatment pharmacopoeia in isolated areas. For example, while rapid diagnostics can confirm malaria, communities may deploy antimalarial plants that are locally available when pharmaceuticals are delayed. Instead of competing philosophies, traditional medicine can be implemented as a first-line approach, with biomedical treatment added when available (Berlowitz et al. 2025; Ramos 2022).

Governments can also formally recognize traditional healers. By working traditional medicine into a community health network, national programs could increase capacity, build community trust, and mitigate any hesitancy to seek care. Such acknowledgment needs to be incorporated in service plans, but the burden of gaps in services will be diminished (Ogorzewsska, 2022; Pesants et al., 2024).

Bridging Traditional and Modern Healthcare Systems

Integration is more than just including plants in official pharmacopeias. Integration is about building bridges between two different systems of knowledge. One model used is "intercultural health," and this takes place in areas of Brazil and Peru. In these areas, clinics may integrate both biomedical practitioners and traditional healers, providing patients a choice and allowing for mutual learning (Berlowitz et al., 2025; Pesantes et al., 2024). Integration of systems also refers to training. An indigenous health agent can be trained in emergency diagnostics utilizing rapid tests and first-line treatments, as well as in community prevention campaigns, and even utilize them for referent points between traditional practices. Biomedial staff can also be trained in local, community-based remedies and cultural constructs of illness, which leads to reducing chances of dismissiveness (Ogorzewska, 2022). Integration as collaboration works best as dialogical processes where healers and doctors share knowledge, negotiate differences and co-create approaches for practice. For instance, the educational messaging regarding mosquito net distribution has met with greater success when framed through local cosmologies of protection, where healers would recommend beds and nets alongside spiritual protection methods (Ramos, 2022). This kind of hybrid model does not take away from either system but builds and strengthens both. It upholds cultural identity and enhances biomedial outcomes (Berlowitz et al., 2025).

Examples of Hybrid Models and Local Innovations

Numerous initiatives in Latin America demonstrate the feasibility of integration. For example, Brazil In the Amazon cities of Acre and Amazonas, intercultural health programs have incorporated traditional practitioners into community-based prevention campaigns, using community gardens to grow medicinal plant species while distributing bed nets (Ramos, 2022). Peru NGOs in Loreto have produced bilingual educational materials to describe malaria transmission that use both biomedical concepts and indigenous cosmologies, showing how alternative avenues of framing prevention messages creates community links (Pesantes et al., 2024).

Colombia University-based initiatives have created new pharmacopeia that have both biomedical medications and validated traditional remedies that can serve as hybrid references for community health agents (Ogorzewska, 2022). These illustrations show that integration is not an abstract policy, but grounded community experimentation. Although still small, collectively they show models that can be sufficiently replicated and expanded through supportive policies.

Potential for Local Production and Distribution of Phytotherapeutics

An additional opportunity exists in developing phytotherapeutics standardized for local production. If local plants with antimalarial activity could be sustainably cultivated and processed locally, it would generate reliable access to care while simultaneously generating new economic opportunities. Tinctures, capsules, or teas could be prepared at small-scale laboratories, generally supported by universities or NGOs, under controlled conditions (Gebara et al., 2023). This would require investment in training to facilitate quality control and regulation; however, this could alleviate some of the reliance on vulnerable pharmaceutical supply chains in remote areas. Local production would also enhance prospects for communities to be the ongoing stewards and beneficiaries of their resources - rather than being simply suppliers of raw product to other markets.

Policy Recommendations

For integration to succeed, policies should

1. Formally recognize indigenous health systems as complementary to biomedical approaches.
2. Ensure benefit-sharing under the Nagoya Protocol for any commercialization of plant-based remedies.
3. Invest in intercultural health training for both biomedical staff and indigenous health agents.
4. Support community gardens and conservation initiatives to safeguard medicinal plant resources.
5. Promote participatory governance, giving indigenous organizations a voice in national malaria strategies (Heinrich et al., 2022; Barreto et al., 2025).

Such measures can transform malaria control from a top-down intervention into a partnership that strengthens resilience, cultural identity, and health outcomes.

Broader Implications and Future Directions

The Amazon region is one of the last main reservoirs of malaria in the Americas, and the work there offers key lessons that apply globally. First, malaria is not only a biomedical problem, it is also an ecological and cultural problem. Control strategies that truly neglect local realities geography, migration, cosmologies will not succeed. The examples from the Amazon region indicate that interventions work when they are culturally grounded and led by the community (Berlowitz et al., 2025; Ramos, 2022).

Second, the Amazonian experience emphasizes the role of biodiversity in drug discovery. Many of the most effective antimalarials came from plants quinine, artemisinin and the Amazon's unparalleled biodiversity means there are likely still medicines to be discovered. Thus, preserving these ecosystems is not only an environmental issue but a global health one (Barreto et al., 2025). Finally, Amazonian collaborations illustrate the idea of indigenous knowledge contributing to health resilience. Indigenous survival strategies that blend plants, ritual, and ecological observation represent potential adaptive health systems that might inform efforts in malaria endemic regions of the world, for example, sub-Saharan Africa or Southeast Asia (Ogorzewska, 2022; Pesantes et al., 2024).

Though malaria is the primary focus, Amazonian ethnomedicine has relevance for non-malaria neglected tropical diseases (NTDs), including leishmaniasis, Chagas, and intestinal parasites. Many communities utilize the same forms of treatment for several NTDs, which is founded in an empirical understanding of symptoms that overlap, and co-infections of NTDs (Berlowitz et al., 2025).

When considering this for global health, it demonstrates that the incorporation of ethnomedicine is not malaria-dependent. Furthermore, some traditional plant based remedies may be considered as newer options, or as broad-spectrum for NTDs within the parasitic and vector-borne diseases. Additionally, the intercultural health frameworks on malaria-related NTDs can be easily translated into other conditions, for instance training indigenous health agents to recognize skin lesions from leishmaniasis, or cardiac symptoms of Chagas while also using traditional remedies that mitigate the symptoms (Pesantes et al., 2024). This broader applicability further supports the idea that ethnomedicine is not marginal or some outdated method of treatment, but an essential component of health work in resource-constrained settings (Berlowitz et al., 2025).

Equity must be at the forefront of future directions in research. Too frequently, indigenous communities have been treated as raw data collectors instead of collaborators. In the future, partnerships must be co-designed with communities developing research questions, determining access to knowledge and, contributing to any benefits (Heinrich et al., 2020; Scott et al., 2023). The need for capacity building is important. For example, creating and training indigenous youth in ethnobotany, lab skills, or public health programming can help ensure that communities are not only participants, but leaders in research. In Brazil and Colombia, some research teams have already created "indigenous ethnobotanists" to collect medicinal plants utilized in their community, both for cultural transmission of knowledge and for preliminary scientific outputs to inform future studies (Ramos, 2022). Equitable partnerships will also require transparency. Agreements regarding intellectual property, sharing of benefits, and publication all need to be established and unit from the beginning. Only then can ethnomedicine add to the healing and health of the world and not further exploit communities in a colonial modelling.

Innovations in Drug Discovery Inspired by Traditional Knowledge

Drug discovery is increasingly shifting towards "biocultural" strategies that fuse insights from ethno-medicine with contemporary drug screen technologies. In lieu of randomizing thousands of compounds without a direction, researchers use plants that have been observed by healers to have anti-fever or anti-infection properties. This reduces the number of compounds unnecessarily tested, optimizes discoverability and, equally important, honors indigenous knowledge (Gebara et al., 2023). The developments in metabolomics, machine learning, and high-throughput screening can significantly amplify this approach. AI models are already trained to analyze plant extracts and identify likelihoods for bioactive compounds, which can radically diminish the time to go from the field to the laboratory. This builds on ethnomedical leads and creating a much more robust pipeline for drug discovery (Berlowitz et al., 2025). The ethics of innovation cannot be overlooked in this process. Any drugs developed from novel compounds or extracts of Amazonian plants should include benefit-share mechanisms, financial or in-kind, for indigenous peoples so that they can receive royalties, healthcare infrastructures, or funding for conservation and stewardship. Otherwise, we risk deepening, rather than alleviating inequalities even with scientific progress.

Future Research Agendas

Future research should prioritize systematic ethnobotanical surveys to document both communities and plants that have not yet been deeply explored, clinical validation studies of cultural-sensitive promising remedies, longitudinal studies examine how environmental change (deforestation, mining, climate) alters malaria dynamics and traditional responses, policy studies to assess intercultural health models and promote larger scale action, and conservation studies linking biodiversity conservation efforts with health security (Barreto et al., 2025). Research effort needs to therefore be interdisciplinary, bridging anthropology, pharmacology, ecology, public health (Ogorzewska, 2022).

CONCLUSION

This chapter has looked into the continuing issue of malaria in the Amazon surrounding ethnomedicine and working with Indigenous groups. Malaria's resilience shows that disease causation is not wholly biological, but is also shaped by the challenging environment, shifting political contexts, and social norms. The literature demonstrates that ethnomedicine is more than a source of plant-based remedies; it is a total pathology-based healing system operating within Amazonian cultures. The literature examining plants such as Cinchona and Aspidosperma demonstrates their medicinal efficacy while simultaneously emphasizing their importance to culture. The partnerships with Indigenous groups demonstrate that trust, reciprocal respect and transparency in communication are essential. These relationships can accomplish more than influence malaria mitigation; they also enhance cultural preservation and self-determination.

Even with its potential, big challenges remain. Factors such as biopiracy, ownership of knowledge, political exclusion, and environmental degradation are real risks that deserve careful consideration. As a result, any policy to leverage traditional knowledge must be based on both science and ethics. An important takeaway is that Indigenous knowledge should not be viewed as a peripheral issue but as central to the emergence of successful and sustainable malaria responses in the region. History reminds us of this, as treatment outcomes like quinine have been extracted from traditional treatment methods and subsequently impacted the global care of malaria historically. The Amazon, with its unique merging of biological and cultural richness, has expressed similar possibilities of new discoveries. In order for us to ethically engage with this knowledge requires a fundamental shift in perspective. Indigenous communities must be regarded as equal partners in research, rather than informers or providers of information.

As a result, it is paramount to protect this knowledge from being appropriated, but do so while honouring its living role in culture and science. Malaria programs that are collaborative, involving traditional healers, training local health care workers, and protecting the source of traditional medicinal plants, will be much more responsive and effective than rigid, top-down models of intervention. Ethical frameworks must ensure equitable benefit-sharing, which recognizes and fairly compensates a community for their knowledge and practice. Finally, sustainability is a non-negotiable requirement in all of our efforts. Programs that marry health objectives with environmental sustainability, for example by investing in community medicinal plant gardens, or establishing sustainable harvesting zones, can deliver double benefits, thus achieving malaria objective-linked outcome measures while contributing

Ultimately, inclusion, sustainability, and ethics are not final luxuries; they are the basic foundation for all progress that lasts. To ignore these principles is to repeat the same social injustices and environmental destruction that have allowed malaria to flourish. Malaria is more than a parasite; it is a sign of broken ecosystems, political failure, and the ignoring of Indigenous knowledge to frame the illness. Conquering malaria lies not only in the advancement of better science but in a deeper commitment to partnership, respect, and equity. The Amazon is not merely a setting for illness but a reservoir of the answers. We can imagine an equity-based future for malaria control that draws on Indigenous knowledge, safeguards its biodiversity, and builds equitable partnerships. This will require us to reconstruct the notion of health as something that can be reflected in the performance of communities and the health of their environment.

REFERENCES

Alum, E. U. (2024). The role of indigenous knowledge in advancing the therapeutic use of medicinal plants: Challenges and opportunities. *Plant Signaling & Behavior, 19*(1), 2439255. DOI: 10.1080/15592324.2024.2439255 PMID: 39652401

Amaral, P. S. T., Klauss, K. S. G., Suárez-Mutis, M. C., Coelho, R. R., Galardo, A. K., Murta, F., Moresco, G. G., Siqueira, A. M., & Gurgel-Gonçalves, R. (2024). Malaria in areas under mining activity in the Amazon: A review. *Revista da Sociedade Brasileira de Medicina Tropical, 57*, e00200–e02024. DOI: 10.1590/0037-8682-0551-2023 PMID: 38922216

Arisco, N. J., Peterka, C., Diniz, C., Singer, B. H., & Castro, M. C. (2024). Ecological change increases malaria risk in the Brazilian Amazon. *Proceedings of the National Academy of Sciences of the United States of America, 121*(44), e2409583121. DOI: 10.1073/pnas.2409583121 PMID: 39432796

Barreto, J. R., Rocha, R., Barlow, J., & Loyola, R. (2025). Indigenous territories safeguard human health in the Brazilian Amazon. *Communications Earth & Environment, 6*(1), 1–9. DOI: 10.1038/s43247-025-02620-7 PMID: 39830897

Bency Baby, T., & Suriyaprakash, T. N. K. (2022). Intellectual Property Rights: Bioprospecting, Biopiracy. *Intellectual Property*, 25.

Berlowitz, I., Cuya-Velásquez, L., Brabec de Mori, B., & Rozin, A. (2025). Towards culturally inclusive healthcare in Peru: Epistemic concepts in Indigenous-Amazonian medicine. *Journal of Ethnobiology and Ethnomedicine, 21*(1), 1–18. PMID: 39794744

Berlowitz, I., Pesantes, M. A., Cárdenas Palacios, C., Martin-Soelch, C., Wolf, U., & Maake, C. (2025). Towards culturally inclusive healthcare in Peru: Mapping epistemic concepts in contemporary Indigenous Amazonian medicine—Traditional healers' perspectives. *PLOS Global Public Health, 5*(1), e0003912. DOI: 10.1371/journal.pgph.0003912 PMID: 39823398

"Biopiracy: the largely lawless plundering of Earth's genetic wealth." (2020, December 15). *Global Landscapes Forum* (opinion piece).

Bussmann, R. W., & Sharon, D. (2022). Ethnobotany in the Andes and the Amazon in a changing world. *Canadian Journal of Botany, 100*(6), 431–444. DOI: 10.1139/cjb-2021-0062

Ceravolo, I. P., Aguiar, A. C., Adebayo, J. O., & Krettli, A. U. (2021). Studies on activities and chemical characterization of medicinal plants in search for new Antimalarials: A ten year review on Ethnopharmacology. *Frontiers in Pharmacology, 12*, 734263. DOI: 10.3389/fphar.2021.734263 PMID: 34630109

Ceravolo, I. P., Arcas, R. D. C. C., & Ursine, A. (2024). Plants from South America: A Systematic Review of Their Antiplasmodial and Antimalarial Activities Based on Ethnopharmacological Use. *Journal of Biomedical Research & Environmental Sciences, 2766*(8), 2276. DOI: 10.37871/jbres1972

Colella, J. P. (2023). Engaging with the Nagoya Protocol on Access and Benefit-Sharing: Implications for noncommercial research. *Journal of Mammalogy, 104*(3), 430–440. DOI: 10.1093/jmammal/gyac122

Colonia, C. B., Vásquez-Rodríguez, A. B., Alexander, N., & de la Hoz Restrepo, F. (2024). Malaria, relationship with climatic variables and deforestation in Colombia, Latin America and the Caribbean from 2000 to 2020: A systematic review. *Malaria Journal, 23*(1), 347. DOI: 10.1186/s12936-024-05140-5 PMID: 39558332

Davis, K., Guimarães, M., Davis, G., & Amarante, L. (2021). Ethnobotanical study of anti-malarial plants among riverine communities, Portel, Pará, Brazil. *Revista Fitos, 15*(4), 498–511. DOI: 10.32712/2446-4775.2021.1156

de Páscoa Júnior, J. G., & Luna de Souza, I. L. (2021). *Medicinal plants used in the Amazon region: A systematic review.* Research. *Social Development, 10*(14), e163101419965.

De Salazar, P. M., Parra-Salazar, A., Niles-Robin, R., Valz, O., James, K., Buckee, C. O., & Cox, H. (2025). Malaria spillover in Indigenous Guyanese communities following a crackdown on illegal gold mining in Brazil. *Lancet Regional Health. Americas, 42*, 42. DOI: 10.1016/j.lana.2024.100969 PMID: 39830894

de Swiet, M. (2023). Cinchona: The source of quinine and quinidine. In *Modern Medicines from Plants* (pp. 93-102). CRC Press.

Dewees, J. (2023). Bittersweet Empire: Clements Robert Markham, Cinchona, and Botanical Exploitation. *PhD diss., Wesleyan University.*

Ferreira, M. U., Gamboa, D., Torres, K., Rodriguez-Ferrucci, H., Soto-Calle, V. E., Pardo, K., Fontoura, P. S., Tomko, S. S., Gazzinelli, R. T., Conn, J. E., Castro, M. C., Llanos-Cuentas, A., & Vinetz, J. M. (2022). Evidence-based malaria control and elimination in the Amazon: Input from the International Center of excellence in malaria research network in Peru and Brazil. *The American Journal of Tropical Medicine and Hygiene*, *107*(4, Suppl), 160–167. DOI: 10.4269/ajtmh.21-1272 PMID: 36228907

Fletcher, I. K., Grillet, M. E., Moreno, J. E., Drakeley, C., Hernández-Villena, J., Jones, K. E., & Lowe, R. (2022). Synergies between environmental degradation and climate variation on malaria re-emergence in southern Venezuela: A spatiotemporal modelling study. *The Lancet. Planetary Health*, *6*(9), e739–e748. DOI: 10.1016/S2542-5196(22)00192-9 PMID: 36087604

Garcia, C. G. R., Ribeiro, B. C., Souza, A. S., Lima, L. J. P., Póvoa, M. M., Laporta, G. Z., & Cunha, M. G. (2025). Assessing the spatial influence of deforestation on malaria incidence in Pará State, Amazon region, Brazil, 2008-2019. *Memorias do Instituto Oswaldo Cruz*, *120*, e240143. DOI: 10.1590/0074-02760240143 PMID: 40531672

Gebara, M. F., Ramcilovic-Suominen, S., & Schmidlehner, M. F. (2023). Indigenous Knowledge in the Amazon's Bioeconomy: Unveiling Bioepistemicide through the case of Kambo Medicine. *Forest Policy and Economics*, *154*, 103012. DOI: 10.1016/j.forpol.2023.103012

Gomes, A. R., Albuquerque, K. C., Brígido, H. P., Correa-Barbosa, J., Dolabela, M. F., & Percário, S. (2021). Development of Antimalarial and Antileishmanial Drugs from Amazonian Biodiversity. [Bentham Science Publishers.]. *Frontiers in Clinical Drug Research-Anti-Infectives*, *7*, 127–172. DOI: 10.2174/9789814998093121070007

Heinrich, M. (2020). Access and Benefit-Sharing under the Nagoya Protocol: Opportunities and challenges in Latin America. *Frontiers in Pharmacology / PMC*. https://www.ncbi.nlm.nih.gov/pmc/articles/PMC7294742/

Heinrich, M., Scotti, F., Andrade-Cetto, A., Berger-Gonzalez, M., Echeverría, J., Friso, F., Garcia-Cardona, F., Hesketh, A., Hitziger, M., Maake, C., Politi, M., Spadafora, C., & Spadafora, R. (2020). Access and benefit sharing under the Nagoya protocol—Quo Vadis? Six Latin American case studies assessing opportunities and risk. *Frontiers in Pharmacology*, *11*, 765. DOI: 10.3389/fphar.2020.00765 PMID: 32581783

Hogan, K. M., Gilmore, M., McCarron, G. P., Griffiths, B. M., Koehler, J. W., García, G. A., & von Fricken, M. E. (2024). Knowledge, attitudes, and practices regarding malaria transmission and prevention in an indigenous Maijuna community: A qualitative study in the Peruvian Amazon. *Malaria Journal, 23*(1), 314. DOI: 10.1186/s12936-024-05121-8 PMID: 39425050

Horackova, J., Chuspe Zans, M. E., Kokoska, L., Sulaiman, N., & Clavo Peralta, Z. M. (2023). Ethnobotanical inventory of medicinal plants used by Cashinahua herbalists in the Peruvian Amazon. *Journal of Ethnobiology and Ethnomedicine, 19*(16). Advance online publication. DOI: 10.1186/s13002-023-00586-4 PMID: 37170108

Khosropour, E., Ahangari, S., & Hakimi, L. (2024). Antimalarial Response, Traditional and Other Potential Uses of Cinchona Genera. In *Antimalarial Medicinal Plants* (pp. 174–187). CRC Press. DOI: 10.1201/9781003378396-11

Kimura, L. T., Andrade, E. R., Nobre, I., Nobre, C. A., De Medeiros, B. A., Riaño-Pachón, D. M., Shiraishi, F. K., Carvalho, T. C. M. B., & Simplicio, M. A.Jr. (2023). Amazon Biobank: A collaborative genetic database for bioeconomy development. *Functional & Integrative Genomics, 23*(2), 101. DOI: 10.1007/s10142-023-01015-1 PMID: 36964864

Lindberg, K., Martvall, A., Lima, M. G. B., & Franca, C. S. (2023). Herbal medicine promotion for a restorative bioeconomy in tropical forests: A reality check on the Brazilian Amazon. *Forest Policy and Economics, 155*, 103058. DOI: 10.1016/j.forpol.2023.103058

Lins, F. S. V., da Silva, V. F., Tavares, J. F., dos Santos, V. L., & da Silva Alves, H. (2021). Bioguided isolation of alkaloids and pharmacological effects of the total alkaloid fraction from *Aspidosperma pyrifolium* Mart. (Apocynaceae). *Plants, 10*(11), 2526. DOI: 10.3390/plants10112526 PMID: 34834889

Middleton, T. (2024). *Quinine's Remains: Empire's Medicine and the Life Thereafter*. University of California Press.

Milliken, W., Walker, B. E., Howes, M. J. R., Forest, F., & Nic Lughadha, E. (2021). Plants used traditionally as antimalarials in Latin America: Mining the tree of life for potential new medicines. *Journal of Ethnopharmacology, 279*, 114221. DOI: 10.1016/j.jep.2021.114221 PMID: 34029639

Nascimento Brandão, D. L., Martins, M. T., Silva, A. O., Almeida, A. D., Aguiar Gomes, A. T., Vasconcelos, F., & Dolabela, M. F. (2020). Anti-malarial activity and toxicity of *Aspidosperma nitidum* Benth: A plant used in traditional medicine in the Brazilian Amazon. *Research. Social Development, 9*(10), e5059108817.

Nosten, F., Richard-Lenoble, D., & Danis, M. (2022). A brief history of malaria. *La Presse Medicale*, *51*(3), 104130. DOI: 10.1016/j.lpm.2022.104130 PMID: 35667599

O'Shaughnessy, D. M., & Berlowitz, I. (2021). Amazonian medicine and the psychedelic revival: Considering the "Dieta". *Frontiers in Pharmacology*, *12*, 639124. DOI: 10.3389/fphar.2021.639124 PMID: 34149407

Ogorzewska, Z. (2022). Intercultural health in the Peruvian Amazon: Problems and potentials. *Anuario Latinoamericano*, *10*(1), 93–111. DOI: 10.17951/al.2022.10.93-111

Ramos, D. P. (2022). Indigenous leadership, anthropology and intercultural initiatives in the Upper Rio Negro, Brazilian Amazon. *Anthropology in Action : Newsletter of the British Association for Social Anthropology in Policy and Practice (BASAPP)*, *29*(1), 59–65. DOI: 10.3167/aia.2022.290105

Ribeiro, G. D. J. G., Rei Yan, S. L., Palmisano, G., & Wrenger, C. (2023). Plant extracts as a source of natural products with potential antimalarial effects: An update from 2018 to 2022. *Pharmaceutics*, *15*(6), 1638. DOI: 10.3390/pharmaceutics15061638 PMID: 37376086

Scott, C. S. (2023). Biopiracy: Using New Laws and Databases to Protect Indigenous Communities. *Rich. JL & Tech.*, *30*, 434.

Silva, J. C. K., Soliani, R. D., Ferreira-Júnior, G. C., de Abreu Freitas, R. G., & Lobão, M. S. P. (2025). Bioeconomy In The Amazon: Challenges, opportunities, and trends for regional development. *Revista de Gestão Social e Ambiental*, *19*(1), 1–16. DOI: 10.24857/rgsa.v19n1-166

Siqueira-Neto, J. L., Wicht, K. J., Chibale, K., Burrows, J. N., Fidock, D. A., & Winzeler, E. A. (2023). Antimalarial drug discovery: Progress and approaches. *Nature Reviews. Drug Discovery*, *22*(10), 807–826. DOI: 10.1038/s41573-023-00772-9 PMID: 37652975

Wetzler, E. A., Marchesini, P., Villegas, L., & Canavati, S. (2022). Changing transmission dynamics among migrant, indigenous and mining populations in a malaria hotspot in Northern Brazil: 2016 to 2020. *Malaria Journal*, *21*(1), 127. DOI: 10.1186/s12936-022-04141-6 PMID: 35439994

Chapter 4
Mechanisms of Action of Phytochemicals Against Plasmodium Parasites

Rahul Kumar
https://orcid.org/0009-0000-1323-2220
Department of Microbiology, Graphic Era University, Dehradun, India

ABSTRACT

Phytochemicals are plant derived bioactive compounds that have emerged as potential contenders in the battle against malaria owing to their versatile mechanisms of action against Plasmodium parasites. This chapter discusses the diverse roles of phytochemicals in interfering with the lifecycle of the parasite, especially at the erythrocytic stages, which are accountable for the clinical presentation of malaria. These include the inhibition of heme polymerization, disruption of parasite invasion and adhesion, induction of apoptosis, and manipulation of the host immune system. Moreover, a number of phytochemicals exhibit synergy when combined with traditional antimalarial drugs, providing new hope for the reversal of drug resistance. In contrast to the issues associated with bioavailability and standardization, current research is still discovering new plant based compounds with significant antiplasmodial activity. This chapter presents a detailed review of these mechanisms and describes the therapeutic potential of phytochemicals and their use in the design of next generation antimalarial strategies.

INTRODUCTION

Malaria is a serious infectious disease caused by protozoan parasites of the genus *Plasmodium*, generally *Plasmodium falciparum*, *Plasmodium vivax*, *Plasmodium*

DOI: 10.4018/979-8-3373-5821-5.ch004

ovale, and *Plasmodium malariae* (Hawadak et al., 2021). Spread to humans by bite of infected female Anopheles mosquitoes, malaria continues to be a major worldwide health issue, especially in the tropics and subtropics regions (Takken et al., 2024). The World Health Organization (WHO) has assessed the number of malaria cases globally in 2021 to be 247 million, causing around 619,000 deaths majority of which were in sub Saharan Africa (Lawal et al., 2024). The children less than five years and pregnant women are particularly susceptible because of their moderately poor immunity (Kumar et al., 2022). Apart from morbidity and mortality malaria also creates high socioeconomic costs in relations of loss of output, healthcare expenses, education, and economic progress in endemic areas (Mezieobi et al., 2025). The clinical syndromes of malaria depend on the *Plasmodium* species that infect the host and the immune status of the host. Fever, chills, headache, lethargy, anemia, cerebral malaria, and multiorgan failure in extreme cases are characteristic of the disease (Salagre et al., 2017). The life cycle of *Plasmodium* includes both erythrocytic (red blood cells) and hepatic (liver) stages, making treatment challenging (Nureye and Assefa, 2020). The malarial treatment is based on antimicrobial drugs such as chloroquine, artemisinin combination therapies (ACTs) and primaquine (van der Pluijm et al., 2021). The development of resistant *Plasmodium* strains notably *P. falciparum* have reduced currently available treatment effects, thus keeping additional findings and complementary treatment techniques (Ward et al., 2022). Over the few decades natural products especially phytochemicals from medicinal plants have emerged as important antimicrobial drugs (Bekono et al., 2020; Kumar et al., 2025). Phytochemicals like terpenoids, alkaloids, polyphenols, and flavonoids have several mechanisms of action against *Plasmodium* inhibition of erythrocytic cycle, inhibition of heme polymerization, damage of parasite metabolic processes and regulation of host immune functions (Onyesom et al., 2022). Phytochemicals are linked to reduced toxicity and poor environments where traditional antimalarial drugs could be limited or too costly (Sokan-Adeaga et al., 2023). The research of phytochemicals valuable to antimalarial use such as quinine from *Cinchona bark* and artemisinin from *Artemisia annua* which remain of therapeutic weapons globally (Ceravolo et al., 2021). The limited of antimalarial therapies is not only in fighting drug resistant malaria but also beneficial worldwide efforts in malaria elimination (Rasmussen et al., 2022). The phytochemical combination involvement with recent treatment has possible to increase value and decrease side effects aid in the formulation of malaria control (Alum, 2024). Malaria is an ongoing public health issues and more effective less expensive that ultimately lower the global malaria burden (Table 8.1)

Table 1. Global Malaria Burden and Need for Alternative Treatments

Parameter	Data Points	Source	References
Annual cases (2021)	~247 million	WHO, 2022	(Chen et al., 2025)
Annual deaths (2021)	~619,000	WHO, 2022	(Cao et al., 2025)
Most affected regions	Sub Saharan Africa, Southeast Asia, South America	Epidemiological data	(Liu et al., 2021)
High risk populations	Children <5 years, pregnant women	WHO, 2022	(Reddy et al., 2023)
Economic impact	Lost productivity, increased healthcare costs, hindered development	Global health reports	(Andrade et al., 2022)
Drug resistance	Chloroquine, sulfadoxine pyrimethamine, ACTs in some regions	WHO Malaria Report, 2022	(Abebe et al., 2025)
Conventional treatments	Chloroquine, Artemisinin based Combination Therapies (ACTs), Primaquine	Clinical guidelines	(Daher et al., 2018)
Limitations of current drugs	Resistance development, toxicity, cost	Multiple studies	(Ippolito et al., 2021)
Alternative approaches	Phytochemicals, plant based extracts, herbal remedies	Pharmacological studies	(Abera et al., 2019)
Mechanisms of phytochemicals	Disrupt erythrocytic cycle, inhibit heme polymerization, impair metabolism, immunomodulation	Literature review	(Soni et al., 2017)
Clinically significant plant derived drugs	Quinine (*Cinchona*), Artemisinin (*Artemisia annua*)	Historical and modern clinical use	(Mohammadi et al., 2020)
Advantages of phytochemicals	Novel targets, lower toxicity, cost effective, accessible	Research evidence	(García et al., 2025)

The *Plasmodium* parasite life cycle is involved both the human host and female Anopheles mosquito as intermediate and definitive hosts. When an infected mosquito inject sporozoites into bloodstream during blood feeding (Brackney et al., 2021). So than sporozoites immediately circulate to liver, to invade hepatocytes and grow into asexual forms that replicate thousands of times to form thousands of merozoites in a process referred to as Schizogony (Gautam et al., 2020). The maturation of merozoites are injected into the blood initiating the erythrocytic cycle by infecting RBCs. Inside RBCs, the parasite develops from a ring to trophozoite to schizont, metabolizing hemoglobin for nutrition and producing toxic heme, which is detoxified to hemozoin. Cyclic lysis of infected RBCs releases merozoites and causes characteristic malarial fever and chills. Other merozoites differentiate into sexual stages known as gametocytes, which are ingested by mosquitoes during a blood meal (Burkot and Graves, 2000). Gametocytes in the mosquito midgut become male and female gametes, fuse to become zygotes, and mature into motile ookinetes.

Ookinetes penetrate the midgut wall to become oocysts, where sporogony gives rise to sporozoites that travel to the salivary glands, poised to infect a new human host. This two host life cycle guarantees the amplification of the parasite in humans and mosquito transmission, supporting the persistence and epidemiology of malaria (Yu et al., 2022). In the RBCs parasites mature into ring shape trophozoites that break down hemoglobin to take nutrient for grow in a parasitophorous vacuoles (Reyes-López et al., 2023). The trophozoite develops into a schizont that experiences repeated nuclear division to yield new merozoites. In this process, the toxic heme released from hemoglobin breakdown is detoxified to hemozoin to avoid oxidative damage. After maturity, the infected RBC break apart, releasing merozoites that infect new erythrocytes and continue the cycle. This repeated invasion, proliferation, and lysis of RBCs cause's typical symptoms of malaria, including fever, chills, anaemia, and weakness (Balaji et al., 2020). The portion of parasites divided into sexual stages termed gametocytes which are ingested by mosquitoes during blood feedings attached to erythrocytic cycle with transmission of finishing off parasite life cycle. The erythrocytic phase is an important target for all antimalarial compounds including phytochemicals which inhibit invasion detoxification of heme and intracellular parasite metabolism (Vaghela et al., 2025).

ANTIMALARIAL COMPOUNDS AS PHYTOCHEMICALS

The antimalarial mixtures has grown in the favour of phytochemicals which are bioactive molecules derivative from medicinal plants because of their operational diversity multitargeting mechanism reduce toxicity level associate to traditional drugs. Traditionally, plant derived molecules, such as quinine from *Cinchona bark* and artemisinin from *Artemisia annua*, have been the cornerstone of contemporary antimalarial therapy, as exemplified by the huge potential of phytochemicals in the fight against malaria (Ain et al., 2024). In addition to direct parasiticidal activity, phytochemicals tend to have immunomodulatory activity, dampen inflammation associated with malaria, and increase host defense mechanisms. Polysaccharides and polyphenolic compounds, for instance, can activate macrophage function and control cytokine production, thereby ameliorating tissue damage caused by the host immune reaction (Sobhani et al., 2021). Phytochemicals also tend to have a synergistic action when mixed together, acting on various pathways, such as heme detoxification, invasion into erythrocytes, and oxidative stress, minimizing the occurrence of drug resistance. Numerous plant species and their bioactive compounds have recently been evaluated for antimalarial activity. *Cinchona officinalis*, *Artemisia annua*, *Azadirachta indica* (neem), *Piper nigrum*, and *Andrographis paniculata* exhibited promising inhibitory activity against *Plasmodium falciparum* and *P. vivax* in *in vitro* and *in vivo* experiments (Kamaraj et al., 2023). Overall, phytochemicals are valuable and green resources for antimalarial drug discovery (Table 8.2). Their complex chemical structures, multitarget activity, and low toxicity potential offer compelling reasons for incorporating plant compounds into malaria prevention strategies, especially in settings of drug resistance and limited access to standard treatments (Fokou et al., 2025).

Table 2. Phytochemicals types and studied of antimalarial activity

Phytochemical Class	Examples	Plant Sources	Mechanism of Action Against *Plasmodium*	Traditional Medicine Use	Notes	References
Alkaloids	Quinine, Berberine, Cryptolepine	*Cinchona officinalis*, *Berberis vulgaris*, *Cryptolepis sanguinolenta*	Inhibit heme polymerization → toxic free heme accumulation; disrupt parasite DNA synthesis	Fever treatment, malaria, digestive disorders	Quinine is the first clinically used antimalarial	(Zhang et al., 2021)
Flavonoids	Quercetin, Kaempferol, Luteolin	*Glycyrrhiza glabra*, *Azadirachta indica*, *Citrus* spp.	Inhibit parasite enzymes (DHFR, LDH), generate ROS, block merozoite invasion	Antipyretic, anti inflammatory, immune modulation	Often synergistic with alkaloids	(Nandi et al., 2022)
Terpenoids / Sesquiterpenes	Artemisinin, Artesunate, Andrographolide	*Artemisia annua*, *Andrographis paniculata*	Produce free radicals → oxidative damage to membranes and organelles	Fever, inflammation, malaria treatment	Artemisinin derivatives are frontline antimalarials	(Shinyuy et al., 2023)
Polyphenols / Tannins	Catechins, Epigallocatechin, Gallic acid	*Camellia sinensis*, *Terminalia chebula*, *Punica granatum*	Disrupt membrane integrity, inhibit protein synthesis, antioxidant → oxidative stress	Antimicrobial, antipyretic, digestive aid	Enhance host immunity and reduce parasite growth	(Wang et al., 2024)
Saponins	Diosgenin, Ginsenosides	*Dioscorea* spp., *Panax ginseng*	Disrupt parasite membranes, interfere with nutrient absorption	Fever, immune booster, general tonic	Often used in decoctions for malaria	(Tiwari et al., 2018)
Coumarins	Scopoletin, Umbelliferone	*Scopolia japonica*, *Ferula* spp.	Interfere with parasite metabolism and enzyme function	Antipyretic, anti inflammatory	Potential for combination therapy	(Abaza, 2024)
Lignans	Podophyllotoxin, Schisandrin	*Podophyllum peltatum*, *Schisandra chinensis*	Inhibit DNA synthesis, oxidative stress induction	Traditional tonics, fever management	Limited studies against *Plasmodium*; emerging interest	(Addissouky et al., 2024)
Terpenophenolics / Phenolic diterpenes	Ferruginol, Carnosic acid	*Rosmarinus officinalis*, *Salvia* spp.	Inhibit parasite replication and induce oxidative damage	Traditional antimicrobial and anti inflammatory	Under study for multi target effects	(Sawerus et al., 2025)

continued on following page

Table 2. Continued

Phytochemical Class	Examples	Plant Sources	Mechanism of Action Against *Plasmodium*	Traditional Medicine Use	Notes	References
Glycosides	Andrographolide glycosides, Stevioside	*Andrographis paniculata, Stevia rebaudiana*	Inhibit parasite growth, immunomodulation	Fever, general health tonic	May enhance erythrocytic stage inhibition	(Hooda et al., 2024)
Essential oils / Volatile compounds	Eugenol, Thymol, Linalool	*Syzygium aromaticum, Thymus vulgaris, Lavandula* spp.	Disrupt membranes, inhibit parasite enzymes	Fever, antimicrobial, digestive disorders	Often used in traditional decoctions and fumigation	(Matte et al., 2023)

ERYTHROCYTIC CYCLE DISRUPTION

Interference with this cycle is one of the main targets of antimalarial treatments, such as phytochemicals. During invasion, merozoites are converted into ring stage trophozoites, which metabolize hemoglobin as a source of nutrients (Sojka et al., 2022). Phytochemicals and drugs interfere with this process via several mechanisms. In general, disruption of the erythrocytic cycle is a multitarget effect that not only lowers parasite load but also alleviates symptoms of malaria, including fever, anaemia, and hemolysis. The multi target activity of phytochemicals renders them good candidates for drug development against malaria, especially against drug resistant strains (Suganya et al., 2022).

Figure 1. Phytochemicals role in Plasmodium stages during disruption

1. INHIBITION OF MEROZOITE INVASION

Certain alkaloids and flavonoids block merozoite attachment and entry into RBCs by interfering with parasite surface proteins or host cell receptors. Preventing invasion halts parasite replication at the earliest erythrocytic stage.

2. INTERFERENCE WITH METABOLISM

Trophozoites rely on enzymes such as lactate dehydrogenase (LDH) and dihydrofolate reductase (DHFR) for energy and nucleotide synthesis. Flavonoids, polyphenols, and alkaloids inhibit these enzymes and reduce parasite growth and proliferation in RBCs.

3. INHIBITION OF HEME DETOXIFICATION

Haemoglobin digestion releases toxic free heme, which *Plasmodium* polymerizes into hemozoin. Alkaloids, such as quinine and certain flavonoids, prevent heme polymerization, leading to oxidative damage and parasite death.

4. OXIDATIVE STRESS INDUCTION

Terpenoids, artemisinin derivatives, and polyphenols generate reactive oxygen species (ROS) inside infected RBCs. Oxidative stress damages parasite membranes, proteins, and organelles, impairing trophozoite and schizont maturation.

5. DISRUPTION OF SCHIZOGONY

The interfering with nuclear division and protein synthesis, phytochemicals prevent trophozoites from developing into schizonts, thereby stopping the release of new merozoites and breaking the cycle of RBC infection.

6. PREVENTION OF GAMETOCYTE FORMATION

Some phytochemicals also inhibit the differentiation of merozoites into gametocytes, reducing the transmission potential when mosquitoes feed on infected individuals.

MECHANISMS BY WHICH PHYTOCHEMICALS DISRUPT PARASITE GROWTH

The development of Plasmodium after interfere with phytochemicals by a range of complementary mechanisms against multiple parasite stage in erythrocytic and hepatic stage (Djokic et al., 2021). Flavonoids act as a metabolic enzyme inhibitors such as dihydrofolate reductase and lactate dehydrogenase by inhibiting parasite replication disrupting nucleotide production and energy metabolism (Sakyi et al., 2025). Terpenoids like as an artemisinin and its produce reactive oxygen species upon heme iron induced activation leading to lipid peroxidation membrane lysis and organelle dysfunction in trophozoites and schizonts. Polyphenols and tannins disrupt the membranes of parasites, halt protein synthesis, cause oxidative stress, and further inhibit intracellular survival (Huang et al., 2024). The parasiticidal action have several phytochemicals immunomodulatory effects that are mediated through activation of macrophages, activation of phagocytosis of infected erythrocytes and modulation of cytokine production which reduces parasite growth and malaria (Wu et al., 2023).

A few of these compounds also inhibit merozoite differentiation into gametocytes, thus decreasing transmission potential. The multi target activity of phytochemicals, with direct cytotoxicity, metabolic inhibition, and immunomodulatory capacities, renders them particularly potent against drug resistant *Plasmodium* species and underlines their potential as alternative or adjuvant antimalarial drugs (Figure 2).

Figure 2. Mechanism by which phytochemical disrupt parasite growth

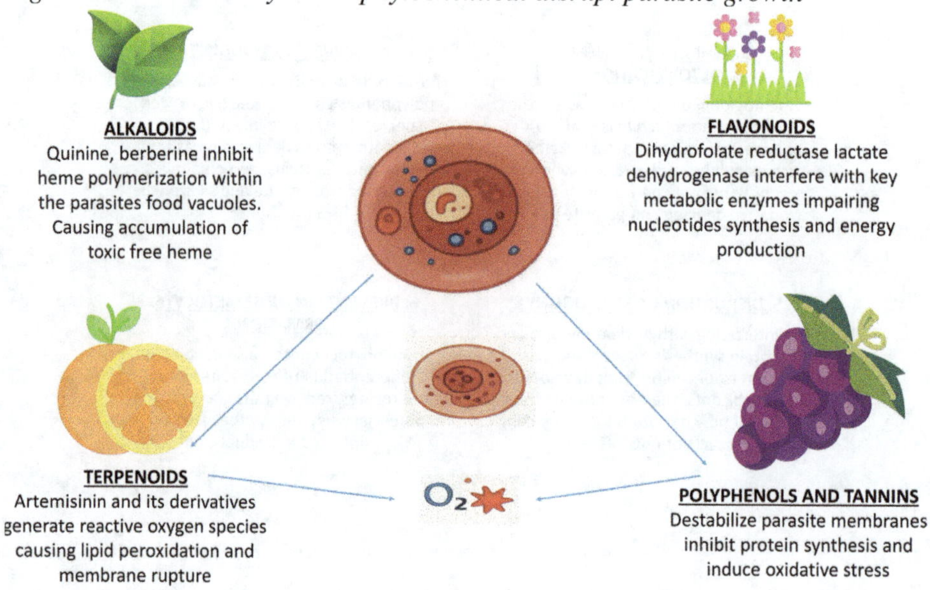

CASE STUDIES OF EFFECTIVE COMPOUNDS AND THEIR MODES OF ACTION

Quinine (Alkaloid)

Quinine, isolated from the bark of Cinchona officinal is a traditional antimalarial drug that primarily acts against the erythrocytic cycle of *Plasmodium falciparum*. The most significant mechanism of action is inhibition of heme polymerization in the food vacuoles of the parasite (Thakur, 2024). When hemoglobin is broken down release heme which is poisonous to the parasite. Quinine inhibits free heme by preventing its formation from hemozoin leading to toxic heme buildup that help oxidative stress and injury to parasite membranes proteins and organelles. This interference detentions parasite growth and replication. Quinine has also been documented to interrupt nucleic acid synthesis, further inhibiting merozoite maturation (Cortez-Maya et al., 2020). Clinically, quinine lowers parasitemia and relieves malaria symptoms such as fever and chills. Its multiple target activity and effectiveness against erythrocytic forms highlights its continuing and past importance, especially in areas where resistance to other antimalarials has developed (Shibeshi et al., 2020).

Artemisinin (Sesquiterpene Lactone)

The artemisinin extract from *Artemisia annua* and its analogs artesunate and artemether are fast acting to antimalarial with their action directed against the erythrocytic stage (Septembre-Malaterre et al., 2020). Their mode of action is mainly iron activated within the heme of the parasite which lead to the formation of ROS. ROS cause lipid peroxidation disrupting parasite membranes and damaging organelles such as endoplasmic reticulum and mitochondria (Pawłowska et al., 2023). Oxidative stress in intracellular homeostasis results in the death of trophozoites and schizonts. Artemisinin derivatives also interfere with metabolic enzymes of parasites and block merozoite growth. They also have synergistic effects when combined with other drugs used in ACTs, which increases their efficacy and minimizes drug resistance (Singh and Yeh, 2017). The fast action, multi target behavior, and efficacy against multidrug resistant *P. falciparum* make artemisinin a pillar of current malaria treatment protocols (Okombo and Fidock, 2025).

Berberine (Isoquinoline Alkaloid)

Berberine, derived from *Berberis vulgaris* and other associated species, has strong antimalarial properties because of the multiple mechanisms acting against the erythrocytic life cycle stages (Rauf et al., 2021). Berberine suppresses heme polymerization, leading to accumulation of cytotoxic free heme, which causes oxidative stress, parasite membrane damage, and intracellular protein damage (Aghili et al., 2024). Berberine also disrupt nucleic acid through blocking the RNA and DNA synthesis mandatory for parasite development. That it inhibit merozoite invasion RBCs thus disrupting the erythrocytic cycle early. Berberine also cause apoptosis like mechanisms in trophozoites further reducing the parasite survival. The mechanism action of multi modal along with its antioxidant and immunomodulatory activities for the through inhibition of parasite growth (Iqbal et al., 2024). The extensive movement and relatively low toxicity of berberine reduce it an attractive for the development of novel antimalarial drugs especially against resistant strain of conventional drugs (Filli et al., 2022).

Quercetin (Flavonoid)

Flavonoid quercetin found in Citrus species *Azadirachta indica* and *Glycyrrhiza glabra* exhibits antimicrobial movement via more mechanisms. It inhibits necessary parasite metabolites enzymes such as lactate dehydrogenase and dihydrofolate reductase damaging energy production and nucleotide synthesis need for replication (Kayamba et al., 2021). Quercetin also produce reactive oxygen species which disrupt the membrane of parasites and organelles in trophozoites and schizonts. Furthermore, it modulates the immune system of the host by promoting phagocytosis of infected erythrocytes by macrophages and the production of cytokines, which inhibits parasite survival and accompanying inflammation (Obeagu, 2024). Quercetin disrupts merozoite invasion, inhibits gametocyte maturation, and restricts replication and transmission. Its direct cytotoxicity, metabolic inhibition, induction of oxidative stress, and immunomodulation make quercetin a potential natural antimalarial drug that can be explored for use in combination therapies against drug resistant *Plasmodium* strains (Ali et al., 2021).

Andrographolide (Diterpenoid)

Andrographolide extract by *Andrographis paniculata* act as several stages of *Plasmodium* development in RBCs. Andrographolide inhibits intracellular metabolism by interfering with protein biosynthesis and redox homeostasis thereby causing oxidative stress that kills trophozoites and schizonts (Mishra et al., 2021). Andrographolide also modulates the parasite's apoptosis like processes, inhibiting its replication and survival. In addition to direct parasiticidal action, it modulates host immunity by inducing macrophages to remove infected erythrocytes and control cytokine production, thereby diminishing the pathology associated with malaria. Some studies have suggested that andrographolide is capable of inhibiting merozoite invasion and disrupting gametocyte development, thus slowing down parasite transmission (Apsari et al., 2025). The synergy of intracellular disturbance, induction of oxidative stress, and immunomodulation makes andrographolide an extremely versatile phytochemical with great promise as a natural antimalarial drug, particularly in regions where drug resistant malarial strains exist (Atwijukire et al., 2025).

Azadirachtin (Triterpenoid / Limonoid)

Azadirachtin, a triterpenoid from *Azadirachta indica* (neem), is an antimalarial agent that inhibits several parasitic processes. Azadirachtin inhibits the invasion of red blood cells by merozoites and inhibits the initiation of the erythrocytic cycle. Azadirachtin also inhibits gametocyte development, thereby decreasing the potential for transmission to mosquitoes (Almadiy et al., 2025). The parasite signalling pathways also disrupt by Azadirachtin that control intracellular growth replication cause to trophozoite and schizont development. The multitargeting action are low toxicity immunomodulatory likely augment host immunity and restrict parasite growth (Nagai and Goto, 2022). Azadirachtin's dual mode of action on the replication and transmission phases renders it a suitable candidate for integrated antimalarial therapy, especially in traditional healing systems, and as a possible adjunct to conventional pharmacological therapy (Su et al., 2023).

INHIBITION OF HEME POLYMERIZATION

Role of heme detoxification in malaria pathogenesis

During the erythrocytic cycle of malaria, *Plasmodium* parasites infect RBCs and metabolize hemoglobin as their sole source of nutrients. Hemoglobin breakdown releases free heme (ferriprotoporphyrin IX), which is extremely toxic because it can catalyze the generation of ROS and destabilize lipid membranes, proteins, and nucleic acids (Haines and Tosaki, 2020). To cope with this poisonous environment, *Plasmodium* developed a unique detoxification mechanism in which free heme is polymerized into an inert crystalline pigment named hemozoin, commonly termed malaria pigment. This is vital for parasite survival and growth, because the build-up of free heme would otherwise cause oxidative stress, membrane lysis, and cell death. Thus, the inhibition of heme detoxification is a major therapeutic target for both antimalarial compounds and phytochemicals (Gupta et al., 2021). Molecules such as quinine, chloroquine, and some flavonoids interact with unbound heme to prevent its polymerization into hemozoin. The consequent accumulation of toxic heme in the food vacuole of the parasite induces oxidative damage, membrane disruption, and eventual parasite lysis. Heme detoxification disruption also impairs the metabolism of nutrients by the parasite, since hemoglobin digestion is at the heart of energy and amino acid acquisition (Mukherjee et al., 2016). The oxidative stress caused by heme buildup can also magnify the host's immune response to exacerbate inflammation and pathology of malaria, as manifested in fever, anemia, and hemolysis. The detoxification is a central mechanism in Plasmodium pathogenesis and modulation of this pathway with drugs or plant based phytochemicals use to antimalarial treatment (Ribbiso et al., 2021).

Inhibit to heme polymerization by phytochemicals

During erythrocytic phase of malaria in RBCs through *Plasmodium* parasites to obtain amino acids and free heme (ferriprotoporphyrin IX) is a by-product (Naser et al., 2024). To prevent self-destruction parasite detoxifies free heme by polymerizing it into an inert crystalline material known as hemozoin. Quinine, berberine and cryptolepine directly interact with free heme to produce stable complexes that cannot polymerize into hemozoin (Duval and Duplais, 2017). The consequent heme toxification cause oxidative stress in the food vacuoles of the parasite leading to lipid peroxidation protein denaturation and membrane lysis. Terpenoids like artemisinin also assist heme induced oxidative damage by discharging free radicals when activated by iron in heme. Through interfering with heme detoxification phytochemicals kill intra erythrocytic parasites suppress merozoite replication and disrupt erythrocytic cycle. The complicated mechanism not only disrupt parasite survival but also inspires to antimalarial activity of plant based medicines and therapeutic drugs (Okoh et al., 2025).

Parasite interfering with invasion and adhesion

Plasmodium merozoites infect RBCs to continue erythrocytic cycle to adhesion of infected RBCs to endothelial surfaces is responsible for more malaria. Phytochemical can interfering process inhibiting parasite develop and disease severity. Flavonoids, alkaloids and saponins block merozoite invasion through disrupting interaction between parasite surface ligands e.g. EBA 175 and MSP 1 and erythrocyte receptors thus blocking entry of the parasite into RBCs (Ezema et al., 2023). Failing invasion stops the erytherythrocytice and bounds parasite replication and parasitemia. The certain phytochemicals control the adhesive features of ill RBCs by prompting the appearance or activity of parasite determined proteins such as PfEMP1, which causes cytoadherence to endothelial cells. The inhibiting adhesion these chemicals minimize microvascular obstruction inflammation and the risk of complication such as cerebral malaria (Beniwal et al., 2025). Overall, the inhibition of invasion and adhesion is an important mechanism by which phytochemicals inhibit antiplasmodial activities, in addition to their intracellular cytotoxic and inhibitory metabolic activities (Zhang et al., 2022).

STRATEGIES EMPLOYED BY PHYTOCHEMICALS TO PREVENT INVASION

Phytochemicals utilize various mechanisms to inhibit merozoite invasion, which is an important process in the erythrocytic cycle of *Plasmodium*. The major mechanism is to inhibit ligand receptor interaction flavonoids and alkaloids interfere with the surface of the parasite like erythrocyte binding antigen 175 (EBA 175) and merozoite surface protein 1 (MSP 1), they cannot bind to erythrocyte receptors (Molina-Franky et al., 2022). Variation of erythrocyte membrane possessions is etra method whereby saponins and some polyphenols affect membrane fluidity or receptor organization to reduce RBCs less permeable to parasite invasion. Phytochemicals may also block parasite signaling cascades involved in merozoite movement and invasion, including calcium dependent protein kinases that control cytoskeletal rearrangement (Kaiser, 2019). Some chemicals also cause oxidative stress or produce reactive oxygen species that damage merozoites before or during invasion. These techniques decrease invasion of merozoites into RBCs curbing parasite proliferation reducing parasitemia and improving malaria symptoms. Through both extracellular inhibition of invasion and intracellular cytotoxic effects phytochemicals deliver a multi target therapeutic method for antimalarial treatment (Sinha et al., 2019).

BLOCKING ADHESION TO HOST CELLS

The cytoadherence of Plasmodium infected red blood cells (iRBCs) to host endothelial cells plays a central role in malaria pathogenesis particularly in severe cases of cerebral malaria. This is facilitated by parasite fixed proteins present on iRBC surface of which Plasmodium falciparum erythrocyte membrane protein 1 (PfEMP1) is the most important (Oleinikov, 2022). PfEMP1 interacts with endothelial receptors, such as ICAM 1, CD36, and CSA, attaching iRBCs to the microvasculature and hindering their removal by the spleen (Jensen et al., 2020). While sequestration shelters the parasite from immune mediated killing, it also causes microvascular obstruction, local hypoxia, and inflammatory reactions, which result in severe complications, such as cerebral malaria, placental malaria, and multi organ failure. Hence, blocking adhesion is an important therapeutic target (Olas et al., 2020). The binding of iRBCs to the vascular endothelium, and enables their circulation and splenic clearance. Through the diminution of microvascular occlusion and inflammation, adhesion blocking chemicals reduce tissue hypoxia, oxidative stress, and immune related damage, thereby alleviating the severity of malaria. Furthermore, indirect inhibition of adhesion decreases the survival and replication of parasites because iRBCs are cleared earlier and would not have a chance to complete the erythrocytic cycle (Boulet et al., 2018). Therefore, adhesion targeting not only counters disease mechanisms, but also synergizes with other antimalarial effects, including invasion inhibition, induction of oxidative stress, and heme detoxification, underlining the significance of multi targeted plant chemical therapies in controlling malaria (Panieri and Saso, 2021).

APOPTOTIC PATHWAYS TARGETED BY PHYTOCHEMICALS

Phytochemicals activate apoptosis like cell death in *Plasmodium* by aiming numerous intracellular pathways serious for parasite survival and replication. One such pathway is mitochondrial impairment, wherein molecules such as flavonoids, alkaloids, and terpenoids disturb the mitochondrial membrane potential, resulting in the release of pro apoptotic factors that trigger parasite cell death (Anchimowicz et al., 2025). The second mechanism is the induction of oxidative stress. ROS designed through phytochemicals cause damage to parasite DNA, lipid membrane, and proteins making apoptosis like pathways. Phytochemical also control like activity in parasite inducing nucleic acid fragmentation and proteolytic breakdown of critical cellular structure (Mallo et al., 2020). Further destabilization of organelle function is also achieved by interference in calcium signaling and redox balance. The concurrently targeting these pathways, phytochemicals inhibit trophozoite and schizont development, merozoite release, and erythrocytic cycle disruption. This multi targeted apoptotic induction augments other antiplasmodial effects, including heme detoxification inhibition, invasion, and adhesion, increasing parasite elimination, and lowering malaria severity (Vijayan et al., 2021).

EVIDENCE OF PROGRAMMED CELL DEATH IN *PLASMODIUM* SPP.

Although classical apoptosis is characteristic of multicellular eukaryotes, various studies have shown that apoptosis like programmed cell death (PCD) is present in *Plasmodium* species, especially when they are in the erythrocytic stage. Evidence comprises DNA fragmentation, by means of TUNEL assays and gel electrophoresis, reflecting controlled nucleic acid breakdown in trophozoites and schizonts (Mutai and Waitumbi, 2010). Loss of mitochondrial membrane possible has been informed with depolarization previous to parasite death parallel to the intrinsic apoptotic pathways in higher eukaryotic cells. Parasite exposed to oxidative stress of antimalarial agents such as phytochemicals shows caspase like protease activation which degrades proteins vital for survival (Memariani et al., 2024). The cells shrinkage chromatin condensation and cytoplasmic vacuolation were observed by microscopic indicating a programmed death process. Experimental representation of *Plasmodium falciparum* and *P. berghei* have recommended that PCD may be encouraged through drug therapy nutrient deprivation or immunologically stress (Timothy and Zininga, 2023). These results emphasize that *Plasmodium* has inherent mechanisms for apoptosis like death that can be therapeutically targeted. Phytochemicals that trigger oxidative stress interfere with mitochondrial function or initiate a caspase like pathway effectively tap into this PCD machinery to curtail the parasite burden and prevent disease progression (Sebghatollahi et al., 2025).

IMMUNE MODULATION AND SYNERGY WITH CONVENTIONAL TREATMENTS

Phytochemicals not only have direct parasiticidal action, but also immunomodulatory action on the host immune system, increasing the clearance of *Plasmodium* and treatment efficacy. Molecules such as flavonoids, polyphenols, alkaloids, and terpenoids can activate macrophage and dendritic cell function, induce phagocytosis of iRBCs and control cytokine production, suppressing overproduction of inflammation while conserving effective immune defense (Iftikhar et al., 2025). Certain phytochemicals activate natural killer (NK) cells and boost the generation of nitric oxide, which is cytotoxic to intracellular parasites. Notably, these immunomodulatory actions synergize with traditional antimalarials, such as chloroquine, artemisinin, and quinine. In combination, phytochemicals can enhance drug potency, decrease the doses needed, and resist the onset of drug resistance by simultaneously acting on multiple parasite pathways (Choudhury, 2022).

PHYTOCHEMICAL RESPONSE TO ENHANCEMENT OF IMMUNE HOST

They also control the production of cytokines to increase the value of pro inflammatory cytokines such as TNF α, IFN γ, and IL 12 to increase killing of parasites while conserving anti-inflammatory cytokines such as IL 10 to avoid the overwhelming destruction of tissues (M'bondoukwé et al., 2022). Phytochemicals also improve the activity of natural killer (NK) cells and cytotoxic T lymphocytes, which kill infected hepatocytes and erythrocytes (Paudel et al., 2023). Through enhanced antigen presentation and adaptive immune response, phytochemicals enable parasite specific immunity to develop, thereby lowering parasite burden and disease intensity. Their capability to act as immunomodulators balances the direct mechanisms of antiplasmodial achievement such as invasion inhibition and oxidative stress in induction of a multi targeted approach to enhance host defense treatment efficacy in malaria (Sarkar et al., 2021).

POTENTIAL FOR COMBINATION THERAPIES WITH EXISTING ANTIMALARIAL

Phytochemicals also show great promise as adjuncts in combination therapy with traditional antimalarial drugs, providing a multi targeted intervention to optimize efficacy and minimize the development of drug resistance. Phytochemicals may complement chloroquine, quinine, and artemisinin derivatives through mechanisms other than those of traditional therapies, such as inhibition of heme polymerization, disruption of merozoite invasion, induction of apoptosis like cell death, and immune modulation (Rudrapal and Chetia, 2021). For instance, flavonoids and alkaloids can increase oxidative stress in infected red blood cells, synergistically complementing artemisinin induced free radical generation to achieve faster parasite clearance. Immunomodulatory phytochemicals can also enhance host immunity by activating macrophages, natural killer (NK) cells, and cytokine responses, complementing the effect of standard medicines to decrease parasitemia and clinical manifestations (Porwal et al., 2021). Critically, the simultaneous targeting of several pathways reduces the potential for resistance development, which is a significant concern in the treatment of malaria (Belete, 2020). The inclusion of phytochemicals in combination regimens offers a promising approach to enhance antimalarial efficacy, optimize patient outcomes, and counter the global threat of drug resistant *Plasmodium* strains (Tarkang et al., 2016).

CHALLENGES AND FUTURE DIRECTIONS

Despite their promising antiplasmodial activities, the therapeutic use of phytochemicals is hindered by numerous bioavailability and pharmacokinetic issues. Chemical classes, such as flavonoids, alkaloids, and terpenoids, have poor solubility in water, low gastrointestinal absorption, fast metabolic turnover, and short plasma half-life, reducing their in vivo therapeutic effects (Yang et al., 2020). The possibility of drug drug interactions when combined with traditional antimalarial also needs to be assessed with caution to prevent adverse reactions. To mitigate these limitations, auspicious research directions are being sought. Nanotechnology based delivery systems, including nanoparticles, liposomes, and solid lipid carriers, have been shown to increase solubility, shield compounds against immediate metabolism, and enhance targeted delivery to infected red blood cells (Yeh et al., 2020). Structural changes and derivatization of natural products have the potential to enhance potency, stability, and bioavailability, while reducing toxicity. High throughput screening, molecular docking, and systems biology strategies can be used to discover new bioactive molecules and explain their multi targeting mechanisms. Additionally, the incorporation of phytochemicals into standardized herbal drugs with established pharmacokinetic profiles will promote clinical translatability. Ongoing work in the areas of pharmacodynamics, toxicity, and mechanism based fine tuning is necessary to fully realize the potential of phytochemicals as effective, sustainable, and adjunctive antimalarial drugs against drug resistant *Plasmodium* parasites (Vanaja et al., 2025).

CONCLUSION

Phytochemicals are an encouraging and multipurpose of antimalarial compounds that can be used to arising from drug resistant *Plasmodium* stains. Their structural diversity agrees to target multiple mechanisms like that inhibiting heme polymerization, interfering with erythrocyte invasion, triggering apoptosis like death and controlling host immune functions. These combinations are lower the parasite burden inhibit pathogenesis and augment the efficacy of standard antimalarial agents. The *in vitro* and *in vivo* clinical research data emphasize the potential of compounds such as artemisinin, quinine, quercetin, berberine, azadirachtin, and andrographolide as effective agents, while also identifying their potential for synergy with conventional therapy for better results. These challenges and benefits are especially in the area of bioavailability, standardization, pharmacokinetics, and clinical validation on a large scale. Improvements in basic modifications, nanotechnology and combination therapies characterize encouraging directions for improving the ability, stability, and targeted delivery of phytochemicals. The investigation through the integration of pharmacological, molecular and immunological perspectives is necessary to appreciate these natural combinations in the form of safe effective and reachable antimalarial involvements. The phytochemical are favourable not only as single treatment but also as assistants in comprehensive malaria control programs and increasing drug resistance.

REFERENCES

Abaza, S. (2024). Recent advances in identification of potential drug targets and development of novel drugs in parasitic diseases: Part V: The value of natural products in drug discovery: Helminths. *Parasitologists United Journal*, *17*(2), 57–73. DOI: 10.21608/puj.2024.292672.1250

Abebe, W., Ashagre, A., Misganaw, T., Dejazmach, Z., Kumie, G., Nigatie, M., Jemal, A., Asmare, Z., Kassahun, W., Gedfie, S., Getachew, E., Gashaw, M., Ayana, S., Gashaw, Y., Sisay, A., Tadesse, S., Eshetu, T., awoke, M., Kassanew, B., & Reta, M. A. (2025). Prevalence of antimalaria drug resistance-conferring mutations associated with sulphadoxine-pyrimethamineine-resistant Plasmodium falciparum in East Africa: A systematic review and meta-analysis. *Annals of Clinical Microbiology and Antimicrobials*, *24*(1), 25. DOI: 10.1186/s12941-025-00795-7 PMID: 40241183

Abera, T., Ashebir, R., Basha, H., Debebe, E., Abebe, A., Meresa, A., & Woldekidan, S. (2019). Phytochemical-constituents, safety and efficacy of commonly used medicinal plants for the treatment of malaria in Ethiopia-a review. *Pharmacy & Pharmacology International Journal*, *7*(6), 284–295. DOI: 10.15406/ppij.2019.07.00266

Addissouky, T. A., El Sayed, I. E. T., Ali, M. M., Alubiady, M. H. S., & Wang, Y. (2024). Schisandra chinensis in liver disease: Exploring the mechanisms and therapeutic promise of an ancient Chinese botanical. *Archives of Pharmacology and Therapeutics*, *6*(1), 27–33. DOI: 10.33696/Pharmacol.6.052

Aghili, Z. S., Magnani, M., Ghatrehsamani, M., Nourian Dehkordi, A., Mirzaei, S. A., & Banitalebi Dehkordi, M. (2024). Intelligent berberine-loaded erythrocytes attenuated inflammatory cytokine productions in macrophages. *Scientific Reports*, *14*(1), 9381. DOI: 10.1038/s41598-024-60103-9 PMID: 38654085

Ain, Q. T., Saleem, N., Munawar, N., Nawaz, R., Naseer, F., & Ahmed, S. (2024). Quest for malaria management using natural remedies. *Frontiers in Pharmacology*, *15*, 1359890. DOI: 10.3389/fphar.2024.1359890 PMID: 39011507

Ain, Q. T., Saleem, N., Munawar, N., Nawaz, R., Naseer, F., & Ahmed, S. (2024). Quest for malaria management using natural remedies. *Frontiers in Pharmacology*, *15*, 1359890. DOI: 10.3389/fphar.2024.1359890 PMID: 39011507

Ali, A. H., Sudi, S., Shi-Jing, N., Hassan, W. R. M., Basir, R., Agustar, H. K., Embi, N., Sidek, H. M., & Latip, J. (2021). Dual anti-malarial and GSK3β-mediated cytokine-modulating activities of quercetin are requisite of its potential as a plant-derived therapeutic in malaria. *Pharmaceuticals (Basel, Switzerland)*, *14*(3), 248. DOI: 10.3390/ph14030248 PMID: 33803419

Almadiy, A. A., Al-Ghamdi, M. S., Abd Al Galil, F. M., & Dar, S. A. (2025). Azadirachtin from Neem (Azadirachta indica): Efficacy and Mechanisms Against Insects and Diseases. In *Natural Pesticides and Allelochemicals* (pp. 261-278). CRC Press.

Alum, E. U. (2024). Phytochemicals in malaria treatment: Mechanisms of action and clinical efficacy. *KIU J. Health Sci*, *4*(2), 71–84. DOI: 10.59568/KJHS-2024-4-2-06

Anchimowicz, J., Zielonka, P., & Jakiela, S. (2025). Plant Secondary Metabolites as Modulators of Mitochondrial Health: An Overview of Their Anti-Oxidant, Anti-Apoptotic, and Mitophagic Mechanisms. *International Journal of Molecular Sciences*, *26*(1), 380. DOI: 10.3390/ijms26010380 PMID: 39796234

Andrade, M. V., Noronha, K., Diniz, B. P., Guedes, G., Carvalho, L. R., Silva, V. A., Calazans, J. A., Santos, A. S., Silva, D. N., & Castro, M. C. (2022). The economic burden of malaria: A systematic review. *Malaria Journal*, *21*(1), 283. DOI: 10.1186/s12936-022-04303-6 PMID: 36199078

Apsari, P. I. B., Suryana, I. K., Satriyasa, B. K., Laksmi, D. A. A. S., Wati, D. K., & Wirasuta, I. M. A. G. (2025). Towards Andrographolide as Antimalarial: A Systematic Review. *Biomedical & Pharmacology Journal*, *18*(1), 499–515. DOI: 10.13005/bpj/3103

Atwijukire, W., Ayogu, E. E., & Onohuean, H. (2025). Immunomodulatory potentials of Andrographis paniculata and Allium sativum in managing plasmodium infections. *Discover Applied Sciences*, *7*(7), 661. DOI: 10.1007/s42452-025-07010-4

Balaji, S. N., Deshmukh, R., & Trivedi, V. (2020). Severe malaria: Biology, clinical manifestation, pathogenesis and consequences. *Journal of Vector Borne Diseases*, *57*(1), 1–13. DOI: 10.4103/0972-9062.308793 PMID: 33818449

Bekono, B. D., Ntie-Kang, F., Onguéné, P. A., Lifongo, L. L., Sippl, W., Fester, K., & Owono, L. C. (2020). The potential of anti-malarial compounds derived from African medicinal plants: A review of pharmacological evaluations from 2013 to 2019. *Malaria Journal*, *19*(1), 183. DOI: 10.1186/s12936-020-03231-7 PMID: 32423415

Belete, T. M. (2020). Recent progress in the development of new antimalarial drugs with novel targets. *Drug Design, Development and Therapy*, *14*, 3875–3889. DOI: 10.2147/DDDT.S265602 PMID: 33061294

Beniwal, P., Joshi, J., & Kaur, S. (2025). A comprehensive review of cerebral malaria. *Journal of Parasitic Diseases : Official Organ of the Indian Society for Parasitology*, *49*(2), 257–272. DOI: 10.1007/s12639-024-01758-z PMID: 40458503

Boulet, C., Doerig, C. D., & Carvalho, T. G. (2018). Manipulating eryptosis of human red blood cells: A novel antimalarial strategy? *Frontiers in Cellular and Infection Microbiology*, *8*, 419. DOI: 10.3389/fcimb.2018.00419 PMID: 30560094

Brackney, D. E., LaReau, J. C., & Smith, R. C. (2021). Frequency matters: How successive feeding episodes by blood-feeding insect vectors influences disease transmission. *PLoS Pathogens*, *17*(6), e1009590. DOI: 10.1371/journal.ppat.1009590 PMID: 34111228

Burkot, T. R., & Graves, P. M. (2000). Malaria, babesiosis, theileriosis and related diseases. In *Medical Entomology: A Textbook on Public Health and Veterinary Problems Caused by Arthropods* (pp. 187–230). Springer Netherlands. DOI: 10.1007/978-94-011-6472-6_7

Cao, Y., Wu, H., Zhang, Y., Wu, X., Li, J., Chen, H., & Gao, W. (2025). Time trends in malaria incidence from 1992 to 2021 in high-risk regions: An age-period-cohort analysis based on the Global Burden of Disease study 2021. *International Journal of Infectious Diseases*, *153*, 107770. DOI: 10.1016/j.ijid.2024.107770 PMID: 39736331

Ceravolo, I. P., Aguiar, A. C., Adebayo, J. O., & Krettli, A. U. (2021). Studies on activities and chemical characterization of medicinal plants in search for new Antimalarials: A ten year review on Ethnopharmacology. *Frontiers in Pharmacology*, *12*, 734263. DOI: 10.3389/fphar.2021.734263 PMID: 34630109

Chen, J., Tian, X., Guo, D., Gu, H., Duan, Y., & Li, D. (2025). Global trends and burdens of neglected tropical diseases and malaria from 1990 to 2021: A systematic analysis of the Global Burden of Disease Study 2021. *BMC Public Health*, *25*(1), 1307. DOI: 10.1186/s12889-025-22477-x PMID: 40197173

Choudhury, A. (2022). Potential role of bioactive phytochemicals in combination therapies against antimicrobial activity. *Journal of Pharmacopuncture*, *25*(2), 79–87. DOI: 10.3831/KPI.2022.25.2.79 PMID: 35837140

Cortez-Maya, S., Moreno-Herrera, A., Palos, I., & Rivera, G. (2020). Old antiprotozoal drugs: Are they still viable options for parasitic infections or new options for other diseases? *Current Medicinal Chemistry*, *27*(32), 5403–5428. DOI: 10.2174/0929867326666190628163633 PMID: 31264538

Daher, A., Pereira, D., Lacerda, M. V., Alexandre, M. A., Nascimento, C. T., Alves de Lima e Silva, J. C., Tada, M., Ruffato, R., Maia, I., dos Santos, T. C., Marchesini, P., Santelli, A. C., & Lalloo, D. G. (2018). Efficacy and safety of artemisinin-based combination therapy and chloroquine with concomitant primaquine to treat Plasmodium vivax malaria in Brazil: An open label randomized clinical trial. *Malaria Journal*, *17*(1), 45. DOI: 10.1186/s12936-018-2192-x PMID: 29361939

Djokic, V., Rocha, S. C., & Parveen, N. (2021). Lessons learned for pathogenesis, immunology, and disease of erythrocytic parasites: Plasmodium and Babesia. *Frontiers in Cellular and Infection Microbiology, 11*, 685239. DOI: 10.3389/fcimb.2021.685239 PMID: 34414129

Duval, R., & Duplais, C. (2017). Fluorescent natural products as probes and tracers in biology. *Natural Product Reports, 34*(2), 161–193. DOI: 10.1039/C6NP00111D PMID: 28125109

Ezema, C. A., Okagu, I. U., & Ezeorba, T. P. C. (2023). Escaping the enemy's bullets: An update on how malaria parasites evade host immune response. *Parasitology Research, 122*(8), 1715–1731. DOI: 10.1007/s00436-023-07868-6 PMID: 37219610

Filli, M. S., Ibrahim, A. A., Kesse, S., Aquib, M., Boakye-Yiadom, K. O., Farooq, M. A., Raza, F., Zhang, Y., & Wang, B. (2022). Synthetic berberine derivatives as potential new drugs. *Brazilian Journal of Pharmaceutical Sciences, 58*, e18835. DOI: 10.1590/s2175-97902020000318835

Fokou, P. V. T., Tali, M. B. T., Mbouna, C. D. J., Yamthe, L. R. T., Sharifi-Rad, J., Calina, D., Radha, , Kumar, M., Tchouankeu, J. C., & Boyom, F. F. (2025). Natural products as transmission-blocking agents against malaria: A comprehensive review of bioactive compounds and their therapeutic potential. *Malaria Journal, 24*(1), 164. DOI: 10.1186/s12936-025-05395-6 PMID: 40420292

García, M., Magi, M. S., & García, M. C. (2025). Harnessing Phytonanotechnology to Tackle Neglected Parasitic Diseases: Focus on Chagas Disease and Malaria. *Pharmaceutics, 17*(8), 1043. DOI: 10.3390/pharmaceutics17081043 PMID: 40871066

Gautam, P. K., Prajapati, B., & Sujatha, R. (2020). Chapter-5 Life Cycle, Pathogenesis and Laboratory Diagnosis of Malaria Parasite. *Chief Editor Dr. Durgadas Govind Naik, 105*, 105.

Gupta, M., Kumar, S., Kumar, R., Kumar, A., Verma, R., Darokar, M. P., Rout, P., & Pal, A. (2021). Inhibition of heme detoxification pathway in malaria parasite by 3-hydroxy-11-keto-β-boswellic acid isolated from Boswellia serrata. *Biomedicine and Pharmacotherapy, 144*, 112302. DOI: 10.1016/j.biopha.2021.112302 PMID: 34678731

Haines, D. D., & Tosaki, A. (2020). Heme degradation in pathophysiology of and countermeasures to inflammation-associated disease. *International Journal of Molecular Sciences, 21*(24), 9698. DOI: 10.3390/ijms21249698 PMID: 33353225

Hawadak, J., Dongang Nana, R. R., & Singh, V. (2021). Global trend of Plasmodium malariae and Plasmodium ovale spp. malaria infections in the last two decades (2000–2020): A systematic review and meta-analysis. *Parasites & Vectors*, *14*(1), 297. DOI: 10.1186/s13071-021-04797-0 PMID: 34082791

Hooda, P., Malik, R., Bhatia, S., Al-Harrasi, A., Najmi, A., Zoghebi, K., Halawi, M. A., Makeen, H. A., & Mohan, S. (2024). Phytoimmunomodulators: A review of natural modulators for complex immune system. *Heliyon*, *10*(1), e23790. DOI: 10.1016/j.heliyon.2023.e23790 PMID: 38205318

Huang, J., Zaynab, M., Sharif, Y., Khan, J., Al-Yahyai, R., Sadder, M., Ali, M., Alarab, S. R., & Li, S. (2024). Tannins as antimicrobial agents: Understanding toxic effects on pathogens. *Toxicon*, *247*, 107812. DOI: 10.1016/j.toxicon.2024.107812 PMID: 38908527

Iftikhar, A., Saleem, M., Raza, S. A., Achuthan, A., Luwor, R., Muhammad, T., & Majeed, U. (2025). Immunomodulatory properties of a methanolic extract of Ficus lyrata mitigate inflammation in Complete Freund's Adjuvant-induced arthritis. *Inflammopharmacology*, *33*(4), 1–14. DOI: 10.1007/s10787-025-01700-6 PMID: 40140117

Ippolito, M. M., Moser, K. A., Kabuya, J. B. B., Cunningham, C., & Juliano, J. J. (2021). Antimalarial drug resistance and implications for the WHO global technical strategy. *Current Epidemiology Reports*, *8*(2), 46–62. DOI: 10.1007/s40471-021-00266-5 PMID: 33747712

Iqbal, T., Altaf, S., Fatima, M., Rasheed, R., Laraib, K., Azam, M., & Usman, S. (2024). A narrative review on effective use of medicinal plants for the treatment of parasitic foodborne diseases. Agrobiological Records 16: 79-92. *Agric Res J*, *16*, 79–92.

Jensen, A. R., Adams, Y., & Hviid, L. (2020). Cerebral Plasmodium falciparum malaria: The role of PfEMP1 in its pathogenesis and immunity, and PfEMP1-based vaccines to prevent it. *Immunological Reviews*, *293*(1), 230–252. DOI: 10.1111/imr.12807 PMID: 31562653

Kaiser, A. (2019). Druggable targets in cyclic nucleotide signaling pathways in apicomplexan parasites and kinetoplastids against disabling protozoan diseases in humans. *International Journal of Molecular Sciences*, *20*(1), 138. DOI: 10.3390/ijms20010138 PMID: 30609697

Kamaraj, C., Ragavendran, C., Prem, P., Naveen Kumar, S., Ali, A., Kazmi, A., Ullah, A., Chandra Satish Kumar, R., Khan, S. U., Luna-Arias, J. P., Mashwani, Z.-U.-R., Balasubramani, G., & Rehman, S. U. (2023). Exploring the therapeutic potential of traditional antimalarial and antidengue plants: A mechanistic perspective. *The Canadian Journal of Infectious Diseases & Medical Microbiology, 2023*(1), 1860084. DOI: 10.1155/2023/1860084 PMID: 37927532

Kayamba, F., Faya, M., Pooe, O. J., Kushwaha, B., Kushwaha, N. D., Obakachi, V. A., Nyamori, V. O., & Karpoormath, R. (2021). Lactate dehydrogenase and malate dehydrogenase: Potential antiparasitic targets for drug development studies. *Bioorganic & Medicinal Chemistry, 50*, 116458. DOI: 10.1016/j.bmc.2021.116458 PMID: 34687983

Kumar, M., Saadaoui, M., & Al Khodor, S. (2022). Infections and pregnancy: Effects on maternal and child health. *Frontiers in Cellular and Infection Microbiology, 12*, 873253. DOI: 10.3389/fcimb.2022.873253 PMID: 35755838

Kumar, R., Pal, O. P., Kamboj, N., & Jaiswal, A. (2025). Phytonutrients in Neuroprotection and Neurodegenerative Disorders. *Current Research in Nutrition and Food Science Journal, 13*(Special Issue Phytonutrients June 2025).

Lawal, L., Buhari, A. O., Jaji, T. A., Alatare, A. S., Adeyemo, A. O., Olumoh, A. O., Yusuff, Y. A., Osborn, G., Mogaji, A. B., Adoto, B. H., Ibrahim, N. G., Saliu, W. O., & Abdul-Rahman, T. (2024). Lingering challenges in malaria elimination efforts in sub-Saharan Africa: Insights and potential solutions. *Health Science Reports, 7*(6), e2122. DOI: 10.1002/hsr2.2122 PMID: 38831778

Liu, Q., Jing, W., Kang, L., Liu, J., & Liu, M. (2021). Trends of the global, regional and national incidence of malaria in 204 countries from 1990 to 2019 and implications for malaria prevention. *Journal of Travel Medicine, 28*(5), taab046. DOI: 10.1093/jtm/taab046 PMID: 33763689

M'bondoukwé, N. P., Moutongo, R., Gbédandé, K., Ndong Ngomo, J. M., Hountohotegbé, T., Adamou, R., Koumba Lengongo, J. V., Pambou Bello, K., Mawili-Mboumba, D. P., Luty, A. J. F., & Bouyou-Akotet, M. K. (2022). Circulating IL-6, IL-10, and TNF-alpha and IL-10/IL-6 and IL-10/TNF-alpha ratio profiles of polyparasitized individuals in rural and urban areas of gabon. *PLoS Neglected Tropical Diseases, 16*(4), e0010308. DOI: 10.1371/journal.pntd.0010308 PMID: 35421083

Mallo, N., Lamas, J., Sueiro, R. A., & Leiro, J. M. (2020). Molecular targets implicated in the antiparasitic and anti-inflammatory activity of the phytochemical curcumin in Trichomoniasis. *Molecules (Basel, Switzerland), 25*(22), 5321. DOI: 10.3390/molecules25225321 PMID: 33202696

Matte, E. H. C., Luciano, F. B., & Evangelista, A. G. (2023). Essential oils and essential oil compounds in animal production as antimicrobials and anthelmintics: An updated review. *Animal Health Research Reviews*, *24*(1), 1–11. DOI: 10.1017/S1466252322000093 PMID: 37401263

Memariani, H., Memariani, M., & Ghasemian, A. (2024). Quercetin as a promising antiprotozoan phytochemical: Current knowledge and future research avenues. *BioMed Research International*, *2024*(1), 7632408. DOI: 10.1155/2024/7632408 PMID: 38456097

Mezieobi, K. C., Alum, E. U., Ugwu, O. P. C., Uti, D. E., Alum, B. N., Egba, S. I., & Michael, E. C. (2025). Economic burden of malaria on developing countries: A mini review. *Parasite Epidemiology and Control*, *30*, 00435. DOI: 10.1016/j.parepi.2025.e00435 PMID: 40519859

Mishra, A., Shaik, H. A., Sinha, R. K., & Shah, B. R. (2021). Andrographolide: A herbal-chemosynthetic approach for enhancing immunity, combating viral infections, and its implication on human health. *Molecules (Basel, Switzerland)*, *26*(22), 7036. DOI: 10.3390/molecules26227036 PMID: 34834128

Mohammadi, S., Jafari, B., Asgharian, P., Martorell, M., & Sharifi-Rad, J. (2020). Medicinal plants used in the treatment of Malaria: A key emphasis to Artemisia, Cinchona, Cryptolepis, and Tabebuia genera. *Phytotherapy Research*, *34*(7), 1556–1569. DOI: 10.1002/ptr.6628 PMID: 32022345

Molina-Franky, J., Patarroyo, M. E., Kalkum, M., & Patarroyo, M. A. (2022). The cellular and molecular interaction between erythrocytes and Plasmodium falciparum merozoites. *Frontiers in Cellular and Infection Microbiology*, *12*, 816574. DOI: 10.3389/fcimb.2022.816574 PMID: 35433504

Mukherjee, S., Mukherjee, N., Gayen, P., Roy, P., Sinha, P., & Babu, S. (2016). Metabolic inhibitors as antiparasitic drugs: Pharmacological, biochemical and molecular perspectives. *Current Drug Metabolism*, *17*(10), 937–970. DOI: 10.2174/1389200217666161004143152 PMID: 27719626

Mutai, B. K., & Waitumbi, J. N. (2010). Apoptosis stalks Plasmodium falciparum maintained in continuous culture condition. *Malaria Journal*, *9*(S3, Suppl 3), S6. DOI: 10.1186/1475-2875-9-S3-S6 PMID: 21144086

Nagai, K., & Goto, Y. (2022). Parasitomimetics: Can we utilize parasite-derived immunomodulatory molecules for interventions to immunological disorders? *Frontiers in Immunology*, *13*, 824695. DOI: 10.3389/fimmu.2022.824695 PMID: 35386686

Nandi, S., Ahmed, S., & Saxena, A. K. (2022). Exploring the role of antioxidants to combat oxidative stress in malaria Parasites. *Current Topics in Medicinal Chemistry*, *22*(24), 2029–2044. DOI: 10.2174/1568026622666220405121643 PMID: 35382719

Naser, R. H., Rajaii, T., Farash, B. R. H., Seyyedtabaei, S., Hajali, V., Sadabadi, F., & Saburi, E. (2024). Hematological changes due to malaria–An update. *Molecular and Biochemical Parasitology*, *259*, 111635. DOI: 10.1016/j.molbiopara.2024.111635 PMID: 38857772

Nureye, D., & Assefa, S. (2020). Old and recent advances in life cycle, pathogenesis, diagnosis, prevention, and treatment of malaria including perspectives in Ethiopia. *TheScientificWorldJournal*, *2020*(1), 1295381. DOI: 10.1155/2020/1295381

Obeagu, E. I. (2024). Role of cytokines in immunomodulation during malaria clearance. *Annals of Medicine and Surgery (London)*, *86*(5), 2873–2882. DOI: 10.1097/MS9.0000000000002019 PMID: 38694310

Okoh, M. P., Egua, M. O., Alli, L. A., Dalu, D., Gundamaraju, R., Singla, R. K., & Shen, B. (2025). Unveiling the Potential of Natural Resources-Derived Therapeutics for Improved Malaria Management: Computational to Experimental Studies. *Advanced Biology*, *9*(2), 2400282. DOI: 10.1002/adbi.202400282 PMID: 39703011

Okombo, J., & Fidock, D. A. (2025). Towards next-generation treatment options to combat Plasmodium falciparum malaria. *Nature Reviews. Microbiology*, *23*(3), 178–191. DOI: 10.1038/s41579-024-01099-x PMID: 39367132

Olas, B., Urbańska, K., & Bryś, M. (2020). Saponins as modulators of the blood coagulation system and perspectives regarding their use in the prevention of venous thromboembolic incidents. *Molecules (Basel, Switzerland)*, *25*(21), 5171. DOI: 10.3390/molecules25215171 PMID: 33172028

Oleinikov, A. V. (2022). Malaria parasite Plasmodium falciparum proteins on the surface of infected erythrocytes as targets for novel drug discovery. *Biochemistry (Moscow)*, *87*(S1, Suppl 1), S192–S202. DOI: 10.1134/S0006297922140152 PMID: 35501996

Onyesom, I., Elu, C. O., Acha, J. O., Ojugbeli, E. T., Ochonogor, E. P., & Udumebraye, L. O. (2022). Evaluation of Antiplasmodial Activity and Inhibitions of Lipid Peroxidation and Parasite Haem Polymerization Activity by Medicinal Phytochemicals of Phyllanthus amarus. *Nigerian Journal of Parasitology*, *43*(2), 293–302. DOI: 10.4314/njpar.v43i2.12

Panieri, E., & Saso, L. (2021). Inhibition of the NRF2/KEAP1 axis: A promising therapeutic strategy to alter redox balance of cancer cells. *Antioxidants & Redox Signaling, 34*(18), 1428–1483. DOI: 10.1089/ars.2020.8146 PMID: 33403898

Paudel, S., Mishra, N., & Agarwal, R. (2023). Phytochemicals as immunomodulatory molecules in cancer therapeutics. *Pharmaceuticals (Basel, Switzerland), 16*(12), 1652. DOI: 10.3390/ph16121652 PMID: 38139779

Pawłowska, M., Mila-Kierzenkowska, C., Szczegielniak, J., & Woźniak, A. (2023). Oxidative stress in parasitic diseases—Reactive oxygen species as mediators of interactions between the host and the parasites. *Antioxidants, 13*(1), 38. DOI: 10.3390/antiox13010038 PMID: 38247462

Porwal, O., Ozdemir, M., Kala, D., & Anwer, E. T. (2021). A review on medicinal plants as potential sources of natural immunomodulatory action. *Journal of Drug Delivery and Therapeutics, 11*(6), 324–331. DOI: 10.22270/jddt.v11i6.5125

Rasmussen, C., Alonso, P., & Ringwald, P. (2022). Current and emerging strategies to combat antimalarial resistance. *Expert Review of Anti-Infective Therapy, 20*(3), 353–372. DOI: 10.1080/14787210.2021.1962291 PMID: 34348573

Rauf, A., Abu-Izneid, T., Khalil, A. A., Imran, M., Shah, Z. A., Emran, T. B., Mitra, S., Khan, Z., Alhumaydhi, F. A., Aljohani, A. S. M., Khan, I., Rahman, M. M., Jeandet, P., & Gondal, T. A. (2021). Berberine as a potential anticancer agent: A comprehensive review. *Molecules (Basel, Switzerland), 26*(23), 7368. DOI: 10.3390/molecules26237368 PMID: 34885950

Reddy, V., Weiss, D. J., Rozier, J., Ter Kuile, F. O., & Dellicour, S. (2023). Global estimates of the number of pregnancies at risk of malaria from 2007 to 2020: A demographic study. *The Lancet. Global Health, 11*(1), e40–e47. DOI: 10.1016/S2214-109X(22)00431-4 PMID: 36521951

Reyes-López, M., Aguirre-Armenta, B., Piña-Vázquez, C., De la Garza, M., & Serrano-Luna, J. (2023). Hemoglobin uptake and utilization by human protozoan parasites: A review. *Frontiers in Cellular and Infection Microbiology, 13*, 1150054. DOI: 10.3389/fcimb.2023.1150054 PMID: 37360530

Ribbiso, K. A., Heller, L. E., Taye, A., Julian, E., Willems, A. V., & Roepe, P. D. (2021). Artemisinin-based drugs target the plasmodium falciparum heme detoxification pathway. *Antimicrobial Agents and Chemotherapy, 65*(4), 10–1128. DOI: 10.1128/AAC.02137-20 PMID: 33495226

Rudrapal, M., & Chetia, D. (2021). Malaria and recent developments in antimalarial drugs. *Neglected tropical diseases and phytochemicals in drug discovery*, 499-542.

Sakyi, P. O., Twumasi, E. B., Twumasi, M. A., Akolgo, G. A., Amewu, R. K., & Osei-Safo, D. (2025). Therapeutic Potential of Natural Products as Innovative and New Frontiers for Combating Parasitic Diseases. *Parasitologia, 5*(3), 49. DOI: 10.3390/parasitologia5030049

Salagre, K. D., Sahay, R. N., Pazare, A. R., Dubey, A., & Marathe, K. K. (2017). A study of clinical profile of patients presenting with complications of acute febrile illnesses during monsoon. *The Journal of the Association of Physicians of India, 65*(9), 37–42. PMID: 29313575

Sarkar, A., Basak, S., Ghosh, S., Mahalanobish, S., & Sil, P. C. (2021). Insights into the relation between oxidative stress and malaria: A mechanistic and therapeutic approach. *Reactive Oxygen Species (Apex, N.C.), 11*, m26–m41. DOI: 10.20455/ros.2021.m.805

Sawerus, M. G., Kamel, H. H., Ahmed, W. M., Ata, E. B., El Amir, D., Mahdi, E. A., Ibrahim, M. A., & Shehata, O. (2025). Antitrypanosomal potential of Salvia officinalis terpenoids-rich fraction in Trypanosoma evansi-infected rat model. *BMC Veterinary Research, 21*(1), 410. DOI: 10.1186/s12917-025-04861-2 PMID: 40571943

Sebghatollahi, Z., Yogesh, R., Mahato, N., Kumar, V., Mohanta, Y. K., Baek, K. H., & Mishra, A. K. (2025). Signaling Pathways in Oxidative Stress-Induced Neurodegenerative Diseases: A Review of Phytochemical Therapeutic Interventions. *Antioxidants, 14*(4), 457. DOI: 10.3390/antiox14040457 PMID: 40298834

Septembre-Malaterre, A., Lalarizo Rakoto, M., Marodon, C., Bedoui, Y., Nakab, J., Simon, E., Hoarau, L., Savriama, S., Strasberg, D., Guiraud, P., Selambarom, J., & Gasque, P. (2020). Artemisia annua, a traditional plant brought to light. *International Journal of Molecular Sciences, 21*(14), 4986. DOI: 10.3390/ijms21144986 PMID: 32679734

Shibeshi, M. A., Kifle, Z. D., & Atnafie, S. A. (2020). Antimalarial drug resistance and novel targets for antimalarial drug discovery. *Infection and Drug Resistance, 13*, 4047–4060. DOI: 10.2147/IDR.S279433 PMID: 33204122

Shinyuy, L. M., Loe, G. E., Jansen, O., Mamede, L., Ledoux, A., Noukimi, S. F., Abenwie, S. N., Ghogomu, S. M., Souopgui, J., Robert, A., Demeyer, K., & Frederich, M. (2023). Secondary metabolites isolated from Artemisia afra and Artemisia annua and their anti-malarial, anti-inflammatory and Immunomodulating properties—pharmacokinetics and pharmacodynamics: A review. *Metabolites, 13*(5), 613. DOI: 10.3390/metabo13050613 PMID: 37233654

Singh, N., & Yeh, P. J. (2017). Suppressive drug combinations and their potential to combat antibiotic resistance. *The Journal of Antibiotics*, *70*(11), 1033–1042. DOI: 10.1038/ja.2017.102 PMID: 28874848

Sinha, S., Batovska, D. I., Medhi, B., Radotra, B. D., Bhalla, A., Markova, N., & Sehgal, R. (2019). In vitro anti-malarial efficacy of chalcones: Cytotoxicity profile, mechanism of action and their effect on erythrocytes. *Malaria Journal*, *18*(1), 421. DOI: 10.1186/s12936-019-3060-z PMID: 31842914

Sobhani, M., Farzaei, M. H., Kiani, S., & Khodarahmi, R. (2021). Immunomodulatory; anti-inflammatory/antioxidant effects of polyphenols: A comparative review on the parental compounds and their metabolites. *Food Reviews International*, *37*(8), 759–811. DOI: 10.1080/87559129.2020.1717523

Sojka, D., Jalovecká, M., & Perner, J. (2022). Babesia, Theileria, plasmodium and hemoglobin. *Microorganisms*, *10*(8), 1651. DOI: 10.3390/microorganisms10081651 PMID: 36014069

Sokan-Adeaga, A. A., Sokan-Adeaga, M. A., Sokan-Adeaga, E. D., Oparaji, A. N., Edris, H., Tella, E. O., Balogun, F. A., Aledeh, M., & Amubieya, O. E. (2023). Environmental toxicants and health adversities: A review on interventions of phytochemicals. *Journal of Public Health Research*, *12*(2), 22799036231181226. DOI: 10.1177/22799036231181226 PMID: 37440795

Soni, R., Sharma, D., Rai, P., Sharma, B., & Bhatt, T. K. (2017). Signaling strategies of malaria parasite for its survival, proliferation, and infection during erythrocytic stage. *Frontiers in Immunology*, *8*, 349. DOI: 10.3389/fimmu.2017.00349 PMID: 28400771

Su, X., Liang, Z., Xue, Q., Liu, J., Hao, X., & Wang, C. (2023). A comprehensive review of azadirachtin: Physicochemical properties, bioactivities, production, and biosynthesis. *Acupuncture and Herbal Medicine*, *3*(4), 256–270. DOI: 10.1097/HM9.0000000000000086

Suganya, T., Packiavathy, I. A. S. V., Aseervatham, G. S. B., Carmona, A., Rashmi, V., Mariappan, S., Devi, N. R., & Ananth, D. A. (2022). Tackling multiple-drug-resistant bacteria with conventional and complex phytochemicals. *Frontiers in Cellular and Infection Microbiology*, *12*, 883839. DOI: 10.3389/fcimb.2022.883839 PMID: 35846771

Takken, W., Charlwood, D., & Lindsay, S. W. (2024). The behaviour of adult Anopheles gambiae, sub-Saharan Africa's principal malaria vector, and its relevance to malaria control: A review. *Malaria Journal*, *23*(1), 161. DOI: 10.1186/s12936-024-04982-3 PMID: 38783348

Tarkang, P. A., Appiah-Opong, R., Ofori, M. F., Ayong, L. S., & Nyarko, A. K. (2016). Application of multi-target phytotherapeutic concept in malaria drug discovery: A systems biology approach in biomarker identification. *Biomarker Research*, *4*(1), 25. DOI: 10.1186/s40364-016-0077-0 PMID: 27999673

Thakur, V. (2024). Food Vacuole as a Drug Target. In *Drug Targets for Plasmodium Falciparum: Historic to Future Perspectives* (pp. 183–199). Springer Nature Singapore. DOI: 10.1007/978-981-19-4484-0_10

Timothy, F. M., & Zininga, T. (2023). Small heat shock proteins as modulators of cell death in Plasmodium falciparum parasites and its human host. *Frontiers in Cell Death*, *2*, 1322780. DOI: 10.3389/fceld.2023.1322780

Tiwari, R., Latheef, S. K., Ahmed, I., Iqbal, H. M., Bule, M. H., Dhama, K., Samad, H. A., Karthik, K., Alagawany, M., El-Hack, M. E. A., Yatoo, M. I., & Farag, M. R. (2018). Herbal immunomodulators-a remedial panacea for designing and developing effective drugs and medicines: Current scenario and future prospects. *Current Drug Metabolism*, *19*(3), 264–301. DOI: 10.2174/1389200219666180129125436 PMID: 29380694

Vaghela, U. P., Jani, B., Tank, T., Kalaria, K., Kanabar, V., Parekh, K., & Yadav, R. (2025). Antimalarial Potential of Medicinal Plants: Phytochemical Insights and Host-Directed Strategies. *The Journal of Communicable Diseases*, *57*(3), 174–181. DOI: 10.24321/0019.5138.202584

van der Pluijm, R. W., Amaratunga, C., Dhorda, M., & Dondorp, A. M. (2021). Triple artemisinin-based combination therapies for malaria–a new paradigm? *Trends in Parasitology*, *37*(1), 15–24. DOI: 10.1016/j.pt.2020.09.011 PMID: 33060063

Vanaja, P., Moorthy, N. H. N., Rajpoot, V. S., Rao, H., Goswami, R. K., Subash, P., Khute, S., & Rao, K. S. (2025). Metabolite profiling, antimalarial potentials of Schleichera oleosa using LC-MS and GC-MS: In vitro, molecular docking and molecular dynamics. *Frontiers in Molecular Biosciences*, *12*, 1543939. DOI: 10.3389/fmolb.2025.1543939 PMID: 40026697

Vijayan, K., Wei, L., Glennon, E. K., Mattocks, C., Bourgeois, N., Staker, B., & Kaushansky, A. (2021). Host-targeted interventions as an exciting opportunity to combat malaria. *Chemical Reviews*, *121*(17), 10452–10468. DOI: 10.1021/acs.chemrev.1c00062 PMID: 34197083

Wang, C., Zhang, H., Wang, X., Wang, X., Li, X., Li, C., Wang, Y., & Zhang, M. (2024). Comprehensive review on fruit of Terminalia chebula: Traditional uses, phytochemistry, pharmacology, toxicity, and pharmacokinetics. *Molecules (Basel, Switzerland)*, *29*(23), 5547. DOI: 10.3390/molecules29235547 PMID: 39683707

Ward, K. E., Fidock, D. A., & Bridgford, J. L. (2022). Plasmodium falciparum resistance to artemisinin-based combination therapies. *Current Opinion in Microbiology*, *69*, 102193. DOI: 10.1016/j.mib.2022.102193 PMID: 36007459

Wu, S., Nie, Q., Tan, S., Liao, G., Lv, Y., Lv, C., Chen, G., & Liu, S. (2023). The immunity modulation of transforming growth factor-β in malaria and other pathological process. *International Immunopharmacology*, *122*, 110658. DOI: 10.1016/j.intimp.2023.110658 PMID: 37467691

Yang, J., Li, K., He, D., Gu, J., Xu, J., Xie, J., Zhang, M., Liu, Y., Tan, Q., & Zhang, J. (2020). Toward a better understanding of metabolic and pharmacokinetic characteristics of low-solubility, low-permeability natural medicines. *Drug Metabolism Reviews*, *52*(1), 19–43. DOI: 10.1080/03602532.2020.1714646 PMID: 31984816

Yeh, Y. C., Huang, T. H., Yang, S. C., Chen, C. C., & Fang, J. Y. (2020). Nano-based drug delivery or targeting to eradicate bacteria for infection mitigation: A review of recent advances. *Frontiers in Chemistry*, *8*, 286. DOI: 10.3389/fchem.2020.00286 PMID: 32391321

Yu, S., Wang, J., Luo, X., Zheng, H., Wang, L., Yang, X., & Wang, Y. (2022). Transmission-blocking strategies against malaria parasites during their mosquito stages. *Frontiers in Cellular and Infection Microbiology*, *12*, 820650. DOI: 10.3389/fcimb.2022.820650 PMID: 35252033

Zhang, L., Ismail, M. M., Rocchetti, G., Fayek, N. M., Lucini, L., & Saber, F. R. (2022). The untargeted phytochemical profile of three meliaceae species related to in vitro cytotoxicity and anti-virulence activity against MRSA isolates. *Molecules (Basel, Switzerland)*, *27*(2), 435. DOI: 10.3390/molecules27020435 PMID: 35056761

Zhang, Y., Alvarez-Manzo, H., Leone, J., Schweig, S., & Zhang, Y. (2021). Botanical medicines Cryptolepis sanguinolenta, Artemisia annua, Scutellaria baicalensis, Polygonum cuspidatum, and Alchornea cordifolia demonstrate inhibitory activity against Babesia duncani. *Frontiers in Cellular and Infection Microbiology*, *11*, 624745. DOI: 10.3389/fcimb.2021.624745 PMID: 33763384

Chapter 5
From Lab to Field Translating Natural Products Into Clinical Candidates

Chinyere Charity Ezeanya-Bakpa
https://orcid.org/0000-0002-7844-7414
Caleb University Lagos, Nigeria

Fisayo Emmanuel Lambe
Caleb University, Lagos, Nigeria

Testimonies Chikanka Adebayo-Olajide
https://orcid.org/0000-0001-9788-3513
Caleb University, Nigeria

Goddidit Esiro Esosa-Enoyoze
https://orcid.org/0000-0003-1369-4171
Edo State University, Uzairue, Nigeria

ABSTRACT

The transition from laboratory research to clinical application in the realm of natural products represents a critical juncture in the development of novel therapeutics. The integration of natural products into modern medicine remains a cornerstone of pharmaceutical innovation. This process involves not only the meticulous isolation and classification of bioactive compounds but also the rigorous assessment of their efficacy and safety through a series of preclinical and clinical trials. There is the need to address the public health threat of malaria, and the invaluable contributions of natural products to clinical candidates is inevitable. This chapter discusses

DOI: 10.4018/979-8-3373-5821-5.ch005

various kinds of natural products with evidence-based antimalarial activity, along with their potential clinical candidacy. It covers the challenges at the preclinical and clinical developmental level in translating natural products to clinical candidates and future prospects.

1.0. INTRODUCTION

Natural products (NPs) are important driver of human development, providing exceptional diversity of chemical and biological activities. Tradition therapy to modern therapeutics, industries such as medicine, agriculture and cosmetics have been significantly influenced by diverse bioactive compounds (Newman and Cragg, 2020). The origin of the compounds are also diverse, including the marine source, metabolite from microorganisms, plants, each of these biochemical offer a unique structural activities relation, mechanism of action that continue to promote discovery and innovation (Newman and Cragg, 2020)

Products from plants and animals have been the basis of natural therapy of man diseases. However, products natural sources remain as vital source of both future medicines and treatment means. Most available drugs are derived from natural products (secondary metabolite) and relative compounds from natural sources. Products from plants and animals provide the pharmaceutical industry with novel compounds which has resulted into the production of different new drugs. These products and their derivative have known for years not only for structural diversity but as drug candidates. Findings revealed that the chemical structure of NP have wide range of diversity of multidimensional structural compounds. This has called for a considerable attention for the use of natural products due to it biological functions (Sircar, 1982). In terms of functional groups, chirality, and structural complexity, natural products are drug like molecules in features (Atanasov et al., 2015; Cragg & Newman, 2013).

1.1. Significance of NPs in drug discovery

Nature serves as natural reservoir in for the discovery of herbal products. The has contributed to the existence of man across the world today. It has been recognized that natural products and its derivatives are major reservoir of health-promoting and of molecular variety. The differences in chemical component of NPs resulted into an advance screening prior to the discovery of new drugs (Lahlou, 2013).

Drug discovery in recent time, natural products contribute one of the major factors in most Pharmaceutical companies have either scaled down or ended their natural products operations. Among the parameters to be considered in the processing natural products include structural elucidation and various separation circles, and it was time consuming. In the early years, many plants have discovered for the their medicinal properties and therapeutic purposes against infections (Ernst et al., 2015; Gozubuyuk et al., 2014; Hotwani et al., 2014; Liu et al., 2011; Mannangatti and Naidu, 2016. Cancer and pathological agents can be treated using plant and animal derived NPs (Blunt et al., 2018; Harvey et al, 2015; Chang et al., 2016). In contrast, herbal drug has been overpowered by modern medicine as means of therapy for human diseases (Tansaz and Tajadini, 2016; Xu et al., 2013; Yuan et al., 2016). Medicinal plants have been used in treating diseases and helath promoting substances for the past decades in many developed countries (Banjari et al., 2017; Yatoo et al., 2017; Thomford et al., 2016). According to Atanasov et al.(2021), compounds derived from natural products and its analogs have placed major role to pharmacotherapy and infections related.

1.2. Overview of the Process from Laboratory Research to Clinical Applications

At every beginning of drug development, a botanical specialists and ethnobotanists are very important in terms of identifying and collecting plant species of therapeutic potential. To ascertain a particular plant species, several sources of information is required especially the traditional knowledge, which indigenous and local people always originate. Therapeutic potential plant with a promising bioactive compounds are often carried out through ethnobotanical and field surveys. This phase plays crucial role in collection of wide range of bioactive chemicals.

Following the collection of the plant material, the bioactive compounds from the plant matrix. To achieve this, different methods. Plants material are collected, the bioactive compounds are extracted from the extracts. These can be achieved through different methods depending on the plant materials (Altemimi et al., 2017). Basic methods of removing bioactive compounds plant include maceration, soxhlet extraction, and super-critical fluid extraction. Maceration involves the process by which the substance i.e. the plant material of interest is immersed in a suitable liquid. Soxhlet method is a simultaneous process of extraction through a suitable fluid. Super-critical fluid extraction extracts phytochemicals through supercritical a suitable liquid. (Jones and Kinghorn, 2012).

Green extraction method commonly known as Eco-extraction techniques promotes environmental sustainability and reduce toxic substances from the environment in the process of phytochemicals from the plant extracts (Vinci et al., 2023). Extraction of Carbodioxide (CO_2) from solvent is carried using superficial fluid extraction at super-critical state. However, it exhibits both a liquid and gas characteristics states (Machado *et al.*, 2013). Super-critical CO_2 evolved due to absence of flammability and toxicity, following its removal during the process, hence it promotes environmental sustainability and substituting the organic solvent (Sapkale et al., 2010).

Also, Phytochemicals can be extracted through steam at 121 °C and 1 atmosphere pressure (Beaufils et al., 2021). It is beneficial by reducing the use of organic solvents and enhance stability of heat sensitive bioactive compounds (Beaufils et al., 2021). Research is on going investigating an alternative to organic solvents without posing any side effects on man and its environment (Calvo-Flores et al., 2018).

Isolation and purification of plant materials is achieved based on chemical characterization, analytical chromatography, a high resolution that performs the functions of sorting and determining molecules and partition chromatography, which compounds are separated based on their individual components. Other purification methods are solvent partitioning and crystallization (Huang et al., 2021). Plant material are composed of varieties of phytochemicals such as bioactive and non-bioactive (Bochkov et al., 2012). in other to have distinct active components, such mixture must pass through both purification and fractionation processes (Bajpai et al., 2016).

Upon the the identification and purification of the phytochemicals, biological test is the next phase involves assessing their therapeutic potential. This can be quantified both *in-vitro* and *in-vivo* study in other to determine its physiological and biochemical action, level of toxicity, and pharmacological potency. Under controlled laboratory condition, *in-vitro* and *in-vivo* biological test is carried out mostly using biochemical systems or cell cultures to find out effect of the substance to a either at molecular or cellular level (Grant, 1994).

Establishing the structural characterization of the target chemical compositions of the substances are important giving an insight on their characteristics and potential in pharmaceutical discovery (Hu et al., 2023). Structural elucidation of substances is determined through nuclear magnetic resonance (NMR) and mass spectrometery (Ezeanya-Bakpa & Adams, 2024). These techniques provide detailed information on the compound to atomic level, and the functional group.

After identifying drug molecules with therapeutic potential, the development of drugs continues to lead optimization. The primary chemicals characteristics is enhanced by the collaboration of Medical chemists and pharmacologists. At this phase, it involves altering the chemical constituents so as to improve the efficacy, target selectivity, drug metabolism. This purpose is aimed to create molecule with promising therapeutically and could fulfil rigorous criteria for a safe and productive drugs (Bregman et al., 2017). All these processes are very important in therapeutic development and effective transformation of bio-products into life-saving pharmaceuticals.

2.0. SYNOPSIS OF NATURAL PRODUCTS

2.1. Sources of NPs

Various organisms have often been the sources of NP, a mainstream of source of medications for the managing various ailment, disorders, mostly pathogenic diseases and cancer (Agarwal et al., 2020; Atanasov et al., 2021). NPs evolved from plants, animals, microbes, and fungi (Singla et al., 2023). NPs or metabolites are compounds derived from organisms. Compounds derived from NPs are composed of various ingredients, especially those in supplements. Natural products have been used by the folk healers in their practice. Mohanraj et al. (2018) described that NPs used in the medical systems are highly documented as in Indian system of medicine.

2.1.1. Microorganisms sources of NP

Marine and terrestrial microbes are screened for drug discovery. Microorganisms were not drug source prior to penicillin was discovered (Woodruff, 1980). Findings showed that microorganisms are known for diverse bioactive compounds resulting to antibacterial agent discovery, including epirubin, carbose and cephalosporin.

2.1.2. Animal sources of NP

NP such as Epibatidine, a poisonous substance found in the skin of Ecuadorian frog is an interesting drug source. This compound is known to be 10 times effective compare to morphine. Animals produce toxins and venoms using for the treatment of numerous disease. For example, Brazilian viper produces teprotide, resulting into the production of cilazapril and captopril, effectively used in treatment of hypertension (Clark, 1996).

2.1.3. Plant as source of NP

Plants contain several phytochemicals, a part of the traditional medicine system used for different treatment for years. Most prescribed drug are derived from plants, this call for further discovery of more plants for curing diseases (Nasim et al., 2022).

Drugs from plant sources are successfully used to address ailment such as inflammatory, diabetic, obesity, malarial, immune-modulators, leshmanial, anti-viral, cardio-vascular and anti-neoplastic properties. Plants such as *Newbouldia laevis* (Umeokoli et al., 2015a) and *Talinum triangulare* (Umeokoli et al., 2015b), has undergone characterization and isolation of bioactive compounds, unveiling the potential NPs from plants in the discovery of novel drugs.

2.2. Chemical structure and complexity of molecule interaction

NPs consist of complex molecular structures, several chiral centers, cyclic semi-rigid scaffolds, with over 5 Hydrogen-bond donors, over 10 Hydrogen-bond receptor, over 5 rotatable Carbon-Carbon bonds, large surface area, high molecular weight above 500. With this diversity and complexity, it may result into low or moderate rate of bio-availability and a corresponding dosage regimens in other to get the required potency, such complex structure may be a latent advantage, as previously highlighted. However, it has been deduced that the complexity has always been known to be a constraint for the average chemical synthesis of natural products-based libraries at a given time and resource frame.

The wide range of secondary metabolites of plants derived natural products have distinctive characteristics which has led to their chemical diversity. The secondary metabolites are made of different phytochemicals including terpernoids, phenols, flavoniods, saponins and alkaloids and so on. The extensive range chemicals found in natural compounds are derived from plant sources, new drug classes are assessed through the process of identification and discovery. These phytochemicals have used for many years as traditional medicines and evaluated for their therapeutic potential, this has resulted into development of novel drugs and diverse treatment of array of health problems (Balandrin et al., 1993 and Lautie et al., 2020).

2.3. Traditional uses and examples of successful drugs derived from nature

Ginkgo biloba commonly called ginkgo, this herbal is derived from the maidenhair tree (Mei et al., 2017). It has been one of the herbal medicine used by the Chinese as a traditional medicine for thousands of years and till date. *Gingkgo biloba* has several benefits because of it contains diversity of active ingredients (Mei et al., 2017). Extracts from the leaf of *Gingko biloba*are used for modern applications, whereas the laves and seeds are used traditionally for teas and tinctures. Also, the raw fruits and toasted seeds can be consumed raw. However, small amount of the seeds are required to be eaten as result of its toxicity. It is known to treat extensive range of ailments such as Cardiovascular risk factors reduction, muscular degeneration mental difficulties, erectile dysfunction and cognitive impairment. But this claim is yet of be proven.

Elderberry is one the ancient traditional medicine typically derived from the cooked fruits of the plant known as *Sambucus nigra.* It is used for the treatment of took ache, viral infections, constipation and relieve headaches. Elderberry is primarily marketed as a therapy for related disease, including flu and common cold. It is now available in the market as a syrup or medicated sweet, but there is specific dosage. Syrup or tea is mostly preferred by some people either by cooking the elderberries with other ingredients such as ginger and honey. Findings in a test-tube showed that its plant chemicals have antioxidant, antiviral properties and antimicrobial activity, but lacks human research (Ezeanya-Bakpa et al., 2022). Study revealed that elderberry shortens the period of flu infections in a few human studies, while larger findings are required to determine if it has more therapeutic efficacy compared to the available convectional antiviral treatment means (Hawkins et al., 2019; Tiralongo et al., 2016).

St. John's wort (SJW) is an ethnomedicine that can be obtained from a flowering plant known as *Hypericum perforatum. H. perforatum* is a small, yellow flowers mostly used to produce juice or tea, and capsules (Klemow et al., 2011). The use of SJW can be traced by the old Greece, it is still frequently prescribed by medical professions by some areas of Europe (Klemow et al., 2011). In the past, SJW was found useful in wound healing and alleviate insomnia, depression, kind of renal and pulmonary disorder, and largely recommended to treat patient with depression (Ng et al., 2017).

Tumeric *(Curcuma longa)* belongs to the family of ginger (Kalman & Hewling, 2017). Tumeric have known long time ago for its medicinal purpose, active ingredient for cooking, and anti-inflammatory properties. The major active compounds in tumeric is Curcumin. It is capable of treating chronic inflammation, metabolic syndrome, pain and anxiety (Kalman & Hewling, 2017*)*. Tumeric and curcumin supplement are less toxic with little side effects including diarrhea, headache, or allergic reaction.

Valerian is sometimes refers to as Valium, a flowering plant whose roots are thought to activate tranquility and a sense of calm. Root of valerian can be dried and fashioned into capsules and produce tea. Its usefulness can be traced backed to the old Greece and Rome, where it was used to relieve restlessness, headaches, palpitations and it often used for insomnia and anxiety therapy (Bučević Popović et al., 2024). Based on a subjective reports from participant, valerian found somewhat found to effective for inducing sleep (Ameer et al., 2024).

2.4. Roles of NPs in modern pharmacology

In human history, the ancient civilization such as Egyptian, Indian and Sumerian knew the value of herbal remedies that are used till date (Chaachouay et al., 2022a). Across the globe, medicinal plants are important recognized their medical therapy for man and animal (Chaachouay et al, 2019; Chaachouay et al., 2022b; Chaachouay et al., 2022c). Plants play a vital role in human development globally. Almost every nation in the worlds has a field of study about the importance of natural remedies. However, the interaction among different cultures have increased pharmacological reference of one group expanding its global recognition and diverse treatment of disease (Chaachouay et al., 2019b). Today, traditional medicine is used globally and its importance has expanded rapidly due to medicinal plants stand out nowadays, especially in economically challenged countries where holistic health services are not available but constitute medicinal plant therapy only. This is common among countries with low levels of education, poor communication network, low available resources and large distances between population centers, high poverty both individual and communal (Karunamoorthi et al., 2013; Sofowora et al., 2013, Ezeanya-Bakpa et al., 2019). Herbs have been used for years as traditional therapy and they are known for their efficacy (Singh & Bharadvaja, 2021). Herbal therapy provides a cost effective option for front line care prior to the absence of convectional healthcare center, side effects, traditional practices, efficacy and selection based on quality. Furthermore, the World Health Organization (WHO) knows the economic values of the traditional medicine, thereby developing policies, guidelines to ensure its quality and purity (Rasoulian & Kheirandish, 2017).

3.0. OPTIMIZATION AND DEVELOPMENT

The voyage from laboratory finding to clinical application is one of the most intricate processes in natural product development. Within the array of evolving therapeutic agents, natural products remain predominant (Bülbül et al., 2025). Their chemical multiplicity reveals an abundant of bioactive compounds with potential clinical applications. The transition from laboratory to the field for successful clinical candidates is faced with numerous challenges. This challenges ranges from biological complexities of optimization to facilitating production.

Natural products are widely known as bioactive compounds derived from sources of natural origins such as plants, marine and microbial organisms. Generally, these natural compounds have contributed significantly to treatment success. A significant number of currently available medicine are derived from natural sources. A typical example is the broad spectrum penicillin produced by the mold *Penicillium chrysogenum*. Also, a well-known anticancer agent of plant-origin - paclitaxel (derived from the Pacific yew tree). The increase in the application of high-throughput screening techniques and mass spectrometry, has widely facilitated the isolation and identification of potential natural bioactive compounds. Nevertheless, isolation is simply the first step in the extensive optimization and development process (Xiao et al., 2016).

3.1. Optimization

An optimization process proceeds an identification of a product of natural origin with therapeutic potential. Here, an encapsulation of enhanced bioactivity, selectivity, and pharmacokinetic properties of the natural compounds while reducing the level of toxicity and adverse side effects occurs. A typical optimization process entails: structural modifications, often proceeding an initially observed biological activity. Given the intricacy of natural products, these structural modifications can be dominant and often require further testing (Tzvetkov et al., 2024).

3.1.1. Structure-Activity Relationship Studies (SAR):

This is a vital stage in the optimization process of natural products. By creating derivatives of the targeted natural compound and evaluating their biological activity, functional groups apt for efficacy and activity are readily identified (Upadhyay & Singh, 2023). The increasingly incorporation of recent computational modeling systems, including but not limited to quantitative structure-activity relationship (QSAR) analysis and molecular docking, provide prediction on the impact of structural changes on biological activity (Kim et al., 2021)

3.1.2. Synthetic Accessibility:

Another vital aspect of the optimization process is the assessment of the synthetic accessibility of the natural compound and its derivatives. Several bioactive compounds of natural origin have complex structure, thus challenging to synthesize in adequate quantities (Singla et al., 2023). The possibility of producing bioactive natural compounds with available synthetic methods is crucial. This is integral in decision making. Usually, analogs with intact biological activity and easy synthesis are mostly considered more readily than complex natural products with difficulty in production (Xiao et al., 2016).

3.1.3. In Vivo and In Vitro Testing:

Following structural modification, in vitro testing aids to assess the effectiveness of an optimized natural bioactive compound. Positive in vitro results, further proceeds to in vivo testing using mostly an animal model. Here, detailed information on potential toxicity, pharmacodynamics, and pharmacokinetics (Hu et al., 2023). Repeated cycles of optimization gradually refines a compound, leading to close similarities with an ideal therapeutic candidates.

3.2. Formulation Development

The translation of natural products into clinical candidates presents intricacies that spans from the laboratory testing of the drug mechanism to its stability in clinical settings. The complexity of the path from laboratory to clinical implementations of a natural bioactive compound is not solely dependent on the active pharmaceutical ingredients' chemical properties but also in their formulation and bioavailability (Domingo-Fernández et al., 2024). Formulation development in drug delivery systems (DDS) is utmost to translating natural products with exhibited range of pharmacological activities and therapeutic potential.

3.2.1. Formulation Development and Drug Delivery

Formulation development represent a template for the therapeutic features of a drug with satisfactory efficacy and safety. The role of formulation defines the following: patient adherence, bioavailability, shelf life, and drug release rates. With natural bioactive compounds known to exhibit a multifaceted mixture of active compounds, formulation possesses to be more challenging. Here, it is important to note that the formulation should aim at preserving the chemical integrity of the bioactive compounds, and boost their delivery to target tissues consequently guaranteeing optimal therapeutic aftermaths (Ezeanya-Bakpa et al., 2023).

Due to the complexity of natural products, rigorous analytical procedures are thus required for an effective formulation development. They include: nuclear magnetic resonance (NMR) spectroscopy, mass spectrometry, and High-Performance Liquid Chromatography (HPLC). These techniques are critical in the identification of bioactive components and subsequently their quantitative evaluation. The designated bioactive compounds undergo certain pre-formulation testing. These testing aid to examine their stability, compatibility, and solubility with different excipients. This principal aspect births an effective and stable formulation (Chen and Kirchmair, 2020).

3.2.2. Stability Concerns in Formulation Development

Stability is a fundamental aspect of formulation development in the translation of natural products. APIs derived from natural sources often possess delicate structures, including alkaloids, flavonoids, and terpenes, that may degrade under extreme temperature fluctuations, humidity, and illumination (Grigalunas et al., 2022). An in-depth stability assessment entails both accelerated stability studies aimed at predicting product performance under challenging circumstances, and long-term stability studies under an ideal storage condition. The stability testing aims to establish shelf life and inform labeling requirements, thus ensuring that the product retains its efficacy and safety over time (Wu & Lu, 2019).

Moreover, excipient interaction can significantly influence the stability profile of a drug formulation. Understanding these interactions requires careful selection of excipients based on their physicochemical properties and their compatibility with the API. The formulation must achieve a delicate balance, ensuring that the excipients enhance, rather than detract from, the stability of the active components. Techniques such as Differential Scanning Calorimetry (DSC) and Thermogravimetric Analysis (TGA) are often employed to evaluate these interactions and thermal properties (Al-Faqeeh, 2023).

3.3. Bioavailability

Bioavailability is the degree and rate at which a substance is absorbed and becomes available at the site of action. This is another basis of formulation development. Natural products can exhibit poor bioavailability due to their low solubility and absorption issues. As such, enhancing bioavailability is crucial for translating these products into effective clinical candidates (Sorkin et al., 2020).

Employing advanced drug delivery systems can significantly improve the bioavailability of natural products. Various strategies such as nano-encapsulation, liposomal formulations, and solid dispersions are being explored to enhance solubility and facilitate controlled release. For instance, nanoparticles can improve the solubility of poorly water-soluble compounds while protecting them from degradation, thereby transcending the limitations posed by traditional formulations (Hedge et al., 2020).

Furthermore, the physicochemical characteristics of the bioactive compounds involved also play a pivotal role in bioavailability. Factors such as molecular weight, lipophilicity, and polarity must be considered during the design of the drug product. In some cases, prodrug strategies may be utilized to improve absorption and lower the metabolic conversion of the compound, further enhancing therapeutic efficiency (Atanasov et al., 2021).

4.0. PRECLINICAL DEVELOPMENT

In pre-clinical development of medication can be considered as drug candidates, a series of laboratory and animal assessment are carried out to determine its safety, toxicity and efficacy before human consumption. Information obtained from these findings would allow a researcher to determine its safety if consumed by man on clinical trials (Shegokar, 2020).

4.1. *In-vitro* and *in-vivo* study to assess safety and efficacy

In-vitro study are established to investigate the potential toxicity of chemical substances and, NPs in the cell culture techniques which determines the interaction between the cells and bioactive compounds/phytochemicals, cell growth and cell apoptosis or destruction. The term Necrosis or apoptosis is the potential of a particular chemical to break down a living cells known as cell cytotoxicity. Researcher in the pharmaceuticals use these as an important marker in other to identify compounds that could be responsible for human risk. The cytoplasm of a living cell where markers are present which could be used to identify living cells either by biological methods (i.e. enzymatic activity) or fluorescent label otherwise called radioactive markers. This is applied onto a living cell to assess its viability (Riss et al., 2019; Uzor et al., 2020). Lactose dehydrogenase is one of the enzyme marker that converts pyruvate to lactate (Xiao et al., 2016). Cell to cell interaction with the fluid matrix found outside the cells are required for cell functioning and developing complex organisms (Candini et al., 2019; Ezeanya-Bakpa et al., 2021).

In-vivo investigation involves the use of animal (I.e. rodent and non-rodent mammal) models which describe pharmacokinetics as ADME (adsorption, distribution, metabolism and excretory), toxicity and safety. In drug discovery process, in-vivo is more beneficial because it mimics natural physiological environment compare to the *in-vitro* study. The use of animal in the clinical trial is as a result of similarity in the metabolic pathway. Statistical data obtained by researcher during the course of this investigation could improve reliability, validity, and generalizability (Laajala et al., 2016).

Table 1. Pre-clinical development of selected natural antimalarials

Plant species	In-vitro assay	In-vivo assay	Reference
Callistemon citrinus	Parasite lactate dehydrogenase (pLDH) assay	Cytotoxicity assay	Larayetan et al., 2019
Cordia Africana	Oral acute toxicity	Four-day suppression test and Chemo-prophylactic tests	Wondafrash et al., 2019
Helianthus annuus	24-well microplate with 1% initial and experimental parasitaemia	Peters' 4-day suppressive test	Ekasari et al., 2019
Andrographis paniculata	Dose-response assays	In-vivo toxicity assay	Dwivedi et al., 2021.

4.2. Challenges

Upon the thorough assessment, many drugs at clinical trial still fail. Most of these drugs failed as result predispose factors include low dissolution rate, unpleasant effects, uneven distribution by the proposed clinical route of pathway, unsustainable production expenses, low therapeutic potential at early clinical trial stage. The investigation of the modern drugs, in terms of toxicity and efficacy of pharmaceuticals are based on the uniformity of the cells or animal model. Heterogeneous cells mostly encounters issues and also requires expensive clinical trials just as in human specifically. In case of can cancer disease, the poor treatment rate requires standard pre-clinical trials to develop target drugs. This evolved from heterogeneity between the animal models and human beings in clinical trial Janghui's, (2010)

4.3. Toxicological assessments

Quantitative Structure-Toxicity Relationship (Q)STR and *in-vitro* models are combine approaches employed in toxicity of natural products screening. *In-silico* and *in-vitro* are two methods on integrating data. Xu et al. (2013) and Ye et al. (2022) describes the prediction (Q)STR models as the combination of both structural data and experimental assay in other to properly evaluate the toxicity and other parameters. The benefit of including additional assay to promote prediction accuracy is uncertain, whereas better accuracy could be achieved with structure alone. *In-vitro* assay and *in-silico* is another approach used to reduce false positive/negative prediction (Chen et al., 2014; Jia et al., 2022). *In-silico* predictions and *in-vitro* data gives insight as computation techniques is combined with experimental analysis, this enables results to be easily interpreted.

5.0. CLINICAL DEVELOPMENT

Clinical trial is described as the process to assess toxicity and potency of a specific pharmaceuticals or device on human (Nayak et al., 2013; Bykerk et al., 2013; Akharaiyi,et al., 2021). Steps involved in clinical trials are approved by the regulatory body after non-clinical data is reviewed and showed satisfactory (Ottinger & Geiselman, 2023).

Figure 1. Overview of Clinical development

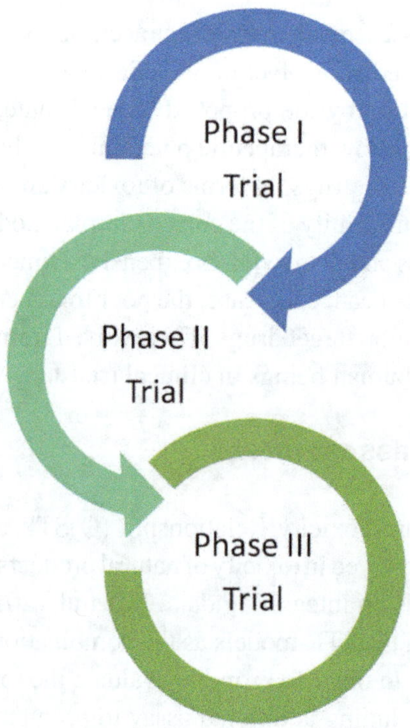

5.1. Phase I trial

Phase I trial is described as the phase at which a successful clinical trial is achieved, however is called the third phase. It accounts for the first phase for research clinical testing. This findings requires experimental testing on human within number (20 - 100). This phase is designed purposely to investigate the risk, acceptability, ADME, effects and mechanisms of actions of therapeutics. Phase I trials are also known as dose magnifying testings, in other to have ideal dose regimen. This research is carried out under clinics known as CPUS (central pharmacological units), medical attention is giving to trial participant for about 24 hours and under the watch of full time clinical staff. However, single ascending dose (SAD) trials, and multiple ascending dose (MAD) are types of Phase trial (FDA, 2010; DeMets et al., 2010). A small trial participants are needed, single dose of the selected pharmaceuticals are administered, and observed for a specific dose. Based on the pharmacokinetics results, if there is no side effects observed it shows that it is safe, the therapeutic dose can be increased to the new volunteers. If the drug produces unfavorable outcome in volunteers, there will be an addition in the volunteers' number. However, in a case where lethal potency is noticed, increase in therapeutic dose is withdrawn, hence the earlier dose is regarded as maximum tolerated dose (MTD) (DeMets et al., 2010).

5.2. Phase II trial

Phase I described the dose arithmetic of the test drug, phase II focuses on assessing if there will be present or absent biological and therapeutic level in such drug (European Medicines Agency, 2020). Phase II trials requires about 100 to 300 participants, it involves the assessment of how drugs functions along with Phase trial I safety with large numbers of volunteers. Phase II is divided into two phases (I.e. Phase IIa and Phase IIb trials). Phase IIa provides insight on therapeutic dose of drugs while Phase IIb describes drug's potency. There are some instances whereby both toxicity and drug's potency combination assessment is carried out. Phase II trials are mostly carried out at universities and hospital clinics (Xiao et al., 2016; Newman and Cragg, 2016).

5.3. Phase III trials

At Phase III trials, this phase evaluates the potency of new pharmaceutical and medicinal effects in the clinical trials. Phase III trials requires larger numbers of participants of about 300 to 3000 in other to investigate new pharmaceuticals and this is compared with available drug standards. This phase is considered mostly to be time consuming and expensive due to the larger numbers of patients required, design and run the process. Proper understanding on progress and timing of disease can allow a researcher to improve on patients' treatment outcome and life quality. After Phase III trial, a comprehensive report on manufacturing methods, trial data, half-life and formulation details are usually submitted to the regulatory body (e.g., National Agency for Food and Drug Administration and Control, Food and Drug Administration). Upon the agency's approval, such drugs can be sold to public but there any report on adverse reaction on such drugs, it can be recalled from the market immediately. The objectives of these is for drugs to meet up with certain treatment means and give less toxicity, if there is challenge such can easily be withdrawn from the market after an approval (Fix, 2013).

6.0. CHALLENGES IN TRANSLATING NATURAL PRODUCTS TO CLINICAL CANDIDATES

6.1. Complexity of natural products

6.1.1. Difficulty in isolation and characterization

Screening of natural products (NPs) utilizes a collection of extracts from natural sources, which often do not work well with traditional target-based assays. It can be difficult to pinpoint the active compounds of interest, so pre-screening methods are needed to prevent rediscovering substances already known. Also, obtaining enough biological material to isolate and study a bioactive product can be a significant challenge. Additionally, leads on drugs from natural products often come from phenotypic screening, making it time-consuming to figure out their exact molecular mechanisms. Fortunately, there have been significant advances in screening methods, such as using induced pluripotent stem cells and gene editing, and improved strategies for identifying how active compounds work (Atanasov et al., 2021).

Natural products often have complex chemical structures. This complexity thwarts the development of throughput methods for synthesis and/or chemical modification necessary for the optimization of clinical candidates. Consequently, it is quite challenging to produce or modify potential natural products, most especially in the case of complex synthetic routes. In contrast, pharmaceutical leads from synthetic libraries are generally easier to generate and modify using simpler chemical approaches (Atanasov et al., 2021).

6.1.2. Pharmacokinetics and bioavailability

Curcumin, the bioactive component of turmeric (*Curcuma longa* L), has been used for medicinal purposes for several years. Today, research has revealed that curcumin influences a wide range of signaling molecules, such as inflammatory molecules, transcription factors, enzymes, protein kinases, protein reductases, carrier proteins, cell survival proteins, drug resistance proteins, adhesion molecules, growth factors, receptors, cell-cycle regulators, chemokines, as well as DNA, RNA, and metal ions (Gupta et al., 2012; Ezeanya-Bakpa et al., 2022). It has also been used in traditional medicine to treat conditions, including skin problems, cancer, inflammation, and diabetes, and it is known to improve blood circulation, reduce blockages, and help ease depression. However, its low bioavailability reduces its effectiveness as a treatment in clinical use, and this is because its water solubility is extremely low (at around 11 ng/mL), it is poorly absorbed in the gut, quickly metabolized, poorly distributed throughout the body, and is rapidly excreted (Ameer et al., 2024; Bučević et al., 2024).

Another challenge is the limited availability of bioactive material, as many natural products occur in low abundance. While trace quantities may be sufficient for preliminary screening, substantially larger amounts are required for structural studies, and preclinical evaluation when a compound demonstrates therapeutic potential. Also, the reliance on wild plant collections (if the source of the NP is a plant) is further constrained by habitat degradation, conservation concerns for endangered species, and pronounced seasonal variations in metabolite profiles, which restrict optimal harvesting periods. Moreover, access to plant materials sourced internationally may be disrupted by geopolitical instability, natural disasters, or fluctuations in trade and export regulations, creating additional barriers to sustained supply (Atanasov et al., 2015).

6.2. Economic considerations

6.2.1. Cost of development and potential financial barriers

Scaling up and developing bioactive products often requires larger and more expensive equipment, as well as additional laboratory space. For instance, products such as Malacidin and Teixobactin, with high potency against resistant gram-positive bacteria like methicillin-resistant *Staphylococcus aureus,* are not yet used in clinics because the cost of producing them in large quantities is high (McCarthy, 2019). Despite exemplary research efforts by groups like Lewis and Boger, the development of novel and potent natural product agents faces a significant threat under the current funding landscape. The high cost of drug development, ranging from approximately 0.5 to over 1 billion U.S. dollars, poses a major barrier. Until regulatory bodies or governments adjust these financial demands, progress in this area of drug discovery may stagnate (Newman and Cragg, 2020).

Also, pharmaceutical companies recognized years ago that the ongoing costs of developing antimicrobial and antifungal agents cannot be justified by the return on investment within existing economic frameworks. Consequently, very few pharmaceutical firms of any size continue to actively pursue natural product-based antibiotics, leading to a decline in industry-driven innovation in this critical field (Newman and Cragg, 2020). Similarly, conducting rigorous clinical trials for the approval of natural product-based drugs poses a significant challenge due to their high costs, often making such trials feasible only with industrial support (Atanasov et al., 2015).

6.3. Regulatory hurdles

6.3.1. Navigating the approval processes and meeting safety requirements

Obtaining intellectual property rights for NPs that show important biological activities can be difficult because unmodified natural compounds are not always eligible for patents. This is partly due to differences and ongoing changes in patent laws across countries (Harrison, 2014).

Another challenge comes from regulations that require sharing benefits with the countries where the biological materials originate. These regulations are based on the United Nations 1992 Convention on Biological Diversity and the Nagoya Protocol, which took effect in 2014, along with recent updates related to the sharing of benefits for marine genetic resources (Heinrich et al., 2020). A worldwide multilateral system has been designed to handle situations where genetic resources and related traditional knowledge cross national boundaries or when obtaining prior informed consent is not possible (CBD, 2018). It aims to conserve biodiversity, use genetic resources sustainably, and share benefits from their use equitably and fairly. While some researchers fear that the protocol might impose stricter regulations that could hinder drug discovery and even negatively impact biodiversity conservation, others believe that if integrated thoughtfully into national laws, the increased legal clarity will encourage more research on plants from biodiversity-rich countries and promote their conservation (Atanasov et al., 2015).

7.0. SPECIFIC CASE STUDIES ON SUCCESSFUL TRANSLATION OF NATURAL PRODUCTS IN CLINICAL APPLICATION

7.1. Successful translations of natural products into therapeutics

7.1.1. Overview of key examples

Natural products are relevant to modern pharmacotherapy as about 35% of consumed medicines are obtained from them, including anticancer medications and antibiotics (Craig and Newman, 2013). Between 1940 and 2014, about 60% of the anticancer medications the FDA approved were either natural products or obtained from them, emphasizing the importance of natural products to cancer research (Newman and Cragg, 2020). Many antibiotics have been produced by bacterial strains, particularly from the genus *Streptomyces*. These include tetracycline from *S. rimosus,* kanamycin from *S. kanamyceticus*, thienamycin from *S. cattleya*, vancomycin from *S. orientalis*, neomycin from *S. fradiae*, erythromycin from *Streptomyces erythraea,* streptomycin from *S. griseus*, and chloramphenicol from *S. venezuelae* (Al-Faqeeh, 2023).

Artemisinin is a sesqui-terpenoid secondary metabolite that was first isolated from the plant *Artemisia annua* L. by Tu Youyou in 1972. Artemisinin-based combination therapy (ACT) is now the World Health Organization's preferred antimalarial agent. Recent research has demonstrated that artemisinin and its derivatives possess broad-spectrum anticancer, antibacterial, and immunomodulatory activities beyond their established antimalarial effects. Additionally, these compounds show therapeutic potential for treating diabetes and pulmonary tuberculosis, highlighting their extensive clinical prospects (Zhao et al., 2022). Artemisinin and its derivatives have demonstrated high efficacy in treating severe malaria. When used in combination with traditional antimalarial drugs, they are particularly effective in combating Plasmodium strains that have developed drug resistance.

Around the year 2000, galanthamine, an alkaloid isolated from various Amaryllidaceae species such as *Leucojum*, *Narcissus*, and *Galanthus*, emerged as an important therapeutic agent to slow neurological degeneration in Alzheimer's disease. This therapeutic development dates back to research initiated in the 1950s in the Soviet Union (Heinrich, 2010).

Morphine, a natural product obtained from *Papaver somniferum,* is an analgesic used in post-surgical care and for patients with cancer for severe pain relief. It binds to opioid receptors, causing an increase in the tolerance of pain and a decrease in pain perception. Paclitaxel is a chemotherapeutic agent used in treating cancers such as lung, breast, and ovarian cancer. It is obtained from *Taxus brevifolia* (Pacific yew tree) that stabilizes microtubules and prevents their depolymerization, thus hindering cell division, which causes apoptosis of cancer cells (Saini et al., 2025). Quinine, which has been used for years in the treatment of malaria, was extracted from cinchona bark.

7.2. Insights into pitfalls and unforeseen challenges

Natural products, which have an extensive clinical use history, can benefit from cutting-edge technologies like single-cell multiomics to precisely reveal their effects at the cellular level, aiding target validation and resistance mechanism studies, especially in complex contexts like tumor microenvironments, thus enhancing the clinical application and understanding of their therapeutic effects (Zhu et al., 2022).

In addition to discovering new natural products with antimicrobial properties, researchers are actively developing and optimizing existing classes of natural products by utilizing advances in biosynthetic engineering, total synthesis, and semi-synthetic strategies (Atanasov et al., 2021).

8.0. FUTURE TRENDS

Plant-based compounds retain their values as an active source that could serve for treatment methods and innovative therapies. The diversity of phytochemicals in plants show its wide range of its therapeutic potentials (Balandrin et al., 1993; Lautie et al., 2020). As new bioactive compounds are being discovered by the scientist, and the mechanisms underlying its action present in plants, therefore the pathway for drug development remains strong. This very important when an alternative and sustainable sources for medication is discovered by researcher. Genomics and Metabolomics are closely related connected towards the improvements following the process of investigating and cultivating NPs. Plant genome sequencing enables researchers to acquire knowledge on the genetic pathways that are responsible for phytochemicals production (Marchev et al., 2021). The small bioactive molecules present in the plant system provides a complete experience through metabolomics.

8.1. Advances in bioengineering

The advances in bioengineering remain topnotch in the use of plant derived NPs. Innovations in bio-production, genetic engineering, and route optimization are required to increase plant extracts. Plant-derived molecules are produced using an enclose device known as bioreactors, provide a sustainable and scalable method. The gene of plants and its pathway could be modified so as to produce desired metabolites of interest are required for drug development (Upadhyay and Singh, 2023; Moon et al., 2019).

The future shows potential for inserting plant-derived phytochemicals into precision medicine and personalized medicines. Through metabolomics and genomics data, scientists will be able to improve patient outcome based on the genetic makeup and health status of individuals (Ottinger and Geiselman, 2023). Assessing the synergistic effects of natural products chemicals and their interaction with the herbal drugs is fast growing field of research. The interaction of natural plant chemicals with synthetic pharmaceuticals has the capability to enhance treatment means, but less toxic, and overcome problem of resistance in a wide range of medical challenge (Yuan et al., 2016).

8.2. The impacts of computational methods in therapeutic innovation

In drug discovery, computational methods including molecular docking, virtual screening, are employed to assume the pharmacological interaction derived from the natural products and the biological targets. Docking study is a computational technique that uses software simulation to determine the behaviour of the molecules and their interactions with other molecules (Dhoundiyal and Alam, 2023). Molecular modelling is used for the examination of the arrangement and operation of biomolecules such as protein, DNA enzymes and others biological elements, and for the development cutting-edge medications and pharmaceuticals. Virtual screening is a computer based method used to discover potential drugs candidates from the wide gathering of bioactive compounds. Molecular modeling and docking simulations to evaluate the binding affinity between the small compounds and the proteins known as the target protein (Xia, 2017; Ambrosino et al., 2019; Singh and Bharadvaja, 2021).

9.0. CONCLUSION

The translation of natural products to clinical candidates represents a pivotal advancement in antimalarial development in the Global South. This process involves systematic preclinical and clinical optimization for drug safety and efficacy. With the continuous exploration of natural products, collaboration between researchers and clinicians has becomes essential for maximizing the therapeutic potential of unique clinical candidates. The translation of Artemisinin, a secondary metabolite from plant into clinical practice has demonstrated high efficacy in treating severe malaria. The successful integration of natural antimalarial products into clinical practice not only enhances treatment options for malaria but also epitomizes the promise of innovative, nature-derived solutions in modern medicine.

REFERENCES

Agarwal, G., Blanco, C. P. J., Addo, E. M., & Kinghorn, A. D. (2020). Current status and contemporary approaches to the discovery of antitumor agents from higher plants. *Biotechnology Advances*, *38*, 107337. DOI: 10.1016/j.biotechadv.2019.01.004 PMID: 30633954

Akharaiyi, F. C., Ezeanya-Bakpa, C. C., & Otumala, S. O. (2021). Inhibition of methicillin resistant *Staphylococcus aureus* (MRSA) with underutilized medicinal plants extracts. *International Medical Journal*, *28*(6), 4953–4964.

Altemimi, A., Lakhssassi, N., Baharlouei, A., Watson, D. G., & Lightfoot, D. A. (2017). Phytochemicals: Extraction, isolation, and identification of bioactive compounds from plant extracts. *Plants*, *6*(4), 42. DOI: 10.3390/plants6040042 PMID: 28937585

Al-Faqeeh, L. A. S. (2023). A comprehensive review of natural products from microbial sources and their applications. *PSM Microbiology*, *8*(2), 30–47.

Ambrosino, L., Tangherlini, M., Colantuono, C., Esposito, A., Sangiovanni, M., Miralto, M., Sansone, C., & Chiusano, M. L. (2019). Bioinformatics for marine products: An overview of resources, bottlenecks, and perspectives. *Marine Drugs*, *17*(10), 576. DOI: 10.3390/md17100576 PMID: 31614509

Ameer, S. F., Mohamed, M. Y., Elzubair, Q. A., Sharif, E. A. M., & Ibrahim, W. N. (2024). Curcumin as a novel therapeutic candidate for cancer: Can this natural compound revolutionize cancer treatment? *Frontiers in Oncology*, *14*, 1438040. Advance online publication. DOI: 10.3389/fonc.2024.1438040 PMID: 39507759

Atanasov, A. G., Waltenberger, B., Pferschy-Wenzig, E. M., Linder, T., Wawrosch, C., Uhrin, P., Temml, V., Wang, L., Schwaiger, S., Heiss, E. H., Rollinger, J. M., Schuster, D., Breuss, J. M., Bochkov, V., Mihovilovic, M. D., Kopp, B., Bauer, R., Dirsch, V. M., & Stuppner, H. (2015). Discovery and resupply of pharmacologically active plant-derived natural products: A review. *Biotechnology Advances*, *33*(8), 1582–1614. DOI: 10.1016/j.biotechadv.2015.08.001 PMID: 26281720

Atanasov, A. G., Zotchev, S. B., Dirsch, V. M., & Supuran, C. T. (2021). Natural products in drug discovery: Advances and opportunities. *Nature Reviews. Drug Discovery*, *20*(3), 200–216. DOI: 10.1038/s41573-020-00114-z PMID: 33510482

Bajpai, V. K., Majumder, R., & Park, J. G. (2016). Isolation and purification of plant secondary metabolites using column-chromatographic technique. *Bangladesh Journal of Pharmacology*, *11*(4), 844–848. DOI: 10.3329/bjp.v11i4.28185

Balandrin, M. F., Kinghorn, A. D., & Farnsworth, N. R. (1993). *Plant-derived natural products in drug discovery and development: An overview.* In American Chemical Society., DOI: 10.1021/bk-1993-0534.ch001

Banjari, I., Misir, A., Savikin, K., Jokic, S., Molnar, M., & Waisundara, V. Y. (2017). Antidiabetic effects of Aronia melanocarpa and its other therapeutic properties. *Frontiers in Nutrition, 4*, 53. DOI: 10.3389/fnut.2017.00053 PMID: 29164127

Blunt, J. W., Carroll, A. R., Copp, B. R., Davis, R. A., Keyzers, R. A., & Prinsep, M. R. (2018). Marine natural products. *Natural Product Reports, 35*(1), 8–53. DOI: 10.1039/C7NP00052A PMID: 29335692

Bochkov, D. V., Sysolyatin, S. V., Kalashnikov, A. I., & Surmacheva, I. A. (2012). Shikimic acid: Review of its analytical, isolation, and purification techniques from plant and microbial sources. *Journal of Chemical Biology, 5*(1), 5–17. DOI: 10.1007/s12154-011-0064-8 PMID: 22826715

Bregman, H., Simard, J. R., Andrews, K. L., Ayube, S., Chen, H., Gunaydin, H., & Huang, X. (2017). The discovery and hit-to-lead optimization of tricyclic sulfonamides as potent and efficacious potentiators of glycine receptors. *Journal of Medicinal Chemistry, 60*(3), 1105–1125. DOI: 10.1021/acs.jmedchem.6b01496 PMID: 28001399

Bučević Popović, V., Karahmet Farhat, E., Banjari, I., Jeličić Kadić, A., & Puljak, L. (2024). Bioavailability of oral curcumin in systematic reviews: A methodological study. *Pharmaceuticals (Basel, Switzerland), 17*(2), 164. DOI: 10.3390/ph17020164 PMID: 38399379

Bülbül, E. F., Bode, H. B., Schmitt, S., & Bozhüyük, K. A. J. (2025). Engineering the future of medicine: Natural products, synthetic biology and artificial intelligence for next-generation therapeutics. *Clinical and Translational Medicine, 15*(2), e70146. DOI: 10.1002/ctm2.70146 PMID: 39856487

Bykerk, V. P., Keystone, E. C., Kuriya, B., Larché, M., Thorne, J. C., & Haraoui, B. (2013). Achieving remission in clinical practice: Lessons from clinical trial data. *Clinical and Experimental Rheumatology, 31*(4), 621–632. PMID: 23622099

Candini, O., Grisendi, G., Foppiani, E. M., Brogli, M., Aramini, B., Masciale, V., Spano, C., Petrachi, T., Veronesi, E., Conte, P., Mari, G., & Dominici, M. (2019). A novel 3D in-vitro platform for pre-clinical investigations in drug testing, gene therapy, and immuno-oncology. *Scientific Reports, 9*(1), 7154. DOI: 10.1038/s41598-019-43613-9 PMID: 31073193

Chaachouay, N., Azeroual, A., Bencharki, B., Douira, A., & Zidane, L. (2022c). Ethnoveterinary medicines plants for animal therapy in the Rif, North of Morocco. *South African Journal of Botany*, *147*, 176–191. DOI: 10.1016/j.sajb.2021.12.037

Chaachouay, N., Azeroual, A., Douira, A., & Zidane, L. (2022b). Ethnoveterinary practices of medicinal plants among the Zemmour and Zayane tribes, Middle Atlas, Morocco. *South African Journal of Botany*, *151*, 826–840. DOI: 10.1016/j.sajb.2022.11.009

Chaachouay, N., Benkhnigue, O., Fadli, M., El Ayadi, R., & Zidane, L. (2019b). Ethnobotanical study of medicinal plants used to treat osteoarticular diseases in the Moroccan Rif, Morocco. *Journal of Pharmacy & Pharmacognosy Research*, *7*(6), 454–470. DOI: 10.56499/jppres19.644_7.6.454

Chaachouay, N., Benkhnigue, O., Fadli, M., El Ibaoui, H., El Ayadi, R., & Zidane, L. (2019a). Ethnobotanical and ethnopharmacological study of medicinal and aromatic plants used in the treatment of respiratory system disorders in the Moroccan Rif. *Ethnobotany Research and Applications*, *18*, 1–16. DOI: 10.32859/era.18.22.1-17

Chaachouay, N., Douira, A., & Zidane, L. (2022a). Herbal medicine used in the treatment of human diseases in the Rif, Northern Morocco. *Arabian Journal for Science and Engineering*, *47*(1), 131–153. DOI: 10.1007/s13369-021-05501-1 PMID: 33842189

Chang, J., Kim, Y., & Kwon, H. J. (2016). Advances in identification and validation of protein targets of natural products without chemical modification. *Natural Product Reports*, *33*(5), 719–730. DOI: 10.1039/C5NP00107B PMID: 26964663

Chen, Y., & Kirchmair, J. (2020). Cheminformatics in natural product-based drug discovery. *Molecular Informatics*, *39*(12), 2000171. DOI: 10.1002/minf.202000171 PMID: 32725781

Clark, A. M. (1996). Natural products as a resource for new drugs. *Pharmaceutical Research*, *13*(8), 1133–1141. DOI: 10.1023/A:1016091631721 PMID: 8865302

Convention on Biological Diversity. (2018). Decision 3/13 on a global multilateral benefit-sharing mechanism (Article 10) (CBD/NP/MOP/DEC/3/13). https://www.cbd.int/doc/decisions/np-mop-03/np-mop-03-dec-13-en.pdf

Cragg, G. M., & Newman, D. J. (2013). Natural products: A continuing source of novel drug leads.

Domingo-Fernández, D., Gadiya, Y., Preto, A. J., Krettler, C. A., Mubeen, S., Allen, A., Healey, D., & Colluru, V. (2024). Natural Products Have Increased Rates of Clinical Trial Success throughout the Drug Development Process. *Journal of Natural Products*, *87*(7), 1844–1851. DOI: 10.1021/acs.jnatprod.4c00581 PMID: 38970498

Dwivedi, M. K., Mishra, S., Sonter, S., & Singh, P. K. (2021). Diterpenoids as potential anti-malarial compounds from Andrographis panculata. *Beni-Suef University Journal of Basic and Applied Sciences*, *10*(1), 7. Advance online publication. DOI: 10.1186/s43088-021-00098-8

DeMets, D. L., Friedman, L., & Furberg, C. D. (2010). *Fundamentals of clinical trials* (4th ed.). Springer., DOI: 10.1021/acs.jnatprod.4c00581

Ekasari, W., Widya Pratiwi, D., Amanda, Z., Suciati, Widyawaruyanti, A. & Arwati H. (2019). Various Parts of *Helianthus annuus* Plants as New Sources of Antimalarial Drugs. *Evidence-Based Complement Alternative Medicine*, .DOI: 10.1155/2019/7390385

Ernst, M., Grace, O. M., Saslis-Lagoudakis, C. H., Nilsson, N., Simonsen, H. T., & Ronsted, N. (2015). Global medicinal uses of Euphorbia L. (Euphorbiaceae). *Journal of Ethnopharmacology*, *176*, 90–101. DOI: 10.1016/j.jep.2015.10.025 PMID: 26485050

European Medicines Agency (2020). Guidelines on Quality of Medicinal Products Derived from Biological Sources.

Tiralongo, E., Wee, S., & Lea, R. (2016, March 24). Elderberry supplementation reduces cold duration and symptoms in air-travellers: A randomized, double-blind placebo-controlled clinical trial. *Nutrients*, *8*(4), 182. DOI: 10.3390/nu8040182 PMID: 27023596

Ezeanya-Bakpa, C. C., Agbakoba, N. R., Enweani, I. B., & Oguejiofor, C. B. (2019). Predominance of cervicitis agents with minimal testing rate within the student population in Benin City, Nigeria. *Journal of Obstetrics & Gynaecology*, *39*(6), 840–844. DOI: 10.1080/01443615.2019.1584888 PMID: 31007108

Ezeanya-Bakpa, C. C., & Adams, A. A. (2024). *In vitro* susceptibility of drug-resistant fungi and urinary bacteria to *Psidium guajava* L. leaf extract. *Nigerian Journal of Biotechnology*, *41*(1), 157–164. DOI: 10.4314/njb.v41i1.17

Ezeanya-Bakpa, C. C., Adetunji, C. O., Enosabata, I. A., & Olori, E. (2021). Lycopene for wound infection: In vitro susceptibility of drug-resistant clinical pathogens. *Tropical Journal of Natural Product Research*, *5*(1), 49–52. DOI: 10.26538/tjnpr/v5i1.4

Ezeanya-Bakpa, C. C., Agbakoba, N. R., Enweani-Nwokelo, I. B., & Oguejiofor, C. B. (2022). Phylogeny-based identification of *Mycoplasma genitalium* in a Nigerian population of apparently healthy sexually active female students. *The Pan African Medical Journal*, *41*, 71–76. PMID: 35382058

Ezeanya-Bakpa, C. C., Akinola, K., Adebayo, O. P., & Akharaiyi, F. C. (2023). Antibacterial combination effect of allicin, lycopene and quercetin on antibiotic-resistant bacteria. *Microbes and Infectious Diseases*, *5*(1), 0. Advance online publication. DOI: 10.21608/mid.2023.253557.1701

Ezeanya-Bakpa, C. C., Inobeme, A., & Adekoya, M. A. (2022). Hospital laundries and their effect on medical textiles. In: Medical Textiles from Natural Resources, Elsevier, United Kingdom, Pp, 767-792. DOI: DOI: 10.1016/B978-0-323-90479-7.00004-X

Fix, J. H. (2013). Fixing a broken drug development process. *Journal of Commercial Biotechnology*, *19*, 5–8.

Gozubuyuk, G. S., Aktas, E., & Yigit, N. (2014). An ancient plant Lawsonia inermis (henna): Determination of in vitro antifungal activity against dermatophytes species. *Journal de Mycologie Médicale*, *24*(4), 313–318. DOI: 10.1016/j.mycmed.2014.07.002 PMID: 25442917

Grant, W. F. (1994). The present status of higher plant bioassays for the detection of environmental mutagens. *Mutation Research*, *310*(2), 175–185. DOI: 10.1016/0027-5107(94)90112-0 PMID: 7523890

Grigalunas, M., Brakmann, S., & Waldmann, H. (2022). Chemical evolution of natural product structure. *Journal of the American Chemical Society*, *144*(8), 3314–3329. DOI: 10.1021/jacs.1c11270 PMID: 35188375

Gupta, S. C., Patchva, S., Koh, W., & Aggarwal, B. B. (2012). Discovery of curcumin, a component of the golden spice, and its miraculous biological activities. *Clinical and Experimental Pharmacology & Physiology*, *39*(3), 283–299. DOI: 10.1111/j.1440-1681.2011.05648.x PMID: 22118895

Harrison, C. (2014). Patenting natural products just got harder. *Nature Biotechnology*, *32*(5), 403–404. DOI: 10.1038/nbt0514-403a PMID: 24811496

Harvey, A. L., Edrada-Ebel, R., & Quinn, R. J. (2015). The re-emergence of natural products for drug discovery in the genomics era. *Nature Reviews. Drug Discovery*, *14*(2), 111–129. DOI: 10.1038/nrd4510 PMID: 25614221

Hawkins, J., Baker, C., Cherry, L., & Dunne, E. (2019). Black elderberry (Sambucus nigra) supplementation effectively treats upper respiratory symptoms: A meta-analysis of randomized, controlled clinical trials. *Complementary Therapies in Medicine, 42*, 361–365. DOI: 10.1016/j.ctim.2018.12.004 PMID: 30670267

Heinrich, M. (2010). Galanthamine from *Galanthus* and other Amaryllidaceae—Chemistry and biology based on traditional use. *The Alkaloids. Chemistry and Biology, 68*, 157–165. DOI: 10.1016/S1099-4831(10)06804-5 PMID: 20334038

Heinrich, M., Scotti, F., Andrade-Cetto, A., Berger-Gonzalez, M., Echeverría, J., Friso, F., Garcia-Cardona, F., Hesketh, A., Hitziger, M., Maake, C., Politi, M., Spadafora, C., & Spadafora, R. (2020). Access and benefit sharing under the Nagoya Protocol—Quo Vadis? Six Latin American case studies assessing opportunities and risk. *Frontiers in Pharmacology, 11*, 765. DOI: 10.3389/fphar.2020.00765 PMID: 32581783

Hotwani, K., Baliga, S., & Sharma, K. (2014). Phytodentistry: Use of medicinal plants. *Journal of Complementary & Integrative Medicine, 11*(2), 233–251. DOI: 10.1515/jcim-2013-0015 PMID: 25153610

Hu, W., Yu, A., Wang, S., Bai, Q., Tang, H., Yang, B., Wang, M., & Kuang, H. (2023). Extraction, purification, structural characteristics, biological activities, and applications of the polysaccharides from Zingiber officinale Roscoe (Ginger): A review. *Molecules (Basel, Switzerland), 28*(11), 4477. DOI: 10.3390/molecules28093855 PMID: 37175266

Huang, Y., Wang, S., Cai, Q., & Jin, H. (2021). Effective methods for isolation and purification of extracellular vesicles from plants. *Journal of Integrative Plant Biology, 63*(9), 2020–2030. DOI: 10.1111/jipb.13181 PMID: 34668639

Karunamoorthi, K., Jegajeevanram, K., Vijayalakshmi, J., & Mengistie, E. (2013). Traditional medicinal plants: A source of phytotherapeutic modality in resource-constrained health care settings. *Journal of Evidence-Based Complementary & Alternative Medicine, 18*(1), 67–74. DOI: 10.1177/2156587212460241

Kim, H. W., Wang, M., Leber, C. A., Nothias, L. F., Reher, R., Kang, K. B., van der Hooft, J. J. J., Dorrestein, P. C., Gerwick, W. H., & Cottrell, G. W. (2021). NP Classifier: A deep neural network-based structural classification tool for natural products. *Journal of Natural Products, 84*(11), 2795–2807. DOI: 10.1021/acs.jnatprod.1c00399 PMID: 34662515

Klemow, K. M., Bartlow, A., Crawford, J., Kocher, N., Shah, J., & Ritsick, M. (2011). Medical attributes of St. John's Wort (*Hypericum perforatum*). In *Herbal Medicine* (2nd ed.). Biomolecular and Clinical Aspects. DOI: 10.1201/b10787-12

Laajala, T. D., Jumppanen, M., Huhtaniemi, R., Väisanen, M. R., Yetukuri, L., Suni, V., & Aittokallio, T. (2016). Optimized design and analysis of preclinical intervention studies in vivo. *Scientific Reports*, *6*(1), 30723. DOI: 10.1038/srep30723 PMID: 27480578

Lahlou, M. (2013). The success of natural products in drug discovery. *Pharmacology & Pharmacy*, *4*(3, 3A), 17–31. DOI: 10.4236/pp.2013.43A003

Larayetan, R., Ololade, Z. S., Ogunmola, O. O., & Ladokun, A. (2019). Phytochemical Constituents, Antioxidant, Cytotoxicity, Antimicrobial, Antitrypanosomal, and Antimalarial Potentials of the Crude Extracts of *Callistemon citrinus*. *Evidence-Based Complementary and Alternative Medicine : eCAM*, *2019*, 1–14. Advance online publication. DOI: 10.1155/2019/5410923 PMID: 31558912

Lautie, E., Russo, O., Ducrot, P., & Boutin, J. A. (2020). Unraveling plant natural chemical diversity for drug discovery purposes. *Frontiers in Pharmacology*, *11*, 397. DOI: 10.3389/fphar.2020.00397 PMID: 32317969

Liu, Q., Lawrence, A. J., & Liang, J. H. (2011). Traditional Chinese medicine for treatment of

Liu, Q., Lawrence, A. J., & Liang, J.-H. (2011, January). alcoholism: From ancient to modern. *The American Journal of Chinese Medicine*, *39*(1), 1–13. DOI: 10.1142/S0192415X11008609 PMID: 21213394

Machado, B. A. S., Pereira, C. G., Nunes, S. B., Padilha, F. F., & Umsza-Guez, M. A. (2013). Supercritical fluid extraction using CO_2: Main applications and future perspectives. *Separation Science and Technology*, *48*(17), 2741–2760. DOI: 10.1080/01496395.2013.811422

Mannangatti, P., & Naidu, K. N. (2016). Indian herbs for the treatment of neurodegenerative disease. *Advances in Neurobiology*, *12*, 323–336. DOI: 10.1007/978-3-319-28383-8_17 PMID: 27651261

Marchev, A. S., Vasileva, L. V., Amirova, K. M., Savova, M. S., Balcheva-Sivenova, Z. P., & Georgiev, M. I. (2021). Metabolomics and health: From nutritional crops and plant-based pharmaceuticals to profiling of human biofluids. *Cellular and Molecular Life Sciences : CMLS*, *78*(15), 6487–6503. DOI: 10.1007/s00018-021-03918-3 PMID: 34410445

McCarthy, M. W. (2019). Teixobactin: A novel anti-infective agent. *Expert Review of Anti-Infective Therapy*, *17*(1), 1–3. DOI: 10.1080/14787210.2019.1550357 PMID: 30449226

Mohanraj, K., Karthikeyan, B. S., Vivek-Ananth, R. P., Chand, R. B., Aparna, S. R., Mangalapandi, P., & Samal, A. (2018). IMPPAT: A curated database of Indian Medicinal P lants, Phytochemistry And Therapeutics. *Scientific Reports*, *8*(1), 4329.

Moon, K. B., Park, J. S., Park, Y. I., Song, I. J., Lee, H. J., Cho, H. S., Jeon, J. H., & Kim, H. S. (2019). Development of systems for the production of plant-derived biopharmaceuticals. *Plants*, *9*(1), 30. DOI: 10.3390/plants9010030 PMID: 31878277

Nayak, C., Oberai, P., Varanasi, R., Baig, H. Ch. R., & Reddy, G. R. (2013). A prospective multi-centric open clinical trial of homeopathy in diabetic distal symmetric polyneuropathy. *Homeopathy*, *102*(2), 130–138. DOI: 10.1016/j.homp.2013.02.004 PMID: 23622263

Newman, D. J., & Cragg, G. M. (2016). Natural Products as Sources of New Drugs over the 30 Years from 1981 to 2010. *Journal of Natural Products*, *79*(3), 629–661. DOI: 10.1021/acs.jnatprod.5b01055 PMID: 26852623

Newman, D. J., & Cragg, G. M. (2020). Natural products as sources of new drugs over the nearly four decades from 01/1981 to 09/2019. *Journal of Natural Products*, *83*(3), 770–803. DOI: 10.1021/acs.jnatprod.9b01285 PMID: 32162523

Ng, X., Venkatanarayanan, N., & Ho, C. Y. (2017). Clinical use of Hypericum perforatum (St John's wort) in depression: A meta-analysis. *Journal of Affective Disorders*, *210*, 211–221. DOI: 10.1016/j.jad.2016.12.048 PMID: 28064110

Ottinger, M. A., & Geiselman, C. (2023). *One Health meets the exposome: Human, wildlife, and ecosystem health*. Elsevier.

Rasoulian, B., & Kheirandish, F. (2017). Herbal medicines: From traditional medicine to modern experimental approaches. *Herbal Medicine Journal*, *2*, 1–2.

Riss, T., Niles, A., Moravec, R., Karassina, N., & Vidugiriene, J. (2019). *Cytotoxicity assays: In-vitro methods to measure dead cells*. Eli Lilly & Company and the National Center for Advancing Translational Sciences.

Saini, A., Kumar, R., & Devi, R. (2025). Natural products in modern drug discovery: Challenges, advances, and emerging opportunities. *International Journal of Pharma Sciences*, *3*(1), 1187–1199. DOI: 10.5281/zenodo.14652293

Shegokar, R. (2020). Preclinical testing—understanding the basics first. In Drug Delivery Aspects (pp. 19–32).

Singh, H., & Bharadvaja, N. (2021). Treasuring the computational approach in medicinal plant research. *Progress in Biophysics and Molecular Biology*, *164*, 19–32. DOI: 10.1016/j.pbiomolbio.2021.05.004 PMID: 34004233

Singla, R. K., De, R., Efferth, T., Mezzetti, B., Uddin, M. S., & Ntie-Kang, F. (2023). The international natural product sciences Taskforce (INPST) and the power of Twitter networking exemplified through #INPST hashtag analysis. *Phytomedicine, 108*, 154520. DOI: 10.1016/j.phymed.2022.154520 PMID: 36334386

Sircar, N. N. (1982). Medicinal plants. *The Eastern Pharmacist, 29*(291), 49–52.

Sofowora, A., Ogunbodede, E., & Onayade, A. (2013). The role and place of medicinal plants in the strategies for disease prevention. *African Journal of Traditional, Complementary, and Alternative Medicines : AJTCAM, 10*(3), 210–229. DOI: 10.4314/ajtcam.v10i5.2 PMID: 24311829

Sorkin, B. C., Kuszak, A. J., Bloss, G., Fukagawa, N. K., Hoffman, F. A., Jafari, M., Barrett, B., Brown, P. N., Bushman, F. D., Casper, S. J., Chilton, F. H., Coffey, C. S., Ferruzzi, M. G., Hopp, D. C., Kiely, M., Lakens, D., MacMillan, J. B., Meltzer, D. O., Pahor, M., & Pauli, G. F. (2020). Improving natural product research translation: From source to clinical trial. [FASEB]. *The FASEB Journal, 34*(1), 41–65. DOI: 10.1096/fj.201902143R PMID: 31914647

Tansaz, M., & Tajadini, H. (2016). Comparison of leiomyoma of modern medicine and traditional Persian medicine. *Journal of Evidence-Based Complementary & Alternative Medicine, 21*(2), 160–163. DOI: 10.1177/2156587215595299 PMID: 26177818

Thomford, N. E., Awortwe, C., Dzobo, K., Adu, F., Chopera, D., Wonkam, A., & Dandara, C. (2016a). Inhibition of CYP2B6 by medicinal plant extracts: Implication for use of efavirenz and nevirapine-based highly active anti-retroviral therapy (HAART) in resource-limited settings. *Molecules (Basel, Switzerland), 21*(2), 211. DOI: 10.3390/molecules21020211 PMID: 26891286

Thomford, N. E., Dzobo, K., Chopera, D., Wonkam, A., Skelton, M., Blackhurst, D., & Dandara, C. (2016b). In vitro reversible and time-dependent CYP450 inhibition profiles of medicinal herbal plant extracts Newbouldia laevis and Cassia abbreviata: Implications for herb-drug interactions. *Molecules (Basel, Switzerland), 21*(7), 891. DOI: 10.3390/molecules21070891 PMID: 27399660

Thomford, N. E., Dzobo, K., Chopera, D., Wonkam, A., Skelton, M., Blackhurst, D., & Dandara, C. (2016c). Pharmacogenomics implications of using herbal medicinal plants on African populations in health transition. *Pharmaceuticals (Basel, Switzerland), 8*(3), 637–663. DOI: 10.3390/ph8030637 PMID: 26402689

Tzvetkov, N. T., Kirilov, K., Matin, M., & Atanasov, A. G. (2024). Natural product drug discovery and drug design: Two approaches shaping new pharmaceutical development. *Nephrology, Dialysis, Transplantation*, *39*(3), 375–378. DOI: 10.1093/ndt/gfad208 PMID: 37708048

Upadhyay, S. K., & Singh, S. P. (2023). *Plants as bioreactors for industrial molecules*. John Wiley & Sons. DOI: 10.1002/9781119875116

U.S. Food and Drug Administration. (n.d.). *How drugs are developed and approved.* Retrieved September 23, 2025, from https://www.fda.gov/drugs/development-approval-process-drugs/how-drugs-are-developed-and-approved

Uzor, P. F., Prasasty, V. D., & Agubata, C. O. (2020). *Natural Products as Sources of Antimalarial Drugs*. Evidence-Based Complement Alternative Medicine., DOI: 10.1155/2020/9385125

Wondafrash, D. Z., Bhoumik, D., Altaye, B. M., Tareke, H. B., & Assefa, B. T. (2019). *Antimalarial Activity of Cordia africana (Lam.) (Boraginaceae) Leaf Extracts and Solvent Fractions in Plasmodium berghei-Infected Mice*. Evidence-Based Complement Alternative Medicine., DOI: 10.1155/2019/8324596

Woodruff, H. B. (1980). Natural products from microorganisms. *Science*, *208*(4449), 1225–1229. DOI: 10.1126/science.7375932 PMID: 7375932

Wu, P., & Lu, J. M. (2019). Stability of Natural Products: Theory and Practice. *Journal of Natural Products*, *82*(2), 267–276.

Xia, X. (2017). Bioinformatics and drug discovery. *Current Topics in Medicinal Chemistry*, *17*(15), 1709–1726. DOI: 10.2174/1568026617666161116143440 PMID: 27848897

Xiao, Z., Morris-Natschke, S. L., & Lee, K. H. (2016). Strategies for the Optimization of Natural Leads to Anticancer Drugs or Drug Candidates. *Medicinal Research Reviews*, *36*(1), 32–91. DOI: 10.1002/med.21377 PMID: 26359649

Xu, Q., Bauer, R., Hendry, B. M., Fan, T. P., Zhao, Z., Duez, P., & Robinson, N. (2013). The quest for modernisation of traditional Chinese medicine. *BMC Complementary and Alternative Medicine*, *13*(1), 132. DOI: 10.1186/1472-6882-13-132 PMID: 23763836

Yatoo, M. I., Dimri, U., Gopalakrishnan, A., Karthik, K., Gopi, M., Khandia, R., & Saxena, A. (2017). Beneficial health applications and medicinal values of Pedicularis plants: A review. *Biomedicine and Pharmacotherapy*, *95*, 1301–1313. DOI: 10.1016/j.biopha.2017.09.041 PMID: 28938521

Yuan, H., Ma, Q., Ye, L., & Piao, G. (2016). The traditional medicine and modern medicine from natural products. *Molecules (Basel, Switzerland), 21*(5), 559. DOI: 10.3390/molecules21050559 PMID: 27136524

Zhao, L., Zhu, Y., Jia, H., Han, Y., Zheng, X., Wang, M., & Feng, W. (2022). From plant to yeast—Advances in biosynthesis of artemisinin. *Molecules (Basel, Switzerland), 27*(20), 6888. DOI: 10.3390/molecules27206888 PMID: 36296479

Zhu, Y., Ouyang, Z., Du, H., Wang, M., Wang, J., Sun, H., Kong, L., Xu, Q., Ma, H., & Sun, Y. (2022). New opportunities and challenges of natural products research: When target identification meets single-cell multiomics. *Acta Pharmaceutica Sinica. B, 12*(11), 4011–4039. DOI: 10.1016/j.apsb.2022.08.022 PMID: 36386472

Chapter 6
Indigenous Knowledge and Antimalarial Enema Therapies:
An Ethnobotanical Survey from Cross River State, Nigeria

Peggy Obaseojei Willie
https://orcid.org/0000-0002-2053-7505
University of Calabar, Nigeria

Effiom Eyo Ita
https://orcid.org/0000-0002-5210-6822
University of Calabar, Nigeria

Mary-Ibenreh Ogaboh Agba
https://orcid.org/0000-0001-8461-4365
University of Calabar, Nigeria

Julius Oyohosuho Phillip
https://orcid.org/0000-0002-0418-9803
University of Calabar, Nigeria

Ibiang Bassey Young
https://orcid.org/0000-0002-4425-5844
University of Calabar, Nigeria

ABSTRACT

This chapter documents the traditional use of antimalarial enemas among the Efik and Qua ethnic groups of Calabar, Cross River State, Nigeria. An ethnobotanical

DOI: 10.4018/979-8-3373-5821-5.ch006

survey was conducted using structured interviews and questionnaires administered to herbal practitioners, elders, and caregivers. Twenty-five medicinal plant species from nineteen families were identified, twelve of which were specifically used in enema preparations for malaria treatment. Frequently cited species included Aspilia africana, Chromolaena odorata, Stachytarpheta cayennensis, Andrographis paniculata, Eremomastax speciosa, and Azadirachta indica. Phytochemical analyses from previous studies revealed that these plants possess alkaloids, flavonoids, tannins, and terpenoids with proven antiplasmodial, anti-inflammatory, and antioxidant activities. The findings underscore the ethnopharmacological relevance of local medicinal knowledge and highlight its potential contribution to natural antimalarial drug discovery and development in the global South.

1. INTRODUCTION

Man dominates his physical environment. In doing so, he faces the challenges of nature, including the sustainable production of food, fuel, fiber, and medicine. The exploration and use of natural resources are among humanity's most outstanding achievements. One major challenge man has had to overcome is illness. Managing common colds, cuts, abdominal pains, fever, and other health problems, including the effects of mosquito bites, has tested man's intelligence. Malaria remains a significant public health concern in Nigeria and across sub-Saharan Africa, contributing significantly to illness and death, particularly among children and pregnant women (Kolawole et al., 2023). According to the World Malaria Report, Nigeria bears the most significant malaria burden, accounting for 27% of the world's estimated cases and 31% of the estimated deaths (WHO, 2023). Alongside modern medical approaches, indigenous medical systems play a key role in primary healthcare, especially in rural and peri-urban communities, because of their affordability, availability, and accessibility. The World Health Organization estimates that up to 80% of the African population relies on traditional medicine for their primary healthcare needs, recognizing traditional medicine as a valuable body of knowledge, skills, and practices rooted in cultural beliefs and local experience that contribute to health maintenance and disease treatment (WHO, 2019; WHO, 2022). Local knowledge of medicinal plants has developed and is intertwined with the history of migration over the years. Although most cultures lack formal documentation of traditional ecological knowledge (TEK) of medicinal plants, this knowledge has been passed down informally through generations. This transfer occurs when community healers train willing individuals to assist in curing community members. In this process, knowledge of medicinal plants is handed down to the younger generation.

Cross River State is located in the southern part of Nigeria. Its geographic location, which includes the largest standing rainforest in Nigeria, ensures its continued abundance of mosquitoes, which cause malaria. In 2021, the state Ministry of Health reported approximately 1,283,000 malaria cases, representing 1.9% of Nigeria's total of 68 million cases (Ugwuibe et al., 2021; WHO, 2022). The rich biodiversity of medicinal plants, combined with limited access to conventional medications, has sustained the use of plant-based remedies. Although these conventional medications may be available in some communities, herbal medicines have nevertheless maintained popularity for historical and cultural reasons, as well as for their lower cost. The use of herbal remedies has increased worldwide in recent years, and the search for new phytochemicals with the potential of being developed as useful drugs for the treatment of malaria and other infectious diseases (Wilcox, 1999). In Nigeria, the medicinal plants used to treat malaria are administered as decoctions or teas, sometimes as ingredients in malaria 'steam therapy', where patients are covered with a thick blanket and made to inhale the vapour from the cooking pot (Adebayo and Krettli, 2011). One traditional method of administration used in the area is the enema, which is employed for various medical conditions, including 'internal heat,' febrile illnesses, and gastrointestinal issues. The use of enemas forms an integral part of the Efik and the Qua traditional medicine. Enema treatments usually involve decoctions or infusions made from leaves, roots, or barks that are administered rectally. Ethnographic and pharmacological research indicate that rectal delivery can offer benefits, including rapid absorption and avoidance of oral bitterness (van Andel et al., 2015). This chapter aims to document traditional practices of antimalarial enemas in Calabar, Cross River State, emphasizing local knowledge, the plant species used, and their potential contributions to global health efforts. Our research questions were:

i. Do you know any plant used as an enema?
ii. Mention their names and the ailments they cure?
iii. How are they prepared for use?

2. CONTEXTUAL BACKGROUND

Africa is renowned for its rich flora and botanical diversity, with diverse ecosystems ranging from rainforests and savannas to deserts and mountains. This biodiversity is reflected in the vast array of medicinal plants utilized by traditional healers and community members across the continent. These plants hold profound cultural significance in African societies, serving not only as sources of healing but also as symbols of spirituality, ancestry, and identity (Lalita Nargawe et al., 2023).

African traditional medicine is the indigenous medicine of Africa, based on traditional indigenous knowledge systems (traditional medicinal knowledge) and passed down by word of mouth, from generation to generation within the particular indigenous community, either along familial lines or through apprenticeships (Sifuna, 2022). It is the total of knowledge, skills, and practices based on the theories, beliefs, and experiences indigenous to different cultures that are used to maintain health, as well as to prevent, diagnose, improve, or treat physical and mental illnesses (WHO, 2008)

Ethnobotany explores how societies utilize and manage plant resources for food, medicine, and culture. Early ethnobotanical studies in Africa established systematic documentation of plant-based traditions (Harshberger, 1896; Schultes, 1960). In Nigeria, surveys such as those by Odugbemi et al. (2017) and Akwaji et al. (2017), and reviews by Erinoso & Aworinde (2018) and Adebayo and Krettli (2011) have shown the continued reliance on medicinal flora for primary healthcare. The historical role of enemas in African healing systems is well-documented. The insertion of herbal extracts through the rectum has been reported among different ethnic groups (van Andel et al., 2015; Dunn et al., 1991). Enema administration is culturally viewed as a purgative, detoxifying, and spiritually cleansing practice (De Smet, 1983). Among the Efik people of Cross River State, enemas remain a respected therapeutic route, often used for malaria, fever, abdominal pain, and menstrual regulation. Cross River State's diverse ecosystems, ranging from tropical rainforests to mangroves, support a high diversity of plant species, many of which are exploited for medicinal use (Benjamin et al., 2021). This ecological and cultural richness forms the basis for a vibrant tradition of ethnomedicine in the region.

3. METHODOLOGY

3.1 Study Area

The research was conducted between September and October 2023 in the Calabar South and Calabar Municipal Local Government Areas of Cross River State, Nigeria. The study area lies approximately between latitude 4.58°N and longitude 8.42°E and is primarily inhabited by the Efik and Qua ethnic groups. Calabar South field sites included Crutech Farm (Ekpo Abasi Street), Creek Town Street, Mbukpa Road, and Mount Zion Road. Calabar municipality field sites included Atekong, Old Ikang, Asim Ikang, Ita Okang, Asuquo Oqua, and Big Qua.

3.2. Study Design

An ethnobotanical survey design was employed. Structured questionnaires and semi-structured interviews were used to elicit information from purposively selected respondents comprising herbal practitioners, elders, household caregivers, and traditional medicine vendors. Interviews were conducted in English, Efik, and Nigerian Pidgin to ensure clarity and cultural sensitivity.

3.3. Data Collection, Identification, and Analysis

Plant specimens were collected with the assistance of informants, labeled by their local Efik names, and later identified at the Department of Plant and Ecological Studies, University of Calabar, Nigeria. Scientific authentication was supported by published floras and regional weed handbooks (Akobundu et al., 2016). A permission letter was obtained from the Cross River State Ministry of Health. Verbal informed consent was obtained from the participants after the purpose and methods of the study had been explained. Since the participants were only asked to describe traditional medicine practices that they were familiar with and mentioned the species used in enema therapies, verbal informed consent was used. Frequency distributions were estimated for the most cited plant family, medicinal plants used in enema therapy, and those cited for malaria enema therapy.

4. FINDINGS

Out of 133 individuals approached, 100 consented to participate, while 33 declined, citing disinterest or lack of knowledge. Respondents included herbal practitioners (6), farmers (27), household caregivers (61), and herbal medicine sellers (6). A total of 26 medicinal plant species were identified as being used in enema preparations. These plants belong to 19 families, such as Asteraceae, Portulacaceae, Verbenaceae, Lamiaceae, Amaranthaceae, Asparagaceae, Rutaceae, Rubiaceae, Stemonuraceae, Fabaceae, Acanthaceae, Meliaceae, Phyllantaceae, Caricaceae, Musaceae, Anacardiaceae, Euphobiaceae, Commelinaceae, and Celastraceae. Asteraceae (also known as the Compositae family) and Acanthaceae were the most dominant plant families (15.4% respectively), followed by Lamiaceae (Figure 1).

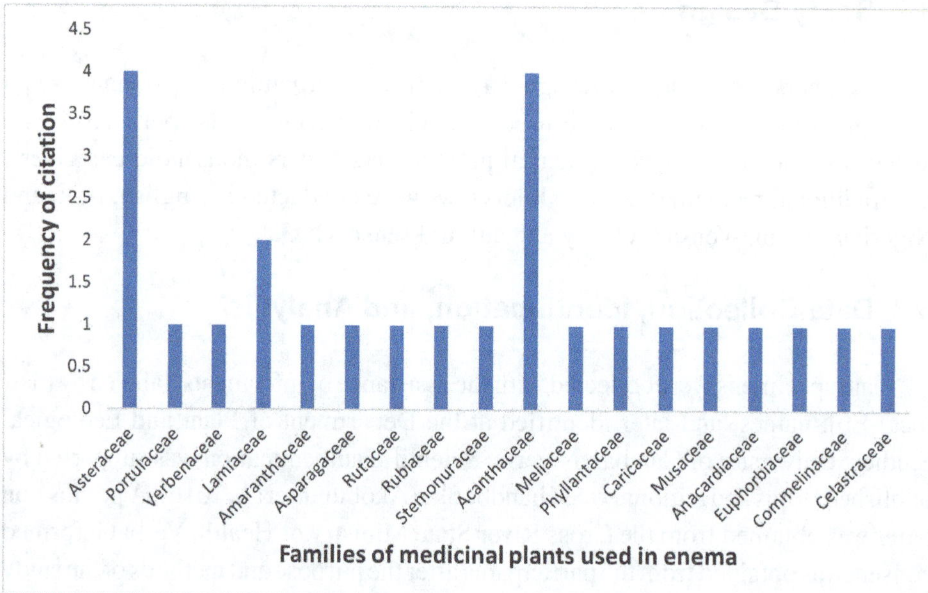

Common ailments treated include malaria, typhoid, fever, constipation, heat, bellyache, and menstrual pain. Preparation methods involved pounding fresh leaves, soaking in cold or warm water, filtering, and rectal administration (Table 1). Some of the plants are reportedly used singly, while some are used in combination with other medicinal plants. Frequently cited species used in enema therapies included Vernonia amygdalina (94%), Talinum triangulare (76%), Carica papaya (94%), Ocimum gratissimum (74%), Lasianthera africana (66%), and Hypoestes rosea (55%) (Figure 2).

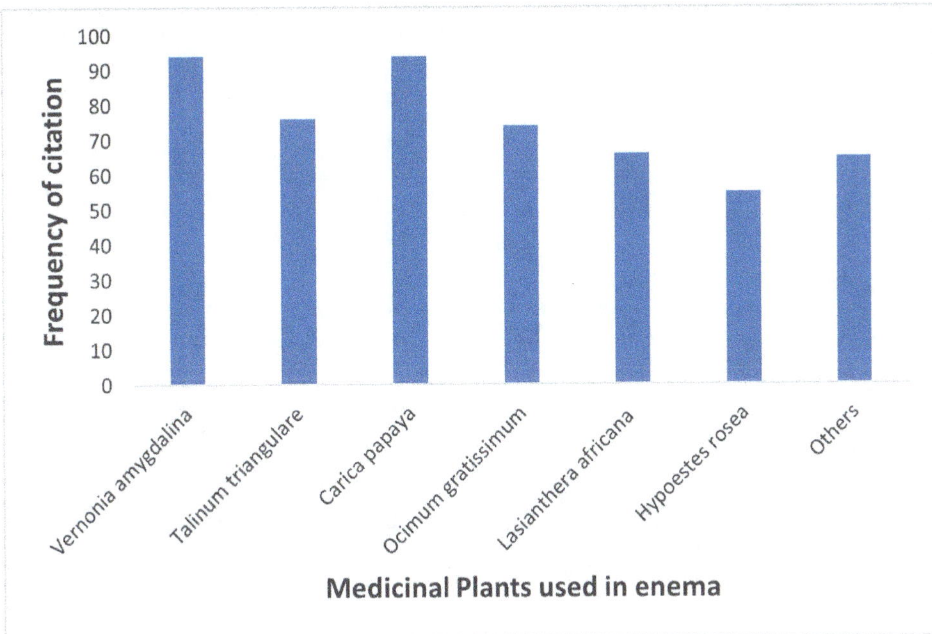

Twelve (12) plants were identified as being used in enemas to treat malaria, and they included Aspilia africana, Chromolaena odorata, Stachytarpheta cayennensis, Androphagis paniculata, Eremomastax speciosa, Hypoestes rosea, Carica papaya, Musa paradisiaca, Mangifera indica, Jatropha tajorensis, Hippocratea africana, and Azadirachta indica (Table 2). Carica papaya (94%) and Hypoestes rosea (55%) were the most cited species used in malaria enema therapies (Figure 3).

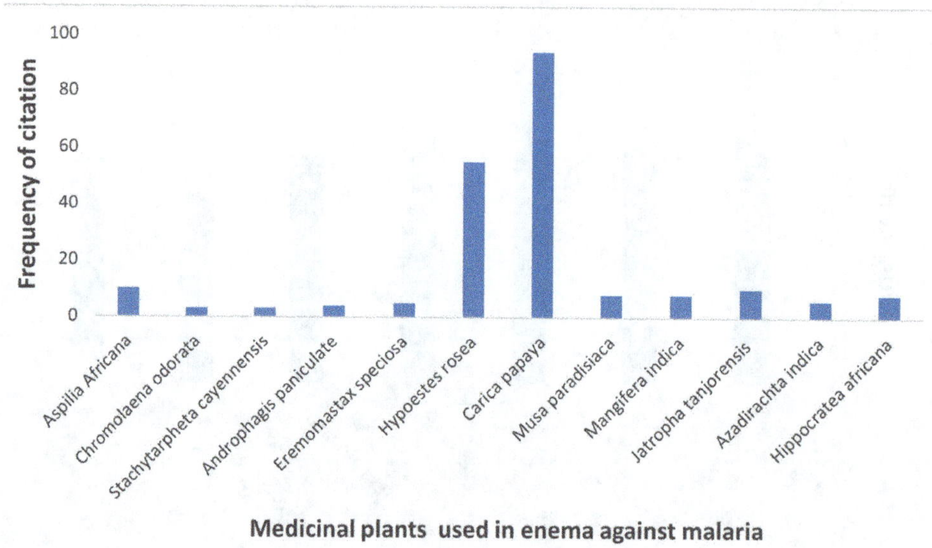

5. ETHNOBOTANICAL AND PHARMACOLOGICAL INSIGHTS

Enema, known in Efik as "ukebe," is a medical practice rooted in the culture and tradition of the Efik people of Cross River State, Nigeria. Knowledge of the use of herbal plants for healing was acquired by traditional healers, native doctors, and spiritualists. For these reasons, enemas, which are a tool used in healing, were considered a ritualistic or spiritual practice based on the belief that they cleanse the body of bad "blood" or heat called "ufiop".

Ethnobotanical knowledge of plants is rooted in tradition and expressed through cultural symbolism (Narzary & Boro, 2025). Others include efficacy and availability. Traditional healers experimented with plants, and their observations were orally transmitted to their protégés, which helped the Efiks develop a rich, unwritten pharmacopeia.

There is growing pharmacological evidence that what the locals perceive as spiritual is no mystery. In fact, the spiritual connotation ascribed to the use in healing is attributed to the phytochemical composition of plants. This is why traditional knowledge of herbal plants used in enema formulations aligns with pharmacological evidence, as shown in various studies. While enemas are usually prepared by a manual extraction process involving cutting, pounding, and soaking in water and absolute alcohol to extract the active ingredients, modern pharmacological methods have improved solvent extraction systems that extract, purify, and obtain the active ingredients, and studies have revealed the optimum dosing for administration.

Table 1. Medicinal plants identified for use in enema preparations in Calabar, reasons for use, and methods of preparation

S/N	Family	Species identified	Local/common name	Ailments indicated	Methods of preparation/ parts used
1	Asteraceae	Aspilia Africana	Edemerong	Malaria and fever	Fresh leaves are cut, ground or pounded, soaked in warm water for a while, and then filtered for use.
		Chromolaena odorata	Mbiet Awolowo	Malaria	Same as in Aspilia Africana
		Vernonia amygdalina	Etidot/bitter leaf	Heat	Fresh leaves are cut, pounded, and filtered with at least 2 cups of cold water, then ready for use.
		Emilia sonchifolia	Awak mmong	Heat and fever	Cut fresh leaves, mix with leaves of Solenostemon monostachyus (ntod ikwot), pound them, add cold water, filter, and use.
2	Portulaceae	Talinum triangulare	Mmong ikong/ waterleaf	Heat in children	Same as in Aspilia Africana
3	Verbenaceae	Stachytarpheta cayennensis	Adan umon	Malaria	Same as in Aspilia Africana
4	Lamiaceae	Ocimum gratissimum	Ntong/ scent leaf	Heat, bowel cleansing	Cut fresh leaves, mix with Oduk mbiet (Achyranthes aspera) leaves, add cold water, filter, and use.
		Solenostemon monostachyus	Ntod ikwot	Heat, menstrual cramps	Cut fresh leaves, pound, add cold water, native egg, and use.
5	Amaranthaceae	Achyranthes aspera	Oduk mbiet	Heat, constipation	Cut and pound fresh leaves with ndom (white chalk), add cold water, filter, and use.
6	Asparagaceae	Dracaena arborea	Okono	Abortion	Same as in Aspilia Africana
7	Rutaceae	Clausena anisate	Mbiet Ekpene	Heat in children	Same as in Aspilia Africana
8	Rubiaceae	Hensia crinata	Atama	Measles in children	Cut and pound fresh leaves, add warm water, filter, add palm kernel oil, and use.
9	Stemonuraceae	Lasianthera africana	Editan	Heat	Same as in Aspilia Africana
10	Fabaceae	Mucuna urens	Ikong Ibaba	Jedi-Jedi in children	Same as in Aspilia Africana

continued on following page

Table 1. Continued

S/N	Family	Species identified	Local/common name	Ailments indicated	Methods of preparation/ parts used
11	Acanthaceae	Eremomastax polysperma	Edem ididuot	Heat	Same as in Aspilia Africana
		Eremomastax speciosa	Nkong-ikong, Ikpo nkong	Malaria and fever	Same as in Aspilia Africana
		Hypoestes rosea	Iyip	Malaria	Cut and pound fresh leaves, mixed with leaves of Solenostemon monostachyus and Emilia sonchifolia, add cold water, filter, and use.
		Andrographis paniculate	Fineka / Vinegar	Malaria, bellyache	Same as in Aspilia Africana
12	Meliaceae	Azadirachta indica	Dogonyaro/neem	Malaria and fever	Same as in Aspilia Africana
13	Phyllantaceae	Phyllanthus amarus	Oyomo k'iso aman k'edem	Heat in children and pregnant women	Cut and pound fresh leaves, add cold water and white chalk, allow to stand for 2 days, filter, and use.
14	Caricaceae	Carica papaya	Mmɔ/Paw-paw	Typhoid and malaria	Cut and pound fresh, green leaves, add cold water, filter, and use for typhoid. For malaria, Cut and pound ripe leaves, add cold water, filter, and use the extract.
15	Musaceae	Musa paradisiaca	Ukɔm/Plantain leaves	Malaria	Cut and pound the ripe, dried leaves, add warm water, filter, and use
16	Anacardiaceae	Mangifera indica	Mango leaf	Malaria	Cut and pound fresh leaves, add cold water, filter, and use.
17	Euphorbiaceae	Jatropha tajorensis	Hospital too far	Malaria improves anemia	Same as in Mangifera indica
18	Commelinaceae	Comelina benghalensis	Wandering Jew	Heat	Cut and pound fresh leaves, mixed with leaves of Solenostemon monostachyus and Emilia sonchifolia, add cold water, filter, and use.
19	Celastraceae	Hippocratea Africana	African paddle-pod	Malaria, fever, and pain	Cut and pound the bark, mix it with fresh leaves of Eremomastax speciosa, add water, filter, and use.

Table 2. Medicinal plants used in enema preparations for the treatment of malaria.

S/N	Plants Identified	Bioactive components and their importance
1	Aspilia Africana	Tannins, phenols, flavonoids, alkaloids, phlobatannins, flavonols, glycosides, anthraquinones, steroids, terpenoids, accounting for its anti-inflammatory, antimicrobial, blood vessel formation, skin regeneration, tissue regeneration, and antioxidant effects (Gerheart et al., 2024; Carvalho et al., 2021; Ibrahim et al., 2018; Vitale et al., 2022)
2	Chromolaena odorata	flavonoids, alkaloids, steroids, tannins, terpenoids, glycosides, and saponins (Nworgu et al., 2022). Reported to have antiplasmodial, antioxidant, antibacterial, wound healing, and haemostatic activities (Elebiyo et al., 2023; Tiamiyu and Okunlade, 2020)
3	Stachytarpheta cayennensis	Alkaloids, tannins, saponins, glycosides, steroids, and phenols (Iwu et al., 2018). Reported to have antimicrobial, anti-plasmodial, and anti-inflammatory effects (Okokon et al., 2008; Adediran et al., 2025)
4	Andrographis paniculate	Diterpenoids, particularly andrographolide, flavonoids and polyphenols, neoandrographolide, and 14-deoxy-11,12-didehydroandrographolide. These compounds contribute to the plant's anti-inflammatory, immunostimulatory, antioxidant, and antibacterial properties (Bhatnagar, 2023; Jayakumar et al., 2013; Chao and Lin, 2010).
5	Eremomastax speciosa	Alkaloids, flavonoids, saponins, tannins, and terpenoids. Its essential oil is rich in volatile compounds like 14β-pregnane, thymol, and fatty acid esters, which are responsible for its antimicrobial, anti-inflammatory, antidiarrheal, antispasmodic, and antioxidant properties (Ibok et al., 2023; Amang et al., 2017)
6	Hypoestes rosea	Alkaloids, flavonoids, saponins, tannins, terpenoids, steroids, and reducing sugars contribute to the plant's anti-inflammatory, antibacterial, and anti-malarial properties (Mensah et al., 2008; Emeribe et al., 2021)
7	Carica papaya	Alkaloids, carotenoids, Flavonoids, and phenolic compounds, which are valuable antioxidants, anti-inflammatory, anticancer properties, and digestive health (Kong et al., 2021; Ugbogu et al., 2023).
8	Musa paradisiaca	Antidiarrheal, anti-dysentery, antihelminthic, anti-ulcerative, antimicrobial, antihyperglycemic, anti-hypertensive, diuretic, anti urolithiatic, wound healing, anti malarial, and anti-snake venom activities (Aziz et al., 2020; Imam & Akter, 2011; Laeliocattleya et al., 2018)
9	Mangifera indica	Contains mangiferin, flavonoids, phenolic acids, and tannins, which have a variety of anti-plasmodial activities and can treat malaria (Yadav, Kumari, and Kumar, 2024).
10	Jatropha tanjorensis	Saponins, flavonoids, alkaloids, tannins, cardiac glycosides, and phenols, which offer various health benefits, including antioxidant, antimicrobial, and anti-inflammatory properties. These compounds can help fight infections and protect against chronic diseases (Okokon et al., 2006; Ndem et al., 2020).
11	Azadirachta indica	limonoids (like azadirachtin), flavonoids (such as quercetin), alkaloids (like nimbin), and phenolic compounds. The limonoids show antimalarial activity (Sandhir, Khurana & Singhal, 2021).
12	Hippocratea Africana	Anti-inflammatory, analgesic, antimalarial, cardioprotective, antioxidant, and antidiabetic properties. (Ndem et al., 2014).

Many of the recorded species possess documented pharmacological properties corroborating their traditional use. Stachytarpheta cayennensis (Aran umon) has been reported to have schizonticidal properties comparable to chloroquine (Okokon, Etteobong & Antia, 2008). Its antiplasmodial properties, as determined by research, have confirmed its use in the traditional unwritten Efik pharmacopeia, which is passed down from parents to their children. An understanding of each of these medicinal plants would suffice.

a. Aspilia africana is known in the Efik/Ibibio language as Edemeron and in some communities as Ndinuene (Respondents). While it is mainly used to prevent haemorrhage, it is also widely used for the treatment of malaria and by traditional birth attendants (TBA) to ease delivery in pregnant women (Okoli et al., 2006). Four essential oils, including sesquiterpenes, monoterpenes, germacrene-d, and alpha-pienene, have been reported in A. africana (Kuiate et al., 1999). These phytochemicals enable the leaf extract to fight the Plasmodium parasite that causes malaria. In addition to its antiplasmodial property, the plant is also utilized to ease the pain of women during the birthing process. The pharmacological properties of A. africana are summarized as antiplasmodial (action against malaria parasites), antimicrobial (for fighting most bacterial infections), anti-inflammatory (easing inflammation caused by infections), and antiulcer (soothing the ulcerations caused by ulcers) (Ezeigbo, Awomukwu & Ezeigbo, 2016; Okello, Lee & Kang, 2020).
b. Chromolaena odorata is commonly known as Awolowo by the Igbos of Nigeria. This name is widely used in Calabar. The decoction of Chromolaena odorata holds significant pharmacological importance in the treatment of malaria due to its multifaceted bioactive properties. Traditionally used in folk medicine, the leaf decoction exhibits potent antimalarial activity by inhibiting the growth and proliferation of Plasmodium species, the parasites that cause malaria. This antiplasmodial activity is attributed to compounds such as flavonoids, alkaloids, and phenolic acids that interfere with the parasite's life cycle (Elebiyo, Oluba & Adeyemi, 2023). The decoction's ability to reduce fever, a key symptom of malaria, further supports its therapeutic use in local malaria treatment in Calabar, making it an accessible and effective remedy for local communities. Beyond its antimalarial properties, Chromolaena odorata decoction also offers additional pharmacological benefits that enhance its treatment efficacy. It possesses potent anti-inflammatory effects, which help in the alleviation of systemic inflammation and tissue damage caused by malaria infection. Moreover, its antimicrobial properties help prevent secondary infections that often complicate malaria cases, while its antioxidant activity protects host cells from oxidative stress induced by the parasite. Collectively, these pharmacological effects make the decoction of Chromolaena odorata a valuable herbal medicine for managing malaria.
c. Stachytarpheta cayennensis is known in Efik as" aran umon". Stachytarpheta cayennensis exhibits significant pharmacological properties that support its traditional use in the treatment of malaria. This has primarily been demonstrated through its potent antimalarial activity in several studies where the ethanolic

leaf extract of S. cayennensis effectively suppressed Plasmodium berghei infection in experimental models, with parasite suppression rates increasing with dosage and comparable survival times to those afforded by chloroquine, a standard antimalarial drug (Okokon et al., 2008; Okoye et al., 2014). The plant's antiplasmodial effects stem from its ability to inhibit blood schizonts during both early and established infections, thereby blocking parasite proliferation and progression of the disease (Ajayi et al., 2024). This aligns and justifies its usage in Efik communities as a natural remedy for malaria. Its safety profile is favourable, with high LD50 values reported, indicating low acute toxicity. Overall, these pharmacological properties make Stachytarpheta cayennensis a valuable herbal agent for the treatment of malaria (Penido et al., 2005).

d. Andrographis paniculata, commonly known as the King of Bitters in Nigeria, is known as Fineka in the Efik/Ibibio language (Ikot et al., 2025). It has demonstrated significant pharmacological potential in malaria treatment, as shown by both in vitro and in vivo studies, which reveal that its methanol leaf extracts effectively inhibit the growth of Plasmodium falciparum, the parasite responsible for malaria (Mishra et al., 2009). This antiplasmodial effect is mainly attributed to andrographolide and related diterpenoids, which exert direct parasiticidal action by interfering with key parasite life cycle stages, such as merozoite invasion and gametocyte formation, and by disrupting energy production processes, such as ATP synthesis. These compounds also inhibit heme polymerization in Plasmodium, which is critical for parasite survival, further enhancing their antimalarial efficacy. Experimental research confirms that andrographolide not only suppresses parasite growth but also induces apoptosis in infected erythrocytes, substantiating its potent direct anti-parasitic mechanism (Mishra et al., 2009; Apsari et al., 2025). In addition to its direct parasiticidal properties, Andrographis paniculata exhibits significant immunomodulatory effects that boost the host's innate and adaptive immune responses, helping to control and eliminate the malaria infection effectively. The extract has been shown to modulate inflammatory mediators without suppressing immune function, unlike some conventional anti-inflammatory drugs, making it well-suited for malaria, where immune competence is critical (Kumar, Singh & Bajpai, 2021).

e. Eremomastax speciosa is known in Efik as Nkong-ikong. The current understanding of the plant's pharmacological profile reveals a rich array of antimicrobial, antioxidant, anti-inflammatory, and antianemia properties. Its phytochemical constituents, such as flavonoids, alkaloids, and tannins, contribute to its effectiveness in reducing fever, combating oxidative stress, and supporting haematological recovery during malaria episodes. Enema administration is preferred locally for its rapid absorption and efficacy, especially when oral intake is difficult due to illness (Ibok et al., 2023).

f. Hypoestes rosea is known as "iyip" in Efik due to its characteristic pinkish colour, which resembles blood (Emeribe et al., 2021). The fresh leaves of Hypoestes rosea are used in traditional medicine to treat various illnesses, including typhoid, anaemia, malaria, hypertension, and others. Hypoestes rosea has been found to possess multiple bioactivities, including anti-inflammatory, antibacterial, and antimalarial (Mensah et al., 2008). These bioactivities are attributed to phytochemicals, such as flavonoids, terpenoids, and tannins, found in the plant's leaves (Bassey et al., 2022).
g. Carica papaya is known as "mmɔ". This plant is mainly used in combination with other plants in enema decoctions. It is rich in phytochemicals, including alkaloids, flavonoids, terpenoids, and saponins. These compounds have demonstrated antiplasmodial activity by inhibiting the growth and replication of Plasmodium parasites. In a study by Titanji et al (2008), they found that papaya leaf extracts can reduce parasitemia levels and improve survival rates in infected animal models. Additionally, Carica papaya supports immune modulation and reduces oxidative stress, which are critical for managing malaria symptoms. Flavonoids and phenolic compounds in the leaves act as antioxidants, helping to neutralize free radicals generated during infection. The plant also contains immunostimulatory agents that enhance white blood cell activity, aiding the body's defense against the parasite (Kong et al., 2021; Ugbogu et al., 2023; Choudhary et al., 2025; Srivastava et al., 2025).
h. Musa paradisiaca, commonly known as "Ukɔm," is a widely used plant with various bioactivities. Abouelfetouh et al. (2024) examined its antimalarial and antioxidant properties. Their findings confirmed significant antimalarial and antioxidant effects, supporting the potential therapeutic use and role in drug discovery. It helps treat malaria by reducing the fever associated with the disease. (Aziz et al., 2020; Imam & Akter, 2011; Laeliocattleya et al., 2018).
i. Azaridachta indica is known as Dogonyaro in Hausa. This name is adopted due to the widespread use of the plant in Northern Nigeria. The antimalarial preparations from neem remain one of the earliest and most widely used remedies for malaria among the Efik/Ibibio ethnic group and in other parts of Africa (Ekanem, 1971). A total of 135 compounds are contained in neem extract, out of which nimbolide, gedunin, and azadirachtin (AZA) have been reported as the compounds that exhibit antimalarial activity (Drabu et al., 2012). Within the general class of active compounds of neem (triterpenes) is the most effective group of compounds called limonoids, for which azadirachtin (AZA) is a member. Neem is reportedly highly effective against chloroquine-resistant and chloroquine-susceptible sexual and asexual stages of human malaria, P. falciparum (Awofego, 2011). In addition, neem exhibits a strong effect against the sexual stages (mature gametocytes) of P. falciparum.

Consequently, the action of neem is different from that of artemisinin because artemisinin only affects the immature stages of the parasite (Adebayo and Krettlie, 2011). Generally, the extracts employ different mechanisms in their antimalarial activities. One is the inhibition of the growth of the malaria parasite. To accomplish this, the extracts stop the malaria parasite from maturing beyond the ring stage by preventing its morphological development. Another is by blocking the transmission of the parasites. To achieve this, the extracts eliminate a high percentage of immature and mature malaria gametocytes (the forms of the parasite that are taken up by mosquitoes), thereby blocking transmission. An essential aspect of the use of neem extract as an antimalarial agent is its advantage in managing high-risk populations consisting of pregnant women, children, and patients with HIV/AIDS. Since the immunity of pregnant women is often compromised, they are more susceptible to severe and complicated malaria (Diala et al., 2013), conditions such as anemia, teratogenicity of the antimalarial drugs, and the risk of undertreatment (Visser et al., 2014). This underscores the complications arising from malaria infection in pregnant women, which can increase the risk of maternal death (Pell et al., 2013). The use of neem extract to manage malaria during pregnancy appears to be most effective in eliminating the risks associated with malaria infection in pregnant women.

Cerebral malaria, which is a severe form of malaria that primarily affects children, is identified as the primary source of neuro-disability among children in areas endemic to malaria (Bedri et al., 2013). A study using *A. indica* ethanolic extract on mice demonstrated neuroprotective effects, which were most likely due to alleviating the edema and adjusting the triggers of neurological apoptosis in mice (Bedri et al., 2013). Although this did not prevent the experimental animal from dying, it opened up a new area for further studies to develop a new treatment regimen for cerebral malaria in children.

Most patients find it challenging to manage HIV and malaria at the same time, as they usually get fatigued and exhausted when they take anti-retrovirals (ARVs) and antimalarials simultaneously (Mangeso et al., 2014). Neem is said to have antiretroviral activity, among many others. It has been demonstrated that neem extract can increase CD4+ cell counts, body weight, and hemoglobin levels (David et al., 2017). This could birth a plausible solution to the pill burden, among the other issues facing HIV patients with malaria. This is because A. indica can serve as both an antimalarial and an antiretroviral (David et al., 2017; Maafoh & Onyedibe, 2024).

j. Mangifera indica: Natives of the Efik/Ibibio ethnic groups have, over the years, incorporated leaf extracts of Mangifera indica in the array of treatment regimens for the management of malaria, either singly or in combination with other medicinal plants such as Azadirachta indica (neem), Artemisia annua (sweet wormwood), or Ocimum sanctum (holy basil) (Ansari et. al., 2022).

This is possible, as the leaf extract of Mangifera indica is safe and non-toxic at concentrations up to 1000mg/kg. Additionally, in another study, Mangifera indica extract reduced parasitemia, achieving a maximum inhibition rate of 93% at 10 mg/ml, comparable to that of the artemether control (96%). The study's findings revealed that M. indica leaf extract holds promise as an affordable and effective candidate for the development of antimalarial drugs (Muhammad et al., 2025).

Mangifera indica has a complex phytochemical makeup, showing activity against Plasmodium and other pathogens. The major bioactive compounds include Mangiferin (a xanthone glycoside), Quercetin and Kaempferol (flavonoids), Gallic Acid and Ellagic Acid (Phenolic acids), Beta-Carotene and Vitamin C. These compounds give the plant its potent antioxidant, anti-inflammatory, antimalarial, antibacterial, and anticancer properties (Ediriweera et. al., 2017; Imran et. al., 2017; Quintana et. al., 2021).

The anti-Plasmodium activity of Mangifera indica operates via different pathways. First is the inhibition of Plasmodium growth and replication. This involves blocking DNA replication and protein synthesis by inhibiting the function of essential enzymes such as dihydrofolate reductase and topoisomerase, suppressing hemozoin formation (parasite toxicity), and the disrupting parasite cell membrane integrity. Second is the interruption of parasite metabolic pathways. This involves inhibiting glycolysis to prevent energy production; blocking the lactate dehydrogenase enzyme, leading to energy depletion; and preventing heme detoxification, resulting in toxic heme accumulation. The third is immune modulatory effects, which involves the activation of immune cells (macrophagocytes, T lymphocytes), boosting cytokine production (IL-12, IL-6, TNF-α), and reduction of oxidative stress, thereby protecting the host cells (Dwivedi et. al., 2013; Yadav et al., 2024). Another mechanism of action of M. Indica's herbal formulation may be as a result of the inhibition of the biosynthesis of fatty acids in the parasite's apicoplast due to the esters of linoleic acids (Kumaratilake et al.,1997). These different approaches ultimately result in the inhibition of Plasmodium growth and enhanced host defense.

k. Jatropha tanjorensis is a medicinal shrub, known for its various pharmacological properties. It is commonly referred to as 'hospital is too far' by locals due to its use in Nigerian traditional medicine. There is no known Efik name for it, but it is usually referred to as "hospital too far" because it is believed to make people well when hospitals are too far to reach. There is documented evidence of the use of the plant in the management of blood sugar due to its antihyperglycemic properties, and it is employed as a traditional remedy for anemia. Studies have shown it has antiplasmodial (antimalarial) and antimicrobial activities. It is also used to lower blood cholesterol and treat related cardiovascular diseases. The plant also exhibits anti-inflammatory effects and is reported to be used for renal problems, hypertension, and as a general tonic (Behl et al., 2021; Obinna et al., 2021; Komolafe et al., 2024; Oseghale et al., 2025).

Jatropha tanjorensis is a rich source of phytochemicals of medicinal importance, which is reflected in its role in traditional folk medicine. Analysis of the phytochemicals of the aqueous leaf extract of J. tanjorensis shows the presence of alkaloids, saponins, tannins, flavonoids, terpenoids, cardiac glycosides, and anthraquinones in appreciable amounts. These bioactive compounds have been reported to have antimalarial and anti-anaemic activities in other plants (Okwu and Okwu, 2004). Thus, the abundance of these compounds in J. tanjorensis has been linked to the antiplasmodial activity observed in the plant. This activity could be due to the effect of a single compound or the synergistic action of several compounds in the plant (Ebenyi et al., 2021).

The immune-boosting properties of the phytochemicals found in J. tanjorensis are considered another potential mechanism for the plant extract's anti-malarial efficacy (Ebenyi et al., 2021). For example, flavonoids are reported to have a potential immune-modulating effect (Deressa et al., 2010), alkaloids are known to intercalate with parasite DNA (Hagazy et al., 2020), while phenolics work by inhibiting protein and fatty acid (FAS II) biosynthesis in the parasite and counteracting the oxidative stress caused by the malaria parasite (Ebenyi et al., 2021).

1. Hippocratea Africana is a perennial plant of the family Celastraceae. It is widely distributed in tropical Africa (Hutchinson and Dalziel, 1973) and used ethnomedically as an antidote and in the treatment of diseases such as malaria and diabetes (Okokon et al., 2006; Ajibesin et al., 2008). The plant has long been used in traditional medicine in Calabar to treat malaria. Its leaves and stem bark are typically prepared as decoctions or infusions to relieve fever and other malaria symptoms. Research on the root extract has shown that it possesses various therapeutic effects, including antimalarial (Okokon et al., 2006; Okokon et al., 2017), anti-edema, antinociceptive, antidiabetic, antioxidant, hypolipidemic, and cardioprotective activities., antidiarrhoeal, antiulcer, hepatoprotective, antimicrobial, antiplasmodial, cytotoxic effects (Okokon et al., 2008; Okokon et al., 2010; Okokon et al.,2022; Okokon et al., 2011; Okokon et al., 2013a; Okokon et al., 2013b; Ndem et al., 2014; Asanga et al., 2025). Research has also reported improved biochemical parameters (cardiac markers) in plasmodial mice with a lethal dosage (LD50) of 2.45 mg/kg body weight (Okokon et al., 2006). Antibacterial and antioxidant activities have also been reported (Folawewo et al., 2017). Also, phytochemical compounds such as δ–3-

carene, α-terpineol (Okokon et al., 2017), monoterpenes, sesquiterpenes, 1,3,7-trihydroxy-6-methoxyxanthone (isoathyriol), and 1,3,6,7-tetrahydroxyxanthone (norathyriol) (Okokon et al., 2013a; Umoh et al., 2021) have been isolated and identified from the plant's leaf extract.

6. DISCUSSION

Before the advent of orthodox medicine, traditional medicine was considered the gold standard for healthcare in many societies (Hosseinzadeh et al., 2015; Jaiswal et al., 2016; Li & Weng, 2017). The medicinal use of plants is primarily attributed to indigenous knowledge passed orally from generation to generation. Although the development of synthetic medicines shifted attention away from traditional practices, many communities have continued to develop and rely on herbal medicines for treating various ailments. The recent global resurgence of interest in ethnobotany can be linked to several factors, including the emergence of drug-resistant pathogens and the high cost of conventional pharmaceuticals. Consequently, traditional medical systems have regained prominence in contemporary health discourse.

This study aimed to document the medicinal plants used as enema therapies by the indigenous people of Calabar. The results revealed 25 plants from 19 families identified for use in enema therapies, out of which 12 plant species from 9 families were identified for use in malaria enema therapies. The implications of these results, including their cultural relevance and possible pharmacological properties, are discussed in detail below.

Asteraceae and Acanthaceae had the highest number of species cited. The dominance of these families has been reported in ethnobotanical studies in Nigeria (Lawal et al., 2022; Odugbemi et al., 2006; Lifongo et al., 2014) and other West African countries such as Ghana and Togo (Agbodeka et al., 2016; Asigbaase et al., 2023).

Within the Efik culture, traditional medicines are administered through diverse routes, including oral ingestion of aqueous or ethanolic leaf extracts, therapeutic baths, and the use of enemas. These methods have been preserved in the unwritten Efik pharmacopeia, reflecting the community's adaptive resilience and deep cultural connection to healing practices. The continued use of enema-based traditional therapies among the Efik people demonstrates how indigenous health systems have endured despite modernization. This integration of cultural beliefs with practical efficacy sustains the relevance of these practices in managing local health challenges such as malaria. The findings of this study align with similar ethnobotanical reports from other regions of West Africa (van Andel et al., 2015). A survey conducted by Agbodeka et al. (2016) in the Plateau region of Togo on medicinal plants used for malaria treatment identified 61 plants. Although they reported the oral route as the most common route of administration for herbal formulations, their findings aligned with this study for some of the identified species, including V. amygdalina, C. papaya, O. gratissimum, M. indica, A. indica, Phyllantus amarus, and Dracaena arborea. However, the differences in the range of species identified could be due to geographical and cultural differences, as well as the method of administration, the parts used, and the concentration of the bioactive components, which may influence the choice of plants for herbal preparations (Truncay, 2023; Kayani et al., 2014).

An ethnobotanical study by Odugbemi et al. (2006) reported the use of similar plant species for malaria therapy in Ondo state, Nigeria. These included Azadirachta indica, Mangifera indica, Chromolaena odorata, Carica papaya, Vernonia amygdalina, and Ocimum gratissimum. Although the respondents in our study identified V. amydalina and O. gratissimum for treating heat, an analysis of their submissions revealed a consistent pattern; most participants referred to treating conditions described as "fever" or "heat." These symptoms are characteristic of malaria, suggesting that many of the local therapies, though symptom-based, are effective antimalarials. This observation underscores the diagnostic framework of traditional medicine, which relies heavily on symptom recognition to guide treatment choices. The geographic proximity and shared sociocultural background of the Efik and Qua ethnic groups likely explain the similarities in the plants used and the methods of preparation employed in enema therapy.

Indigenous and traditional uses of medicinal plants can significantly enrich modern drug discovery and development. Traditional knowledge systems, refined over centuries, often embody detailed understandings of the therapeutic potential and preparation of plant-based remedies (Tshali et al., 2024). However, despite their efficacy, challenges persist, including issues of contamination, incorrect dosing, and the potential misuse of herbal preparations. These underscore the importance of pharmacovigilance, standardization, and public health education. Bridging indigenous wisdom with modern pharmacological validation not only enhances the safety and efficacy of herbal treatments but also promotes cultural preservation.

The overlap between traditional and modern pharmacopoeias demonstrates that indigenous practices remain a valuable resource for future natural product research, particularly in the development of new antimalarial agents. The integration of ethnobotanical knowledge into formal health systems could thus accelerate the discovery of novel bioactive compounds, contribute to sustainable health innovation, and reaffirm the relevance of indigenous knowledge in global health.

7. LIMITATIONS OF THE STUDY

The ethnobotanical information presented was primarily self-reported, based on respondents' recollections and interpretations of traditional practices. As such, the findings may be subject to recall bias or selective reporting. Additionally, the study did not conduct pharmacological or toxicological validation of the reported enema formulations, making it difficult to ascertain their efficacy, standard dosage, and safety profiles. Future research should include controlled laboratory and clinical studies to validate the therapeutic claims and ensure safe integration into modern healthcare frameworks.

8. CONCLUSION

This chapter emphasizes the significance of indigenous medicinal knowledge in malaria management among communities in Cross River State, Nigeria. The identification of 26 medicinal plant species used in enema-based therapies reflects a rich cultural and ecological heritage. While the persistence of these traditional practices highlights their perceived efficacy, bridging them with scientific inquiry is essential. Collaborative efforts between ethnobotanists, pharmacologists, and public health experts are necessary to validate and optimize these remedies for broader application. Overall, this study provides a valuable baseline for further research into the development of safe, plant-based antimalarial formulations and drug discovery.

8.1 Future Perspectives

The findings of this study provide an opportunity to investigate and discover novel bioactive compounds from indigenous medicinal plants. In addition, several of the identified species warrant detailed phytochemical testing and structural activity studies, which could lead to the development of locally available antimalarial products. This transformation will require strengthening cooperation among traditional healers, research institutions, and the pharmaceutical industry. By combining traditional enema therapy with modern biotechnology and pharmacological approaches, future research can enhance safety, reproducibility, and consumer confidence through quality control frameworks and standardization protocols. This will promote sustainable health solutions, contributing to both local healthcare and economic development.

REFERENCES

Abouelfetouh, M., metwaly., Ali., Marwan., Khan, I., & Shaker, E. (2024). Phytochemical analysis, antimalarial and antioxidant activities of Musa paradisiaca rhizome. Journal of Advanced Pharmacy Research, 8(4), 188–197. doi:10.21608/aprh.2024.291519.1272DOI: 10.21608/aprh.2024.291519.1272

Adebayo, J. O., & Krettli, A. U. (2011). Potential antimalarials from Nigerian plants: A review. Journal of Ethnopharmacology, 133(2), 289–302. doi:10.1016/j.jep.2010.11.024 PubMedDOI: 10.1016/j.jep.2010.11.024 PMID: 21093570

Agbodeka, K., Gbekley, H. E., Karou, S. D., Anani, K., Agbonon, A., Tchacondo, T., Batawila, K., Simpore, J., & Gbeassor, M. (2016). Ethnobotanical Study of Medicinal Plants Used for the Treatment of Malaria in the Plateau Region, Togo. Pharmacognosy Research, 8(5, Suppl 1), S12–S18. doi:10.4103/0974-8490.178646 PubMedDOI: 10.4103/0974-8490.178646 PMID: 27114686

Ajayi, O., Balogun, O., Fakola, E., Olawuni, I., October, N., & Adewole, A. (2024). Evaluation of Antioxidant & Antidiabetic Activities of Iridoid glycoside Isolated from Stachytarpheta cayennensis (Rich) Vahl Leaf Extract: In vitro combined with molecular docking approach. South African Journal of Botany, 176, 184–196. doi:10.1016/j.sajb.2024.11.008DOI: 10.1016/j.sajb.2024.11.008

Ajibesin, K. K., Ekpo, B. A., Bala, D. N., Essien, E. E., & Adesanya, S. A. (2008). Ethnobotanical survey of Akwa Ibom State, Nigeria. Journal of Ethnopharmacology, 115(3), 387–408. doi:10.1016/j.jep.2007.10.021 PubMedDOI: 10.1016/j.jep.2007.10.021 PMID: 18053664

Akobundu, I. O., Ekeleme, F., Agyakwa, C. W., & Ogazie, C. A. (2016). A handbook of West African weeds (3rd ed.). International Institute of Tropical Agriculture. Nigeria, OfKAR Publishing Company Limited. Pp 381

Akwaji, P. I., Eyam, E. O., & Bassey, R. A. (2017). Ethnobotanical survey of medicinal plants in Northern Cross River State, Nigeria. World Scientific News, 70(2), 140–157.

Amang, A. P., Mezui, C., Siwe, G. T., Emakoua, J., & Tan, P. V. (2017). Healing and antisecretory effects of aqueous extract of Eremomastax speciosa (Acanthaceae) on unhealed gastric ulcers. Evidence-Based Complementary and Alternative Medicine : eCAM, 2017(1), 1924320. doi:10.1155/2017/1924320 PubMedDOI: 10.1155/2017/1924320 PMID: 29234676

Ansari, P., Akther, S., Hannan, J. M. A., Seidel, V., Nujat, N. J., & Abdel-Wahab, Y. H. (2022). Pharmacologically active phytomolecules isolated from traditional antidiabetic plants and their therapeutic role for the management of diabetes mellitus. Molecules (Basel, Switzerland), 27(13), 4278. doi:10.3390/molecules27134278 PubMedDOI: 10.3390/molecules27134278 PMID: 35807526

Apsari, P. I. B., Suryana, I. K., Satriyasa, B. K., Laksmi, D. S., Wati, D. K., & Wirasuta, I. M. G. (2025). Towards Andrographolide as Antimalarial: A Systematic Review. Biomedical & Pharmacology Journal, 18(1), 499–515. doi:10.13005/bpj/3103DOI: 10.13005/bpj/3103

Asanga, E. E., Noah, K. U., Okokon, J. E., Ekeleme, C. M., Udoh, I. E., Bassey, A., Anagboso, M. O., & Inyang, A. N. (2025). Integrative investigation on Hippocratea africana root: Insights from cardio-protective, antioxidative stress activities, isolation, GC/MS, and pharmacological significance profiling. BMC Complementary Medicine and Therapies, 25(1), 200. doi:10.1186/s12906-025-04941-8 PubMedDOI: 10.1186/s12906-025-04941-8 PMID: 40468373

Asigbaase, M., Adusu, D., Anaba, L., Abugre, S., Kang-Milung, S., Acheamfour, S. A., Adamu, I., & Ackah, D. K. (2023). Conservation and economic benefits of medicinal plants: Insights from forest-fringe communities of Southwestern Ghana. Trees, Forests and People, 14, 100462. doi:10.1016/j.tfp.2023.100462DOI: 10.1016/j.tfp.2023.100462

Aziz, S. M. A., Ahmed, O. M., El-Twab, S. M. A., Al-Muzafar, H. M., Amin, K. A., & Abdel-Gabbar, M. (2020). Antihyperglycemic Effects and Mode of Actions of Musa paradisiaca Leaf and Fruit Peel Hydroethanolic Extracts in Nicotinamide/Streptozotocin-Induced Diabetic Rats. Evidence-based Complementary and Alternative Medicine, 2020(1). https://doi.org/doi:10.1155/2020/9276343DOI: 10.1155/2020/9276343

Bassey, N. O., Eteng, O. E., Nelson, V. A., Essien, N. M., Udo, E. P., Ogar, B. A., & Udosen, E. O. (2022). Proximate And Phytochemical Screening: Evaluation of Minerals And Vitamin Composition Of (Hypoestes rosea) Plant Harvested In Calabar, Cross River State, Nigeria. FUDMA Journal of Sciences, 5(4), 229–234. doi:10.33003/fjs-2021-0504-809DOI: 10.33003/fjs-2021-0504-809

Bedri, S., Khalil, E. A., Khalid, S. A., Alzohairy, M. A., Mohieldein, A., Aldebasi, Y. H., Etet, P. F. S., & Farahna, M. (2013). Azadirachta indica ethanolic extract protects neurons from apoptosis and mitigates brain swelling in experimental cerebral malaria. Malaria Journal, 12(1), 298. doi:10.1186/1475-2875-12-298 PubMedDOI: 10.1186/1475-2875-12-298 PMID: 23984986

Behl, T., Kumar, K., Brisc, C., Rus, M., Nistor-Cseppento, D. C., Bustea, C., Aron, R. A. C., Pantis, C., Zengin, G., Sehgal, A., Kaur, R., Kumar, A., Arora, S., Setia, D., Chandel, D., & Bungau, S. (2021). Exploring the multifocal role of phytochemicals as immunomodulators. Biomedicine and Pharmacotherapy, 133, 110959. doi:10.1016/j.biopha.2020.110959 PubMedDOI: 10.1016/j.biopha.2020.110959 PMID: 33197758

Bhatnagar, A. (2023). Chemical constituents of Andrographis paniculata (Burm. F) Nees: A review. International Journal of Pharmaceutical Sciences and Research, 14(7), 3238–3245.

Carvalho, M. T., Araújo-Filho, H. G., Barreto, A. S., Quintans-Júnior, L. J., Quintans, J. S., & Barreto, R. S. (2021). Wound healing properties of flavonoids: A systematic review highlighting the mechanisms of action. Phytomedicine, 90, 153636. doi:10.1016/j.phymed.2021.153636 PubMedDOI: 10.1016/j.phymed.2021.153636 PMID: 34333340

Chao, W. W., & Lin, B. F. (2010). Isolation and identification of bioactive compounds in Andrographis paniculata (Chuanxinlian). Chinese Medicine, 5(1), 17. doi:10.1186/1749-8546-5-17 PubMedDOI: 10.1186/1749-8546-5-17 PMID: 20465823

Choudhary, R., Kaushik, R., Akhtar, A., Manna, S., Sharma, J., & Bains, A. (2025). Nutritional, Phytochemical, and Antimicrobial Properties of Carica papaya Leaves: Implications for Health Benefits and Food Applications. Foods, 14(2), 154. doi:10.3390/foods14020154 PubMedDOI: 10.3390/foods14020154 PMID: 39856820

David, P. E., Luis, B. S. G., Alma, D. E. A., Martha, P. N. H., & Mariadel, C. V. M. (2017). HIV-1 Infection Inhibition by Neem (Azadirachta indica A. Juss.) leaf extracts and azadirachtin. Indian Journal of Traditional Knowledge, 16, 437–441.

De Smet, P. A. G. M. (1983). A multidisciplinary overview of intoxicating enema rituals in the Western Hemisphere. Journal of Ethnopharmacology, 9(2-3), 129–166. doi:10.1016/0378-8741(83)90031-4 PubMedDOI: 10.1016/0378-8741(83)90031-4 PMID: 6677814

Deressa, T., Mekonnen, Y., & Animut, A. (2010). In-vivo antimalarial activities of Clerodendrum myricoides, Dodonea angustifolia, and Aloe debrana against Plasmodium berghei. The Ethiopian Journal of Health Development, 24(1), 25–29. doi:10.4314/ejhd.v24i1.62941DOI: 10.4314/ejhd.v24i1.62941

Diala, C. C., Pennas, T., Marin, C., & Belay, K. A. (2013). Perceptions of intermittent preventive treatment of malaria in pregnancy (IPTp) and barriers to adherence in Nasarawa and Cross River States in Nigeria. Malaria Journal, 12(1), 342. doi:10.1186/1475-2875-12-342 PubMedDOI: 10.1186/1475-2875-12-342 PMID: 24059757

Drabu, S., Khatri, S., & Babu, S. (2012). Neem: Healer of all ailments. Research Journal of Pharmaceutical, Biological and Chemical Sciences, 3, 120–126.

Dunn, J. P., Krige, J. E. J., Wood, R., Bornman, P. C., & Terblanche, J. (1991). Colonic complications after toxic tribal enemas. British Journal of Surgery, 78(5), 545–548. doi:10.1002/bjs.1800780510 PubMedDOI: 10.1002/bjs.1800780510 PMID: 2059802

Dwivedi, G. R., Tripathi, P., & Mishra, S. K. (2013). Repurposing quercetin as a potential anti-malarial: In vitro and in silico studies. Journal of Biomolecular Structure & Dynamics, 31(4), 400–410.

Ebenyi, L. N., Yongabi, K. A., Ali, F. U., Ominyi, M. C., Anyanwu, C. B., Benjamin, E., & Ogbanshi, M. E. (2021). Effect of aqueous leaf extract of Jatropha tanjorensis on parasitaemia and haematological parameters in mice infected with Plasmodium berghei. Nigerian Journal of Biotechnology, 38(1), 146–153. doi:10.4314/njb.v38i1.17DOI: 10.4314/njb.v38i1.17

Ediriweera, M. K., Tennekoon, K. H., & Samarakoon, S. R. (2017). A review on ethnopharmacological applications, pharmacological activities, and bioactive compounds of Mangifera indica (Mango). Evidence-Based Complementary and Alternative Medicine : eCAM, 6949835(1), 6949835. Advance online publication. doi:10.1155/2017/6949835 PubMedDOI: 10.1155/2017/6949835 PMID: 29456572

Elebiyo, T. C., Oluba, O. M., & Adeyemi, O. S. (2023). Anti-malarial and haematological evaluation of the ethanolic, ethyl acetate, and aqueous fractions of Chromolaena odorata. BMC Complementary Medicine and Therapies, 23(1), 402. Advance online publication. doi:10.1186/s12906-023-04200-8 PubMedDOI: 10.1186/s12906-023-04200-8 PMID: 37946127

Emeribe, A. U., Anyanwu, S. O., Isong, I. K., Bassey, U. R., Inyang, I. J., Ibeneme, E. O., Asemota, E. A., Okhormhe, Z., Icha, B., & Abdullahi, I. N. (2021). Phytochemical analysis and toxicological evaluation of the ethanolic Leaves extract of Hypoestes rosea on the morphology and biochemical indices of the Kidneys of albino Wistar Rats. Saudi Journal of Biological Sciences, 28(12), 6748–6755. doi:10.1016/j.sjbs.2021.07.045 PubMedDOI: 10.1016/j.sjbs.2021.07.045 PMID: 34866973

Erinoso, S. M., & Aworinde, D. O. (2018). Current outlook and future promise of ethnobotany in Nigeria: A review and personal observation. African Journal of Plant Science, 12(4), 73-80. • https://doi.org/doi:10.5897/AJPS2017.1571DOI: 10.5897/AJPS2017.1571

Ezeigbo, O., Awomukwu, D., & Ezeigbo, I. (2016). The Antimicrobial and Phytochemical Analysis of the Leaves of Aspilia africana on Clinical Isolates. European Journal of Medicinal Plants, 15(2), 1–6. doi:10.9734/EJMP/2016/26481DOI: 10.9734/EJMP/2016/26481

Folawewo, A. D., Madu, A. N., Agbaje-Daniels, F. V., Faboyede, A. O., & Coker, A. R. (2017). Phytochemical screening and antibacterial activities of the root bark extracts of Hippocratea africana (Willd.) Loes. ex Engl. European Journal of Medicinal Plants, 19(1), 1–8. doi:10.9734/EJMP/2017/32765DOI: 10.9734/EJMP/2017/32765

Gerheart, W. A., Edward, E. K., Mohammed, A., Prince, N. A., Jeremiah, A. S., & Boansi, A. A. (2024). Comparative analysis of phytochemical constituents in different parts of Aspilia africana: A potential medicinal plant for therapeutic applications. Phytomedicine Plus : International Journal of Phytotherapy and Phytopharmacology, 4(4), 100656. Advance online publication. doi:10.1016/j.phyplu.2024.100656DOI: 10.1016/j.phyplu.2024.100656

Hagazy, K., Sibhat, G. G., Karim, A., Tekulu, G. H., Periasamy, G., & Hiben, M. (2020). Antimalarial activity of Meriandra dianthera leaf extracts in Plasmodium berghei-infected mice. Evidence-Based Complementary and Alternative Medicine : eCAM, 12(1), 8980212. doi:10.1155/2020/8980212 PubMedDOI: 10.1155/2020/8980212 PMID: 32104197

Harshberger, J. W. (1896). The purposes of ethno-botany. Botanical Gazette (Chicago, Ill.), 21(3), 146–154. doi:10.1086/327316DOI: 10.1086/327316

Hosseinzadeh, S., Jafarikukhdan, A., Hosseini, A., & Armand, R. (2015). The application of medicinal plants in traditional and modern medicine: A review of Thymus vulgaris. International Journal of Clinical Medicine, 6(9), 635–642. doi:10.4236/ijcm.2015.69084DOI: 10.4236/ijcm.2015.69084

Hutchinson, J., & Dalziel, J. M. (1973). Flora of West Tropical Africa (2nd ed., Vol. 1, Pt. 2. Crown Agents for Overseas Governments and Administrations.

Ibok, M. G., Odeja, O. O., Okpala, E. O., Eghwubare, J. E., & Anifalaje, E. O. (2023). Eremomastax speciosa (Hochst.): GC/MS profiling, antioxidant and antimicrobial activities of stem essential oil. Future Journal of Pharmaceutical Sciences, 9(1), 51. doi:10.1186/s43094-023-00501-4DOI: 10.1186/s43094-023-00501-4

Ibrahim, N. I., Wong, S. K., Mohamed, I. N., Mohamed, N., Chin, K. Y., Ima-Nirwana, S., & Shuid, A. N. (2018). Wound healing properties of selected natural products. International Journal of Environmental Research and Public Health, 15(11), 2360. doi:10.3390/ijerph15112360 PubMedDOI: 10.3390/ijerph15112360 PMID: 30366427

Ikot, M., Mbong, E., Akpabio, K., & Uyoh, V. (2025). Morpho-statistical variation and taxonomic characterization of Andrographis paniculata (Burm. F.) Nees population obtained from selected locations within Southern Nigeria. Dutse Journal of Pure and Applied Sciences, 10(4c), 14–23. doi:10.4314/dujopas.v10i4c.2DOI: 10.4314/dujopas.v10i4c.2

Imam, M. Z., & Akter, S. (2011). Musa paradisiaca L. and Musa sapientum L.: A phytochemical and pharmacological review. Journal of Applied Pharmaceutical Science, 1(5), 14–20.

Imran, M., Arshad, M. S., Butt, M. S., Kwon, J. H., Arshad, M. U., & Sultan, M. T. (2017). Mangiferin: A natural miracle bioactive compound against lifestyle-related disorders. Lipids in Health and Disease, 16(1), 1–17. doi:10.1186/s12944-017-0449-y PubMedDOI: 10.1186/s12944-017-0449-y PMID: 28464819

Iwu, I. C., Onu, U. L., Ukaoma, A. A., & Oze, R. N. (2018). Phytochemical, antimicrobial, and Gc/Ms analysis of the root of Stachytarpheta cayennensis (L. Vahl) grown in Eastern Nigeria. International Research Journal of Natural Sciences., 6(2), 1–14. 10.37745/irjns.13

Jaiswal, Y., Liang, Z., & Zhao, Z. (2016). Botanical drugs in Ayurveda and Traditional Chinese Medicine. Journal of Ethnopharmacology, 194, 245–259. doi:10.1016/j.jep.2016.06.052 PubMedDOI: 10.1016/j.jep.2016.06.052 PMID: 27394388

Jayakumar, T., Hsieh, C. Y., Lee, J. J., & Sheu, J. R. (2013). Experimental and Clinical Pharmacology of Andrographis paniculata and Its Major Bioactive Phytoconstituent Andrographolide. Evidence-Based Complementary and Alternative Medicine : eCAM, 846740, 1–16. Advance online publication. doi:10.1155/2013/846740 PubMedDOI: 10.1155/2013/846740 PMID: 23634174

Kayani, S., Ahmad, M., Zafar, M., Sultana, S., Khan, M. P. Z., Ashraf, M. A., Hussain, J., & Yaseen, G. (2014). Ethnobotanical uses of medicinal plants for respiratory disorders among the inhabitants of Gallies–Abbottabad, Northern Pakistan. Journal of Ethnopharmacology, 156, 47–60. doi:10.1016/j.jep.2014.08.005 PubMedDOI: 10.1016/j.jep.2014.08.005 PMID: 25153021

Kolawole, E., Ayeni, E., Abolade, S., Ugwu, S., Awoyinka, T., Ofeh, A., & Okolo, B. (2023). Malaria endemicity in sub-Saharan Africa: Past and present issues in public health. Microbes and Infectious Diseases, 4(1), 242-251. https://doi.org/10 .21608/mid.. 2022.150194.1346

Komolafe, C. J., Adetoyinbo, I. I., Alao, F. O., & Ogunsola, J. F. (2024). Phytochemical Analyses and Antibacterial Activities of Jatropha tanjorensis J. L. Ellis and Saroja leaves extract against clinical pathogens. Asian Journal of Applied Chemistry Research, 15(4), 79–93. doi:10.9734/ajacr/2024/v15i5298DOI: 10.9734/ajacr/2024/v15i5298

Kong, Y. R., Jong, Y. X., Balakrishnan, M., Bok, Z. K., Weng, J. K. K., Tay, K. C., Goh, B. H., Ong, Y. S., Chan, K. G., Lee, L. H., & Khaw, K. Y. (2021). Beneficial Role of Carica papaya Extracts and Phytochemicals on Oxidative Stress and Related Diseases: A Mini Review. Biology (Basel), 10(4), 287. doi:10.3390/biology10040287 PubMedDOI: 10.3390/biology10040287 PMID: 33916114

Kuiate, J. R., Amvam-Zollo, P. H., Lamaty, G., Menut, C., & Bessiere, J. M. (1999). Composition of the Essential Oils from the Leaves of two varieties of Aspilia africana (Pers). C.D. Adams from Cameroon. Flavour and Fragrance Journal, 14(3), 167–169. doi:10.1002/(SICI)1099-1026(199905/06)14:3<167::AID-FFJ802>3.0.CO;2-ODOI: 10.1002/(SICI)1099-1026(199905/06)14:3<167::AID-FFJ802>3.0.CO;2-O

Kumar, S., Singh, B., & Bajpai, V. (2021). Andrographis paniculata (Burm.f.) Nees: Traditional uses, phytochemistry, pharmacological properties, and quality control/quality assurance. Journal of Ethnopharmacology, 275, 114054. doi:10.1016/j.jep.2021.114054 PubMedDOI: 10.1016/j.jep.2021.114054 PMID: 33831465

Kumaratilake, L. M., Ferrante, A., Robinson, B. S., Jaeger, T., & Poulos, A. (1997). Enhancement of the neutrophil-mediated killing of Plasmodium falciparum asexual blood forms by fatty acids: Importance of fatty acid structure. Infection and Immunity, 65(10), 4152–4157. doi:10.1128/iai.65.10.4152-4157.1997 PubMedDOI: 10.1128/iai.65.10.4152-4157.1997 PMID: 9317021

Laeliocattleya, R. A., Estiasih, T., Griselda, G., & Muchlisyiyah, J. (2018). The bioactive compounds and antioxidant activity of ethanol and ethyl acetate extracts of CandiBanana (Musa paradisiaca). IOP Conference Series. Earth and Environmental Science, 131, 012013. doi:10.1088/1755-1315/131/1/012013DOI: 10.1088/1755-1315/131/1/012013

Lalita Nargawe, G. Malathi, Vidhya C. S., Lalit Upadhyay. (. (2023). Ethnobotanical Survey of Medicinal Plants Used in Traditional Medicine in Africa. Plant Science Archives, 26-28. Advance online publication. doi:10.51470/PSA.2023.8.4.26DOI: 10.51470/PSA.2023.8.4.26

Lawal, I. O., Rafiu, B. O., Ale, J. E., Majebi, O. E., & Aremu, A. O. (2022). Ethnobotanical Survey of Local Flora Used for Medicinal Purposes among Indigenous People in Five Areas in Lagos State, Nigeria. Plants, 11(5), 633. doi:10.3390/plants11050633 PubMedDOI: 10.3390/plants11050633 PMID: 35270103

Li, F., & Weng, J. (2017). Demystifying traditional herbal medicine with modern approach. Nature Plants, 3(8), 17109. Advance online publication. doi:10.1038/nplants.2017.109 PubMedDOI: 10.1038/nplants.2017.109 PMID: 28758992

Lifongo, L. L., Simoben, C. V., Ntie-Kang, F., Babiaka, S. B., & Judson, P. N. (2014). A bioactivity versus ethnobotanical survey of medicinal plants from Nigeria, West Africa. Natural Products and Bioprospecting, 4(1), 1–19. doi:10.1007/s13659-014-0005-7 PubMedDOI: 10.1007/s13659-014-0005-7 PMID: 24660132

Maafoh, C., & Onyedibe, K. (2024). Alternative first-line malaria treatment. Annals of African Medicine, 23(1), 5–12. doi:10.4103/aam.aam_35_23 PubMedDOI: 10.4103/aam.aam_35_23 PMID: 38358164

Mensah, J. K., Okoli, R. I., Ohagu-Obodo, J. O., & Lifediyi, K. (2008). Phytochemical, nutritional, and medicinal properties of some leafy Vegetables consumed by the Edo people of Nigeria. African Journal of Biotechnology, 7(3), 2304–2309. 10.4314/ajb.v7i14.58988

Mishra, K., Dash, A. P., Swain, B. K., & Dey, N. (2009). Anti-malarial activities of Andrographis paniculata and Hedyotis corymbosa extracts and their combination with curcumin. Malaria Journal, 8(1), 26. Advance online publication. doi:10.1186/1475-2875-8-26 PubMedDOI: 10.1186/1475-2875-8-26 PMID: 19216765

Muhammad, R. H., Sanusi, F. S., & Safiyanu, M. (2025). In-vitro Anti-Plasmodial Activity of Mangifera indica Leaves Against Plasmodium falciparum. Bima Journal of Science and Technology Gombe, 9(2B), 295–301. doi:10.64290/bima.v9i2B.1300DOI: 10.64290/bima.v9i2B.1300

Narzary, D., & Boro, I. (2025). Plants in Bodo Folklore and Ritual Practices: An Ethnobotanical Perspective. International Journal for Multidisciplinary Research, 7(4), 53553. Advance online publication. doi:10.36948/ijfmr.2025.v07i04.53553DOI: 10.36948/ijfmr.2025.v07i04.53553

Ndem, J., Uwah, A., Effiong, B., Bassey, U., Umanah, B., & Chukwudike, C. (2020). Ethanol leaf extract of Jatropha tanjorensis ameliorates hepatorenal toxicity of Plasmodium berghi-berghi infected mice treated with Hippocratea africana root bark extract. The Journal of Phytopharmacology, 9(5), 374–377. doi:10.31254/phyto.2020.9515DOI: 10.31254/phyto.2020.9515

Ndem, J. I., Eteng, M. U., & Uwah, A. F. (2014). Effect of Hippocratea Africana Root Bark Extract on Lipid Profile of Female and Male Albino Wistar Rats. Journal of Scientific Research and Reports, 3(19), 2574–2583. doi:10.9734/JSRR/2014/12491DOI: 10.9734/JSRR/2014/12491

Ndem, J. I., Eteng, M. U., & Uwah, A. F. (2014). Effect of Hippocratea africana Root Bark Extract on Lipid Profile of Female and Male Albino Wistar Rats. Journal of Scientific Research and Reports, 3(19), 2574–2583. doi:10.9734/JSRR/2014/12491DOI: 10.9734/JSRR/2014/12491

Nworgu, C. O., Elele, K., & Adikwu, E. (2022). Toxicity and antiplasmodial assessments of Chromolaena odorata leaf extract on Plasmodium berghei-infected mice. Journal of Infectious Diseases and Epidemiology, 8(8), 276. doi:10.23937/2474-3658/1510276DOI: 10.23937/2474-3658/1510276

Obinna, A., Onyedikachi, U., Alaebo, P., Odo, C., Okechukwu, G., & Omodamiro, O. (2021). Methanol leaf extract of Jatropha tanjorensis Ellis and Saroja possesses phytoconstituents with free radical scavenging activity. FUDMA Journal of Sciences, 5(3), 286–293. doi:10.33003/fjs-2021-0503-660DOI: 10.33003/fjs-2021-0503-660

Odugbemi, T. O., Akinsulire, O. R., Aibinu, I. E., & Fabeku, P. O. (2006). Medicinal plants useful for malaria therapy in Okeigbo, Ondo State, Southwest Nigeria. African Journal of Traditional, Complementary, and Alternative Medicines : AJTCAM, 4(2), 191–198. doi:10.4314/ajtcam.v4i2.31207 PubMedDOI: 10.4314/ajtcam.v4i2.31207 PMID: 20162091

Okello, D., Lee, J., & Kang, Y. (2020). Ethnopharmacological Potential of Aspilia africana for the Treatment of Inflammatory Diseases. Evidence-Based Complementary and Alternative Medicine : eCAM, 2020(1), 1–11. doi:10.1155/2020/8091047 PubMedDOI: 10.1155/2020/8091047 PMID: 32733588

Okokon, J. E., Akpan, H. D., Umoh, E. E., & Ekaidem, I. S. (2011). Antidiarrhoeal and antiulcer activities of Hippocratea africana root extract. Pakistan Journal of Pharmaceutical Sciences, 24(2), 201–205. PubMed PMID: 21454170

Okokon, J. E., Antia, B. S., Umoh, E. E., & Etim, E. I. (2010). Antidiabetic, cardioprotective, and hypolipidaemic activities of Hippocratea africana. International Journal of Drug Development Research, 2, 501–506.

Okokon, J. E., Chinyere, P. C., Amaechi, P., Bassey, A. L., & Thomas, P. S. (2022). Antioxidant, antidiabetic, and hypolipidemic activities of ethanol root extract and fractions of Hippocratea africana. Tropical Journal of Natural Product Research, 6(3), 446–453.

Okokon, J. E., Dar, A., & Choudhary, M. I. (2013b). Immunomodulatory, cytotoxic, and antileishmanial activities of Hippocratea africana. Journal of Natural Pharmaceuticals, 4(2), 81–85.

Okokon, J. E., Ettebong, E., & Antia, B. S. (2008). In vivo antimalarial activity of ethanolic leaf extract of Stachytarpheta cayennensis. Indian Journal of Pharmacology, 40(3), 111–113. doi:10.4103/0253-7613.42303 PubMedDOI: 10.4103/0253-7613.42303 PMID: 20040937

Okokon, J. E., Ita, B. N., & Udokpoh, A. E. (2006). The In Vivo Antimalarial Activities of Uvariae chamae and Hippocratea africana. Annals of Tropical Medicine and Parasitology, 100(9), 585–590. doi:10.1179/136485906X118512 PubMedDOI: 10.1179/136485906X118512 PMID: 16989684

Okokon, J. E., Nwafor, P. A., Charles, U., Dar, A., & Choudhary, M. I. (2013a). The antioxidative burst and hepatoprotective effects of ethanolic root extract of Hippocratea africana against paracetamol-induced liver injury. Pharmaceutical Biology, 51(7), 872–880. doi:10.3109/13880209.2013.768273 PubMedDOI: 10.3109/13880209.2013.768273 PMID: 23530960

Okokon, J. E., Okokon, P. J., & Sahal, D. (2017). In vitro antiplasmodial activity of some Nigerian medicinal plants. International Journal of Herbal Medicine, 5(5), 102–109.

Okoli, C., Akah, P. A., Nwafor, S. V., Anisiobi, A. I., Ibegbunam, I. N., & Erojikwe, O. (2006). Anti-inflammatory activity of hexane leaf extract of Aspilia africana C.D. Adams. Journal of Ethnopharmacology, 109(2), 219–225. doi:10.1016/j.jep.2006.07.037 PubMedDOI: 10.1016/j.jep.2006.07.037 PMID: 16950582

Oseghale, I. D., Ikokwu, G. M., Ralph-Okhiria, O. H., Odunvbun, P., & Adedotun, A. M. (2025). Comprehensive ethnomedicinal and phytopharmacological review of Jatropha tanjorensis. Asian Journal of Research in Biochemistry, 15(4), 62–76. doi:10.9734/ajrb/2025/v15i4407DOI: 10.9734/ajrb/2025/v15i4407

Pell, C., Meñaca, A., Afrah, N. A., Manda-Taylor, L., Chatio, S., Were, F., Abraham Hodgson, A., Hamel, M. J., Kalilani, L., Tagbor, H., & Pool, R. (2013). Prevention and management of malaria during pregnancy: Findings from a comparative qualitative study in Ghana, Kenya, and Malawi. Malaria Journal, 12(1), 427. doi:10.1186/1475-2875-12-427 PubMedDOI: 10.1186/1475-2875-12-427 PMID: 24257105

Penido, C., Costa, K., Futuro, D., Paiva, S., Kaplan, M., Figueiredo, M. R., & Henriques, M. G. M. O. (2005). Anti-inflammatory and anti-ulcerogenic properties of Stachytarpheta cayennensis (L.C. Rich) Vahl. Journal of Ethnopharmacology, 104(1–2), 225–233. doi:10.1016/j.jep.2005.09.006 PubMedDOI: 10.1016/j.jep.2005.09.006 PMID: 16219439

Quintana, S. E., Salas, S., & García Zapateiro, L. A. (2021). Bioactive compounds of mango (Mangifera indica): A review of extraction technologies and chemical constituents. Journal of the Science of Food and Agriculture, 101(15), 6186–6192. doi:10.1002/jsfa.11455 PubMedDOI: 10.1002/jsfa.11455 PMID: 34324201

Sandhir, R., Khurana, M., & Singhal, N. K. (2021). Potential benefits of phytochemicals from Azadirachta indica against neurological disorders. Neurochemistry International, 146, 105023. doi:10.1016/j.neuint.2021.105023 PubMedDOI: 10.1016/j.neuint.2021.105023 PMID: 33753160

Schultes, R. E. (1960). Tapping our heritage of ethnobotanical lore. Economic Botany, 14(4), 257–262. https://www.jstor.org/stable/4252190. doi:10.1007/BF02908034DOI: 10.1007/BF02908034

Sifuna, N. (2022). African Traditional Medicine: Its Potential, Limitations and Challenges. J Healthcare, 5(1), 141–150. doi:10.36959/569/475DOI: 10.36959/569/475

Srivastava, R., Jaiswal, N., Kharkwal, H., Dubey, N. K., & Srivastava, R. (2025). Phytomedical Properties of Carica papaya for Boosting Human Immunity Against Viral Infections. Viruses, 17(2), 271. doi:10.3390/v17020271 PubMedDOI: 10.3390/v17020271 PMID: 40007026

Tiamiyu, M., & Okunlade, O. A. (2020). Benefits and detriments of Siam weed (Chromolaena odorata): A review. Biochemistry and Biotechnology Research (Delta), 8(2), 21–28.

Titanji, V. P. K., Zofou, D., & Ngenenya, M. N. (2008). The antimalarial potential of medicinal plants used for the treatment of malaria in Cameroonian folk medicine. (2008, April 10). PubMed. https://pubmed.ncbi.nlm.nih.gov/20161952/

Ugbogu, E. A., Dike, E. D., Uche, M. E., Etumnu, L. R., Okoro, B. C., Ugbogu, O. C., Adurosakin, O. E., Chinma, C. E., Ohaeri, E., & Iweala, E. J. (2023). Ethnomedicinal uses, nutritional composition, phytochemistry, and potential health benefits of Carica papaya. Pharmacological Research. Modern Chinese Medicine, 7, 100266. doi:10.1016/j.prmcm.2023.100266DOI: 10.1016/j.prmcm.2023.100266

Ugwuibe, C. O., Onah, F. N., & Olise, C. N. (2021). Flood disasters in Aba North Local Government Area of Abia State, Nigeria: Policy options. In Economic effects of natural disasters (pp. 373-380). Academic Press. https://doi.org/doi:10.1016/B978-0-12-817465-4.00023-6DOI: 10.1016/B978-0-12-817465-4.00023-6

Umoh, U. F., Thomas, P. S., Essien, E. E., Okokon, J. E., De Leo, M., Ajibesin, K. K., Flamini, G., & Eseyin, O. A. (2021). Isolation and characterization of bioactive xanthones from Hippocratea africana (Willd.)Loes.ex Engl. (Celastraceae). Journal of Ethnopharmacology, 280, 114031. doi:10.1016/j.jep.2021.114031 PubMedDOI: 10.1016/j.jep.2021.114031 PMID: 33737141

Van Andel, T., Onselen, S. B., Myren, B., Towns, A., & Quiroz, D. (2015). "The medicine from behind": The frequent use of enemas in Western African traditional medicine. Journal of Ethnopharmacology, 174, 637–643. doi:10.1016/j.jep.2015.06.040 PubMedDOI: 10.1016/j.jep.2015.06.040 PMID: 26133063

Visser, B. J., van Vugt, M., & Grobusch, M. P. (2014). Malaria: An update on current chemotherapy. Expert Opinion on Pharmacotherapy, 15(15), 2219–2254. doi:10.1517/14656566.2014.944499 PubMedDOI: 10.1517/14656566.2014.944499 PMID: 25110058

Vitale, S., Colanero, S., Placidi, M., Di Emidio, G., Tatone, C., Amicarelli, F., & D'Alessandro, A. M. (2022). Phytochemistry and biological activity of medicinal plants in wound healing: An overview of current research. Molecules (Basel, Switzerland), 27(11), 3566. doi:10.3390/molecules27113566 PubMedDOI: 10.3390/molecules27113566 PMID: 35684503

WHO. Fact sheet N°134, (2008), https://www.who.int/mediacentre/factsheets/2003/fs134/en/

WHO. (2019). WHO global report on traditional and complementary medicine. https://www.who.int/publications/i/item/978924151536

WHO. (2022). Report on Malaria in Nigeria 2022. Pp 195. ISBN: 978-929023498-2

WHO. World Malaria Report (2023). Geneva, World Health Organization, 2023. https://www.who.int/teams/global-malaria-programme/reports/world-malaria-report-2023. Accessed: January 8, 2024.

World Health Organization. (2002). WHO traditional medicine strategy 2002-2005. In the WHO traditional medicine strategy 2002-2005 (pp. 61-61).

Chapter 7
AI and Computational Chemistry in Phytochemical Drug Discovery

P. Selvakumar
https://orcid.org/0000-0002-3650-4548
Department of Science and Humanities, Nehru Institute of Technology, Coimbatore, India

T.C. Manjunath
https://orcid.org/0000-0003-2545-9160
Rajarajeswari College of Engineering, Bangalore, India

R. Mythili
SRM Institute of Science and Technology, Chennai, India

ABSTRACT

The landscape of modern drug discovery is undergoing a paradigm shift, with computational tools at the forefront of transforming the way new therapeutics are identified, developed, and optimized. Traditional methods of drug discovery, often reliant on serendipity and lengthy experimental trials, are being revolutionized by the integration of computational approaches such as artificial intelligence (AI), machine learning (ML), and computational chemistry. These technologies not only enhance efficiency and accuracy but also open previously inaccessible avenues in biomedical research. Computational methods are enabling researchers to process vast and complex datasets, model intricate biological systems, predict molecular interactions, and accelerate the identification of novel drug candidates with un-

DOI: 10.4018/979-8-3373-5821-5.ch007

precedented precision. In this context, computational tools are not just auxiliary assets—they are becoming indispensable engines of innovation in pharmaceutical sciences.

INTRODUCTION

The landscape of modern drug discovery is undergoing a paradigm shift, with computational tools at the forefront of transforming the way new therapeutics are identified, developed, and optimized. Traditional methods of drug discovery, often reliant on serendipity and lengthy experimental trials, are being revolutionized by the integration of computational approaches such as artificial intelligence (AI), machine learning (ML), and computational chemistry. These technologies not only enhance efficiency and accuracy but also open previously inaccessible avenues in biomedical research. Computational methods are enabling researchers to process vast and complex datasets, model intricate biological systems, predict molecular interactions, and accelerate the identification of novel drug candidates with unprecedented precision. In this context, computational tools are not just auxiliary assets—they are becoming indispensable engines of innovation in pharmaceutical sciences. One of the most compelling developments in this digital revolution is the convergence of computational technologies with traditional medicine, particularly phytochemistry—the study of bioactive compounds derived from plants. Historically, natural products, especially phytochemicals, have been a rich source of therapeutic agents. Compounds such as paclitaxel, artemisinin, and morphine exemplify the profound medical value embedded in nature. However, the process of isolating, characterizing, and optimizing these compounds has traditionally been time-intensive and resource-demanding. Today, computational tools are bridging this gap by digitizing ethnobotanical knowledge, systematizing phytochemical databases, and modeling biological interactions in silico. This allows researchers to screen thousands of natural compounds against disease targets, predict their pharmacokinetic and toxicological properties, and even suggest structural modifications to enhance efficacy and safety—all before a single compound is synthesized or tested in vitro.

Artificial intelligence, particularly machine learning and deep learning algorithms, plays a pivotal role in this transformation. These technologies excel in recognizing patterns, analyzing high-dimensional data, and making predictive models based on training datasets derived from experimental or clinical studies. In drug discovery, AI can be deployed to identify target proteins, classify disease types, suggest lead compounds, and even forecast the clinical success of candidate molecules(Abbas, 2024). When applied to phytochemical research, AI can integrate data from diverse sources—traditional medicinal texts, ethnobotanical surveys, genomic repositories, chemical structure databases—and derive actionable insights for drug development. For instance, neural networks can predict the biological activity of a phytochemical based on its molecular structure, while reinforcement learning algorithms can iteratively improve compound design based on predefined therapeutic goals. Computational chemistry complements AI by providing the theoretical and simulation-based framework to understand molecular interactions at atomic and subatomic levels. Tools such as molecular docking, molecular dynamics simulations, quantum mechanics/molecular mechanics (QM/MM) models, and density functional theory (DFT) calculations allow researchers to visualize and quantify the binding affinity, conformational stability, and reactivity of drug candidates. These methods are particularly useful in studying phytochemicals, which often exhibit complex structures with multiple stereocenters, diverse functional groups, and non-linear conformations. Through computational modeling, researchers can explore the pharmacophoric features of these compounds, assess their interaction with specific protein targets, and estimate ADMET (Absorption, Distribution, Metabolism, Excretion, and Toxicity) profiles with remarkable accuracy.

Furthermore, the integration of omics technologies—such as genomics, transcriptomics, proteomics, and metabolomics—into computational workflows has enriched phytochemical research by enabling a systems-level understanding of plant-derived compounds. With the help of bioinformatics tools, scientists can correlate the presence of specific phytochemicals with gene expression patterns, protein-protein interaction networks, and metabolic pathways involved in disease pathophysiology(Amit Kadan et al., 2024). Importantly, computational tools also offer a platform for preserving and validating traditional medicinal knowledge, which is often orally transmitted and at risk of being lost(Arora et al., 2024). By digitizing and systematizing this information, AI and machine learning can identify patterns and correlations that are not readily apparent through anecdotal evidence. For example, AI can reveal which plant species are commonly used for similar ailments across different cultures, suggesting a shared pharmacological basis that merits further investigation. This approach not only validates the therapeutic potential of traditional remedies but also respects and preserves the cultural heritage of indigenous communities, fostering a more inclusive and ethical framework for drug discovery. Moreover, the growing field of explainable AI (XAI) enhances the interpretability and trustworthiness of machine learning models in drug discovery. Unlike traditional "black-box" algorithms, XAI models can provide human-understandable rationales for their predictions—explaining, for instance, why a certain phytochemical is predicted to bind strongly to a cancer-related receptor. This transparency is crucial in regulatory settings, clinical applications, and multidisciplinary collaborations, where understanding the logic behind predictions can inform experimental design, guide ethical decision-making, and build stakeholder confidence.

Interdisciplinary collaboration is another cornerstone of this digital transformation. The fusion of botany, pharmacology, data science, bioinformatics, and chemistry fosters a holistic approach to drug discovery that leverages the strengths of each domain. Pharmacognosists contribute knowledge of medicinal plants; computational chemists model molecular behavior; AI specialists develop predictive algorithms; and clinicians provide insights into disease mechanisms and patient needs(Beccari & Vistoli, 2022). This synergy accelerates the translation of phytochemicals from traditional uses to validated therapeutics, embodying a true bench-to-bedside approach. In addition, regulatory bodies and academic institutions are increasingly recognizing the value of computational approaches in phytochemical drug development. Regulatory science is evolving to accommodate data-driven submissions, virtual screening data, and in silico toxicity models. Academic curricula are incorporating bioinformatics and computational chemistry modules, equipping the next generation of scientists with the skills needed to thrive in this hybrid landscape of tradition and technology. To conclude, the integration of computational tools in modern drug discovery represents a transformative shift in the biomedical sciences. In the realm of phytochemical research, it bridges centuries-old traditional medicine with the cutting-edge capabilities of AI and computational chemistry. This convergence not only accelerates the discovery of novel therapeutics but also ensures that natural products—once limited by empirical methods—can be explored, validated, and optimized with scientific rigor and digital precision. As computational power continues to grow and datasets become richer, the role of AI and computational methods in unlocking the therapeutic potential of nature will only expand, heralding a new era of holistic, efficient, and ethically grounded drug discovery.

Phytochemical Libraries and Data Curation

In the digital age of pharmaceutical innovation, the creation and maintenance of phytochemical libraries—comprehensive digital repositories of plant-derived compounds—have become a cornerstone in natural product research and modern drug discovery. These libraries serve as structured databases containing the chemical structures, biological activities, pharmacokinetic properties, and ethnomedicinal uses of phytochemicals sourced from plants across diverse geographical and cultural backgrounds. Phytochemical libraries play a dual role: they preserve centuries-old ethnopharmacological wisdom and simultaneously render it accessible for high-throughput computational modeling, virtual screening, and artificial intelligence (AI)-driven drug design. By digitizing the immense molecular diversity found in nature, particularly within medicinal plants, researchers can systematize, analyze, and exploit this resource using modern computational tools, accelerating the transition from traditional remedies to scientifically validated therapeutics. The construction of these repositories is rooted in decades of botanical surveys, phytochemical isolation, and empirical medicinal practice. However, unlike synthetic compound libraries, which are typically generated in controlled laboratory settings with standard formats and descriptors, phytochemical libraries must capture the natural heterogeneity of plant secondary metabolites—terpenoids, flavonoids, alkaloids, lignans, polyphenols, and more(Boldini et al., 2024). These compounds are structurally diverse, biologically potent, and often difficult to synthesize artificially, making their digital documentation all the more valuable. With this in mind, numerous curated databases have emerged to centralize and organize this information, offering a vital bridge between traditional medicine and digital bioinformatics platforms.

One of the most notable examples is NPASS (Natural Product Activity and Species Source Database), a publicly accessible database that catalogs over 35,000 natural compounds with experimentally verified biological activity. NPASS not only documents molecular structures and source species but also links compounds to quantitative bioactivity data (e.g., IC_{50}, EC_{50} values) and targets(Chen & Kirchmair, 2020). This makes it particularly suitable for machine learning algorithms and virtual screening applications, which require high-quality, annotated data for training predictive models. NPASS stands out for its comprehensive cross-referencing with other databases like PubChem, ChEMBL, and BindingDB, enabling broader integrative analyses and compound-target interaction predictions. AfroDb is another specialized resource that focuses on the vast phytochemical diversity of Africa's medicinal flora. It compiles around 1,000 natural products derived from African medicinal plants, including structural, physicochemical, and pharmacokinetic descriptors. What makes AfroDb unique is its regional specificity—tailoring its content to an underrepresented yet pharmaceutically rich continent. This empowers African scientists and pharmacognosists to explore indigenous plants with new technological tools and fosters inclusive drug discovery that respects biodiversity and cultural knowledge.

IMPPAT (Indian Medicinal Plants, Phytochemistry And Therapeutics) is a critically important database dedicated to the Indian ethnopharmacological tradition. It curates data on over 1,700 Indian medicinal plants, approximately 10,000 phytochemicals, and 1,100 therapeutic uses. IMPPAT is structured to support computational workflows by including chemical structure files (e.g., SMILES, InChI), molecular descriptors, and drug-likeness evaluations based on Lipinski's Rule of Five and ADMET profiles. This database is invaluable for researchers investigating Ayurveda-inspired compounds and serves as a key resource for AI-driven drug repurposing, QSAR (Quantitative Structure–Activity Relationship) modeling, and molecular docking studies. Other noteworthy databases include TCM-Mesh (Traditional Chinese Medicine database for mechanism-oriented research), NAPRALERT (Natural Products Alert), Dr. Duke's Phytochemical and Ethnobotanical Databases, and SuperNatural II, each contributing to a global effort to digitize and centralize natural product data. These repositories differ in focus—some emphasize pharmacological data, others prioritize structural diversity, and still others catalog ethnobotanical uses. Yet, they all converge on a common objective: to make phytochemical data searchable, interoperable, and computable(Chihomvu et al., 2024). However, these NLP models must be context-aware and sensitive to cultural semantics to avoid misinterpretation or over-simplification (Choudhury, Murugan & Priyakumar, 2022).

Figure 1. Artificial intelligence for antiviral drug discovery

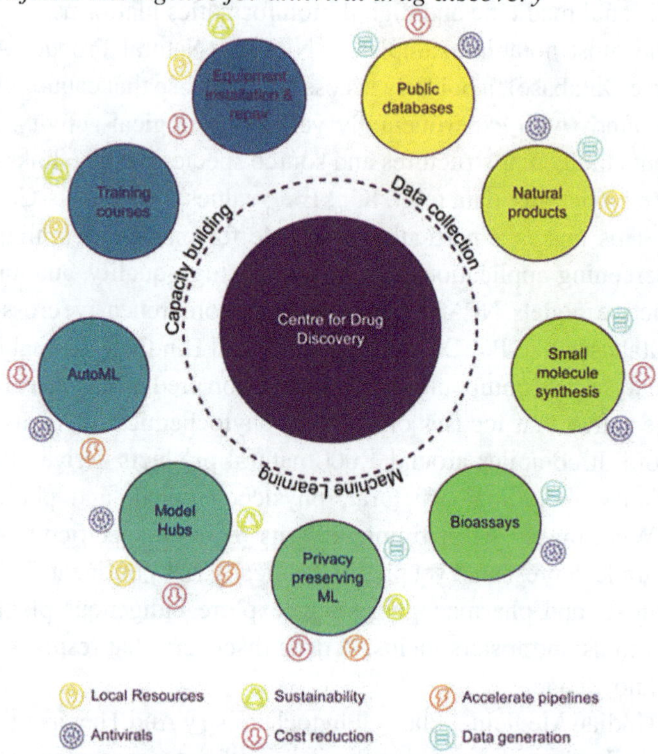

Additionally, linking phytochemical data to biological targets remains a formidable task. While some natural products have well-characterized mechanisms of action, many others lack experimental target annotations. Computational approaches such as target fishing, inverse docking, and proteochemometric modeling are increasingly used to infer likely targets based on structural similarity, binding pocket predictions, and bioactivity profiles. Integration with omics data, protein interaction networks, and pathway databases like KEGG or Reactome allows for a systems pharmacology view of phytochemical effects—crucial for understanding polypharmacology and potential side effects. Moreover, intellectual property (IP) rights and benefit-sharing must be ethically managed during data curation. Many indigenous communities have historically been excluded from the commercialization of their traditional knowledge. Therefore, efforts to digitize and use such knowledge in drug discovery must include frameworks for ethical sourcing, consent, benefit-sharing, and acknowledgment of knowledge holders. Initiatives like the Nagoya Protocol advocate for the equitable sharing of benefits arising from the utilization of genetic resources and associated traditional knowledge, guiding how data should be collected and shared responsibly. In conclusion, phytochemical libraries and data curation are pivotal components of the evolving intersection between traditional medicine and modern computational drug discovery. Through the meticulous aggregation, validation, and digitization of natural product data, these repositories empower AI and bioinformatics tools to harness the therapeutic potential of nature with scientific precision and scale(Dara et al., 2022). Despite the inherent challenges in standardizing and interpreting traditional knowledge, ongoing advancements in NLP, taxonomy reconciliation, cheminformatics, and ethical data governance are enhancing the quality, usability, and inclusivity of these digital resources. As a result, phytochemical libraries are not merely data repositories—they are living bridges connecting ancient wisdom with contemporary biomedical science, fueling the next generation of plant-based therapeutics.

Molecular Docking and Virtual Screening

In the evolving landscape of drug discovery, molecular docking and virtual screening have emerged as essential computational techniques that leverage structural biology and cheminformatics to identify novel drug candidates with high precision and reduced cost. Rooted in the principles of structure-based drug design (SBDD), these methodologies facilitate the prediction of how small molecules (ligands) interact with biological macromolecules (typically proteins), enabling rational lead identification and optimization. Unlike traditional high-throughput screening that relies on experimental assays to test thousands of compounds, virtual screening uses computer-aided models to prioritize candidates for experimental validation, thereby saving time, resources, and labor. Within the context of antimalarial drug discovery, these tools are particularly invaluable given the urgent need to combat emerging drug-resistant strains of Plasmodium falciparum—the most lethal species of malaria-causing parasites(Dou et al., 2023). The core principle of molecular docking involves predicting the optimal binding orientation, conformation, and affinity of a ligand within the active site of a biological target, typically a protein receptor or enzyme. This process is underpinned by biophysical theories of molecular recognition, including hydrogen bonding, hydrophobic interactions, electrostatics, and van der Waals forces. The success of a docking simulation depends on the accuracy of the protein structure (experimental or modeled), the chemical representation of the ligand, and the computational scoring function that ranks potential binding modes. When scaled to large compound libraries, docking becomes part of virtual screening, allowing researchers to scan hundreds of thousands of molecules against a single or multiple targets to identify high-probability binders—termed "hits"—that warrant further investigation.

Molecular Dynamics (MD) Simulations

A fundamental prerequisite for effective docking and virtual screening is the careful selection of druggable targets, which in the case of Plasmodium parasites, includes enzymes and proteins that are essential for parasite survival, replication, or transmission. Several validated and emerging molecular targets in Plasmodium falciparum are widely studied: Dihydrofolate reductase (DHFR): A key enzyme in the folate biosynthesis pathway, DHFR is crucial for DNA synthesis and cell replication. Resistance mutations in DHFR are a primary cause of resistance to antifolate drugs like pyrimethamine. Consequently, docking studies targeting both wild-type and mutant DHFR have been instrumental in designing new antifolates with improved binding affinity and resistance-evasion capabilities. PfATP6: This is the P. falciparum homolog of the sarco/endoplasmic reticulum Ca^{2+}-ATPase (SERCA). It is hypothesized to be the primary target of artemisinin, a frontline antimalarial. Molecular docking against PfATP6 is often used to study the binding of artemisinin derivatives and to design novel inhibitors that mimic or enhance its mechanism of action. Falcipains (especially falcipain-2 and falcipain-3): These are cysteine proteases involved in hemoglobin degradation during the parasite's erythrocytic stage. Inhibiting falcipains disrupts the parasite's nutrient acquisition process, making them attractive targets for antimalarial compounds. Molecular docking facilitates the identification of specific inhibitors that bind to the active or allosteric sites of falcipains, with selectivity over human homologs(Fromer & Coley, 2024). The workflow of a molecular docking and virtual screening campaign typically involves a series of integrated computational steps, beginning with ligand preparation. This stage involves assembling a virtual library of candidate compounds from in-house collections, commercial databases (e.g., ZINC, ChemDiv), or natural product repositories (e.g., NPASS, IMPPAT). These molecules undergo energy minimization, protonation state assignment (e.g., using Epik or OpenBabel), tautomer enumeration, and stereoisomer generation to ensure accurate and chemically realistic input for docking. Additionally, compounds may be filtered based on Lipinski's Rule of

Five and other drug-likeness or ADMET (Absorption, Distribution, Metabolism, Excretion, and Toxicity) parameters to improve hit quality.

However, scoring functions are often approximate and may yield false positives or negatives. As a result, post-docking refinement steps—such as molecular dynamics (MD) simulations, MM-GBSA/MM-PBSA free energy calculations, or consensus scoring across multiple docking platforms—are often employed to enhance prediction reliability (Gangwal et al., 2024a). The final step involves hit identification, where top-ranked ligands are subjected to in silico validation. This approach has led to the identification of unexpected antimalarial activity in molecules originally designed for cancer, inflammation, or cardiovascular conditions(Gangwal et al., 2024b). Virtual screening of such libraries can yield fast-tracked drug leads with known safety profiles, greatly accelerating the development pipeline. Despite its many strengths, molecular docking is not without limitations. Protein flexibility, solvation effects, entropic contributions, and induced fit phenomena are often inadequately captured by static docking protocols. This can lead to overestimation or underestimation of binding affinity. To mitigate this, hybrid approaches combining docking with MD simulations, free energy perturbation (FEP), or AI-driven scoring are increasingly employed.

Pharmacophore Modeling and QSAR Studies

In the computational drug discovery pipeline, pharmacophore modeling and quantitative structure–activity relationship (QSAR) studies represent two cornerstone techniques for rationalizing and accelerating the identification of bioactive molecules, particularly in the context of antimalarial drug development. These ligand-based strategies are invaluable when structural data of biological targets are unavailable or incomplete, allowing researchers to extrapolate the essential chemical features and quantitative descriptors required for biological activity based solely on compound libraries and experimental data. As malaria continues to pose a global health threat—compounded by the rise of resistance to frontline therapies like artemisinin—the ability to harness computational models for predicting activity of novel, structurally diverse compounds, including phytochemicals, has become a critical facet of modern research. Pharmacophore modeling involves the identification of a 3D arrangement of molecular features that are necessary for a compound to interact with a specific biological target. These features typically include hydrogen bond donors and acceptors, hydrophobic regions, aromatic rings, and charged or ionizable groups(Gorantla et al., 2024). A pharmacophore hypothesis is typically generated from a set of known active compounds (training set) by aligning their structures and identifying common spatial features associated with activity. In antimalarial drug discovery, pharmacophore models have been developed for a range of validated targets including dihydrofolate reductase (DHFR), falcipain-2, plasmepsins, and PfATP6, even when the crystal structure of the protein is unavailable or unreliable. Tools such as LigandScout, PHASE (Schrödinger), Discovery Studio, and MOE are widely employed to generate and validate pharmacophore hypotheses. These tools align a training set of known inhibitors and define consensus pharmacophoric elements which are then used as 3D queries to screen compound libraries for novel candidates that fulfill the same interaction pattern.

Following pharmacophore screening, QSAR modeling provides a complementary, quantitative approach to predict biological activity. QSAR models establish mathematical relationships between the molecular descriptors of compounds (e.g., electronic, topological, steric, hydrophobic properties) and their experimentally measured biological activities, such as IC_{50} or EC_{50} values. The success of a QSAR model depends heavily on the quality of the dataset, the selection of relevant descriptors, and the modeling algorithm employed. Common descriptor types include constitutional descriptors (e.g., number of atoms, molecular weight), topological indices (e.g., Wiener index, Kier–Hall index), electronic descriptors (e.g., HOMO–LUMO gap, partial charges), and physicochemical properties (e.g., logP, polar surface area). Software packages such as QSARINS, MOE, KNIME, Dragon, PaDEL, and ADMET Predictor enable descriptor calculation, feature selection, model building, and validation using techniques such as multiple linear regression (MLR), partial least squares (PLS), support vector machines (SVM), random forest (RF), and artificial neural networks (ANNs). In antimalarial research, QSAR models have been successfully applied to numerous compound classes, including 4-aminoquinolines, trioxanes, and chalcones, predicting their inhibitory activities against both sensitive and resistant Plasmodium falciparum strains. Notably, QSAR has proven effective even in scenarios where structural data for the target protein is unavailable, enabling early-stage prioritization of hits from high-throughput screening or ethnopharmacological studies(Gu et al., 2024).

A standard QSAR workflow begins with data collection and curation, where compound activity data is gathered from literature, databases (e.g., ChEMBL, PubChem BioAssay, BindingDB), or in-house assays. Data preprocessing involves removing duplicates, standardizing structures, and correcting inconsistencies in activity units. Descriptor calculation is followed by feature selection, often using genetic algorithms, principal component analysis (PCA), or recursive feature elimination to reduce dimensionality and enhance model interpretability. The model is then trained and validated using cross-validation techniques (e.g., leave-one-out, k-fold), and its predictive power is assessed through statistical metrics such as R^2 (coefficient of determination), Q^2 (cross-validated R^2), RMSE (root mean square error), and MAE (mean absolute error). An externally validated QSAR model can then be used to predict the activity of untested phytochemicals, guiding selection for experimental validation. When combined, pharmacophore modeling and QSAR studies provide a synergistic strategy for antimalarial drug discovery. Pharmacophore modeling acts as a qualitative filter, ensuring that molecules possess the spatial and functional prerequisites for target engagement, while QSAR offers a quantitative prediction of potency based on statistical models. This dual approach enables the efficient prioritization of compounds for synthesis or testing, particularly in resource-constrained environments where experimental validation must be highly focused. In integrated platforms, pharmacophore hits are passed through QSAR filters, or vice versa, to identify leads with both favorable interaction profiles and predicted bioactivity(Horne et al., 2024). Furthermore, machine learning advancements are enhancing both pharmacophore modeling and QSAR. In conclusion, pharmacophore modeling and QSAR studies offer powerful, complementary approaches for rational antimalarial drug discovery, particularly when targeting structurally diverse phytochemicals(Hubballi et al., 2025). These techniques enable the efficient extraction of biologically relevant features, prediction of compound efficacy, and prioritization of leads for experimental testing.

Machine Learning and Deep Learning in Lead Optimization

The process of lead optimization is a critical phase in drug discovery wherein promising hit compounds are refined to enhance their pharmacological efficacy, safety, and drug-like properties. In recent years, machine learning (ML) and deep learning (DL) approaches have revolutionized this phase by enabling the rapid and accurate prediction of biological activity, ADMET properties (Absorption, Distribution, Metabolism, Excretion, and Toxicity), and other relevant pharmacokinetic and pharmacodynamic parameters. These models serve as computational filters and predictive engines, guiding medicinal chemists in the strategic selection and structural optimization of candidate molecules, particularly from large and diverse phytochemical libraries(Wang et al., 2024). This is especially valuable in natural product-based drug discovery, where the chemical diversity and complexity of plant-derived compounds often make exhaustive in vitro and in vivo screening impractical. ML and DL models learn from historical bioactivity and physicochemical data to generate predictive functions that map chemical structure to biological effect. These models utilize various types of molecular descriptors (e.g., topological indices, physicochemical properties, fingerprints) as input features, with outputs typically being numerical values (e.g., IC_{50}) or categorical labels (e.g., active/inactive, toxic/nontoxic). In lead optimization, such models are trained to assess a compound's potential to bind to specific targets (e.g., Plasmodium falciparum enzymes like PfDHFR, PfATP6, or falcipains), predict off-target effects, or flag ADMET liabilities. Popular algorithms include support vector machines (SVM), random forests

(RF), k-nearest neighbors (k-NN), Naïve Bayes, gradient boosting machines (e.g., XGBoost, LightGBM), and deep neural networks (DNNs). Deep learning models, especially graph convolutional networks (GCNs) and recurrent neural networks (RNNs), are particularly adept at learning complex nonlinear patterns and handling high-dimensional data without the need for manual feature engineering.

The selection of an appropriate algorithm and training dataset is crucial for model performance. High-quality, diverse, and well-annotated datasets are essential. Public repositories like ChEMBL, PubChem BioAssay, BindingDB, and DrugBank, as well as specialized natural product databases like NPASS, AfroDb, and IMPPAT, provide rich sources of training data. In addition, proprietary data from laboratory experiments or collaborative research initiatives can be used to build custom models tailored to specific targets or compound classes. Preprocessing steps typically include data cleaning, normalization, descriptor calculation, feature selection or dimensionality reduction (e.g., using PCA or recursive feature elimination), and splitting into training, validation, and test sets. Data imbalance (e.g., few active vs. many inactive compounds) is often addressed using techniques like SMOTE (Synthetic Minority Over-sampling Technique) or cost-sensitive learning. Case studies highlight the tangible benefits of AI-driven approaches in lead optimization (Kao et al., 2022). For instance, ML-based models have been used to optimize derivatives of artemisinin, chalcones, and flavonoids, improving their efficacy against both chloroquine-sensitive and resistant Plasmodium strains. In one study, random forest classifiers were trained on bioactivity data of flavonoids and used to predict novel antimalarial analogs with favorable binding to PfATP6. Another investigation employed deep learning to model the ADMET profiles of terpenoid derivatives, revealing candidates with significantly reduced hepatotoxicity and improved bioavailability. Moreover, ensemble learning models that combine multiple base algorithms (e.g., RF + SVM + DNN) often outperform individual models by capturing complementary information. Hybrid models that integrate ligand-based features with structure-based docking scores further improve prediction accuracy and reliability, creating a multidimensional framework for lead refinement.

Another innovative strategy involves the use of generative models like variational autoencoders (VAEs) and generative adversarial networks (GANs) to design novel compounds with optimized properties. These models learn latent representations of molecular structures and can generate new, synthetically accessible analogs of known phytochemicals, expanding the chemical space explored during lead optimization. Reinforcement learning (RL)-based methods can also be employed to iteratively modify compounds to maximize predicted activity or ADMET desirability, using scoring functions derived from ML models. Interpretability of ML models has also advanced with the adoption of explainable AI (XAI) techniques. Tools such as SHAP (Shapley Additive Explanations), LIME (Local Interpretable Model-Agnostic

Explanations), and counterfactual analysis help identify which features (e.g., specific functional groups, substructures) are most influential in predicting activity or toxicity. This not only enhances the trustworthiness of predictions but also provides actionable insights for medicinal chemists, guiding rational structural modifications. In the specific context of phytochemical lead optimization, machine learning offers several key advantages. Firstly, it compensates for the scarcity of high-throughput experimental data by extrapolating from limited known actives. Secondly, it enables prioritization of compounds based on multi-objective optimization—maximizing efficacy while minimizing toxicity and enhancing drug-likeness(Keith et al., 2021). Thirdly, it supports de novo design, helping to scaffold-hop from natural products to novel derivatives with improved synthetic tractability. Furthermore, the ability of deep learning models to learn from raw molecular graphs means that even stereochemically complex phytochemicals—often challenging for traditional descriptor-based methods—can be effectively modeled.

Real-world examples demonstrate that AI-assisted lead optimization can reduce the time and cost of antimalarial drug development. For example, a collaborative study between an academic lab and a biotech startup used an ensemble of SVM and RF models trained on antimalarial screening data to identify 20 prioritized compounds from over 10,000 phytochemicals. Of these, five showed sub-micromolar activity against P. falciparum and acceptable in vitro ADMET profiles, validating the model predictions. Such studies exemplify the capacity of AI to act as a force multiplier in natural product-based drug discovery efforts. Importantly, integration with multi-omics data—such as transcriptomics, proteomics, and metabolomics—can further refine ML-driven optimization. For instance, correlating compound activity with Plasmodium gene expression profiles or metabolic signatures may uncover context-specific vulnerabilities, enabling the design of precision antimalarials. In such systems-level approaches, machine learning models serve as integrative frameworks that synthesize heterogeneous data to reveal actionable patterns and guide compound development. Despite these advances, challenges remain(Kotte, Attaluri & Selvakumar, 2025). Model generalizability to novel chemical scaffolds is a persistent issue, especially for natural products with underrepresented structural motifs. Biases in training data, lack of experimental validation, and insufficient representation of ADMET endpoints (e.g., transporter interactions, chronic toxicity) can limit the utility of predictions. Addressing these issues requires ongoing curation of high-quality datasets, the development of transfer learning frameworks that adapt pre-trained models to new data domains, and the incorporation of active learning strategies, wherein models iteratively query for the most informative new data points to improve their predictions. In conclusion, machine learning and deep learning are redefining the landscape of lead optimization in phytochemical-based antimalarial drug discovery. Through accurate prediction of bioactivity and ADMET properties, intelligent compound selection, and automated design of novel analogs, these computational approaches dramatically accelerate the path from hit to lead to candidate drug. As these technologies continue to evolve—driven by algorithmic innovation, expanding datasets, and interdisciplinary collaboration—their role in delivering safe, effective, and affordable antimalarial agents from nature's bounty will only deepen, offering transformative potential in the global fight against malaria.

Molecular Dynamics (MD) Simulations

Molecular Dynamics (MD) simulations have emerged as a cornerstone of modern computational drug discovery, offering a detailed, atomistic view of biomolecular systems over time. Unlike static methods such as molecular docking, which provide a snapshot of ligand–receptor interactions, MD simulations capture the full dynamism of molecular interactions, accounting for atomic motion, solvent effects, temperature, and pressure. This time-dependent modeling enables researchers to observe the stability of ligand–protein complexes, monitor conformational changes in proteins, evaluate binding affinities, and identify crucial molecular determinants of biological activity(Maheswaran et al., 2025). In the context of phytochemical-based drug discovery, particularly against challenging targets like Plasmodium falciparum proteins involved in malaria, MD simulations provide critical insights into the real-world behavior of promising compounds identified through virtual screening or docking studies. The core principle of MD simulation is rooted in classical mechanics, where Newton's equations of motion are applied iteratively to all atoms in a system. Each atom is treated as a particle with defined mass, velocity, and position, and their trajectories are calculated based on the forces derived from empirical force fields. The most commonly used force fields include AMBER, CHARMM, GROMOS, and OPLS, each parameterized for biomolecules like proteins, nucleic acids, lipids, and small molecules. During simulation, atoms interact through bonded (bond, angle, dihedral) and non-bonded (van der Waals, electrostatics) forces, and their behavior is recorded over femtosecond (fs) time steps for durations ranging from nanoseconds (ns) to microseconds (μs) or longer. The trajectory data generated is subsequently analyzed to assess the stability and behavior of the molecular system.

One of the key applications of MD simulations in drug discovery is the refinement of molecular docking results. While docking provides an initial estimate of how a ligand might bind to a protein active site, it often neglects protein flexibility, water molecules, and long-range electrostatics. MD simulations bridge this gap by allowing the protein and ligand to adapt to each other dynamically, thereby validating and potentially improving upon the docked pose. During the simulation, root mean square deviation (RMSD) and root mean square fluctuation (RMSF) metrics are commonly employed to assess structural stability and atomic mobility, respectively. A stable RMSD value over time indicates a well-converged system, while RMSF can identify flexible regions of the protein, such as loops or binding pockets. Another important output of MD simulations is the radius of gyration (Rg), which reflects the compactness of the protein structure, and hydrogen bond analysis, which quantifies the number and persistence of hydrogen bonds between the ligand and the protein. Persistent hydrogen bonding is often indicative of strong ligand binding and contributes significantly to overall affinity. Solvent-accessible surface area (SASA) analysis helps to assess ligand exposure and potential interaction with the aqueous environment(Min et al., 2024). Moreover, interaction energy calculations, such as molecular mechanics Poisson–Boltzmann surface area (MM-PBSA) and molecular mechanics generalized Born surface area (MM-GBSA), are employed post-simulation to estimate the binding free energy of the ligand–protein complex. These methods combine molecular mechanics energy terms with solvation and entropy contributions to yield a more accurate estimate of binding affinity, which can be compared across multiple ligands for prioritization.

In the specific context of Plasmodium enzymes like PfDHFR, PfATP6, falcipains, and Plasmepsins, MD simulations have provided valuable insights into the mechanism of inhibition by phytochemicals. For example, simulations of quercetin binding to PfATP6 revealed that the ligand forms a stable hydrogen bond network with key residues like Glu255 and Phe256, maintaining a consistent binding mode over 100 ns. Similarly, simulations of curcumin analogs against falcipain-2 demonstrated conformational shifts in the active site loop that enhanced ligand accommodation. Such analyses not only confirm binding site compatibility but also elucidate induced-fit effects and allosteric interactions, which are difficult to capture through docking alone. MD simulations also facilitate the identification of allosteric sites and transient pockets that may not be visible in crystallographic structures. These cryptic sites can be exploited for novel mechanism-of-action drugs, offering an opportunity for phytochemical scaffolds to act in unique and synergistic ways. For instance, simulations of artemisinin derivatives have shown that they may bind preferentially to flexible regions of PfATP6, suggesting allosteric modulation. Such findings are vital for overcoming drug resistance—a major hurdle in antimalarial therapy—by designing inhibitors that avoid common resistance-conferring mutations. The implementation of MD simulations relies heavily on sophisticated software tools. GROMACS is one of the most widely used MD packages, known for its speed and versatility, supporting GPU acceleration and a variety of force fields. It is particularly suited for biomolecular systems and includes tools for extensive post-simulation analysis. AMBER, originally developed for simulating proteins and nucleic acids, offers high-accuracy force fields and supports advanced techniques like replica exchange MD and constant pH simulations. NAMD, designed for high-performance parallel computing, is ideal for large-scale simulations and long timescales(Moshawih,

2022). All these platforms interface with molecular visualization tools such as VMD, PyMOL, and Chimera, allowing researchers to visually inspect trajectories, analyze interactions, and generate publication-quality graphics.

The success of MD simulations depends not only on software and force field selection but also on rigorous system preparation. This includes protein structure optimization (e.g., adding missing atoms/residues, assigning protonation states), ligand parameterization using tools like Antechamber, ACPYPE, or CGenFF, solvation in explicit water models (e.g., TIP3P), and neutralization with appropriate counterions. Equilibration stages—typically including energy minimization, heating, and pressure equilibration—are crucial to ensure the system is free from steric clashes and thermal instability before production runs begin. The duration of the production simulation depends on the system's complexity and the phenomena being studied; for ligand binding stability, 100–200 ns is commonly sufficient, while conformational transitions may require microsecond-scale simulations. Recent advances in MD methodologies further enhance the depth and breadth of insight. Enhanced sampling techniques such as metadynamics, accelerated MD, and replica exchange allow for the exploration of rare events and large conformational changes that may not be accessible on standard simulation timescales. Coarse-grained MD models simplify the system by grouping atoms into pseudo-particles, enabling the simulation of very large systems or longer durations at the cost of atomic detail. AI-assisted MD simulations—where machine learning is used to predict regions of interest or guide adaptive sampling—are emerging as powerful tools to increase efficiency and focus computational resources where they matter most. In phytochemical research, MD simulations also support structure–activity relationship (SAR) studies by validating hypotheses about critical binding interactions(Nahal et al., 2024). For example, if a certain hydroxyl group on a flavonoid is thought to enhance activity, MD can reveal whether this group forms stable interactions during simulation or merely increases polar surface area without real binding contribution. This can inform synthetic derivatization efforts and guide the rational design of improved analogs. Furthermore, in multi-target drug design, MD can help assess how a single phytochemical interacts with multiple Plasmodium proteins, identifying potential polypharmacological effects.

While MD simulations are powerful, they are computationally intensive and require high-performance computing infrastructure. Cloud-based platforms and GPU-accelerated clusters have made simulations more accessible, but proper parameterization, validation, and interpretation of results still demand expertise. Moreover, care must be taken to avoid overinterpreting short simulations or assuming that stability equates to efficacy without supporting experimental validation. In conclusion, Molecular Dynamics simulations provide an indispensable bridge between molecular modeling and experimental biology, enabling detailed exploration of ligand–receptor interactions over time. Their application in antimalarial phytochemical research allows for a deeper understanding of how natural compounds engage with essential Plasmodium targets, informs lead optimization, and supports the discovery of novel mechanisms of action. As computational power continues to grow and simulation methods become more sophisticated, MD simulations will play an ever-increasing role in rational drug design, accelerating the development of effective, safe, and resistance-resilient antimalarial therapies derived from the rich biodiversity of nature.

Integration of Multi-Omics and Systems Biology

The integration of multi-omics data with systems biology approaches has transformed the landscape of drug discovery, particularly in the study of phytochemicals and their therapeutic potential. This integrative framework enables a holistic view of biological systems by capturing the complexity of molecular interactions across different layers—transcriptomics, proteomics, metabolomics, and epigenomics—and linking them with the mechanistic action of plant-derived compounds. Rather than focusing on single-target interactions, multi-omics approaches facilitate the understanding of multi-target and polypharmacological effects, aligning closely with the pharmacodynamic nature of many phytochemicals, which often exert their therapeutic activity through modulation of several biological pathways concurrently. This comprehensive strategy is particularly valuable in tackling complex diseases such as malaria, cancer, neurodegenerative disorders, and metabolic syndromes, where network perturbations rather than isolated molecular defects are central to pathogenesis. Transcriptomics reveals changes in gene expression profiles upon treatment with phytochemicals, enabling the identification of upregulated or downregulated genes and elucidating how these compounds influence cellular transcriptional networks(Zhang et al., 2024). Nuclear magnetic resonance (NMR), gas chromatography-mass spectrometry (GC-MS), and liquid chromatography-mass spectrometry (LC-MS) are frequently used to detect changes in metabolite levels following treatment with phytochemicals. These metabolic signatures can reflect perturbed biochemical pathways, such as glycolysis, lipid metabolism, or amino acid synthesis, particularly in parasites like Plasmodium, which exhibit unique metabolic traits. For example, certain triterpenoids and quinones have been found to disrupt heme detoxification pathways or mitochondrial respiration, mechanisms that are readily traceable through metabolomic shifts.

The integration of these omics datasets—termed multi-omics analysis—provides a powerful tool for constructing systems-level models of cellular response. Using bioinformatics pipelines and statistical modeling, researchers can correlate changes in gene expression with protein activity and downstream metabolite flux, reconstructing the flow of information through cellular pathways(Oliveira et al., 2023). This enables the identification of critical nodes, or "hubs," in regulatory networks that are disproportionately affected by treatment, which are potential therapeutic targets or resistance checkpoints. Tools like Ingenuity Pathway Analysis (IPA), Cytoscape, MetaboAnalyst, and OmicsNet are commonly employed to visualize these complex interactions and support data-driven hypothesis generation. Network pharmacology, a central aspect of systems biology, expands on this integration by modeling drug–target–disease relationships within a graph-theoretical framework. Here, phytochemicals are treated as nodes connected to their potential targets, which are further linked to biological processes and disease phenotypes. This modeling allows the identification of shared targets among multiple compounds or diseases, highlighting pleiotropic effects and synergistic interactions. Such network-based approaches have been used to demonstrate how compounds like berberine or resveratrol interact with multiple targets involved in inflammation, metabolism, and cell proliferation, making them suitable candidates for polypharmacological strategies. Moreover, network topology metrics such as betweenness centrality or degree distribution can be used to prioritize drug targets based on their influence within the biological system.

In the context of phytochemical research, network pharmacology facilitates the rationalization of traditional medicinal knowledge by mapping herbal formulas or plant extracts onto biological networks. This approach is particularly relevant for Ayurvedic and Traditional Chinese Medicine (TCM), where combinations of herbs are prescribed based on empirical efficacy. By identifying shared targets or common pathways influenced by multiple phytochemicals, systems biology validates these traditional practices and provides a scientific basis for combination therapy. Furthermore, reverse pharmacology—starting from clinical observations to dissecting molecular mechanisms—is increasingly guided by multi-omics and network analyses. Another significant contribution of systems biology is the identification of multi-target phytochemicals capable of modulating several key pathways simultaneously. These compounds, often described as "network-targeting agents," are particularly valuable for diseases with multifactorial etiologies, where single-target drugs may prove insufficient or lead to resistance. For example, curcumin, epigallocatechin gallate (EGCG), and andrographolide have been shown to regulate transcription factors (e.g., NF-κB, AP-1), kinases (e.g., MAPKs), and epigenetic modulators across multiple disease contexts. Through modular analysis, researchers can dissect how a single compound influences clusters of interconnected proteins or genes, enhancing its appeal as a broad-spectrum therapeutic. Pathway mapping, the process of aligning omics data to canonical biological pathways (e.g., KEGG, Reactome, WikiPathways), is instrumental in interpreting phytochemical action. This mapping reveals which cellular routes are activated, inhibited, or reprogrammed in response to treatment. For instance, if metabolomics shows an accumulation of intermediates in the pentose phosphate pathway and transcriptomics shows upregulation of glucose-6-phosphate dehydrogenase (G6PD), it can be inferred that a compound enhances cellular antioxidant defenses. Similarly, if proteomics indicates downregulation of cyclins and transcriptomics confirms decreased expression of CDKs, one can conclude that a phytochemical induces cell cycle arrest, relevant for anticancer mechanisms.

A growing number of case studies illustrate the power of multi-omics integration in phytochemical drug discovery (Paliwal et al., 2024). For instance, a systems biology study on Withania somnifera extracts showed that withaferin A modulates NF-κB signaling, inhibits proteasome activity, and alters redox metabolism in cancer cells—findings corroborated across transcriptomic, proteomic, and metabolomic platforms. Similarly, studies on artemisinin derivatives revealed modulation of parasite calcium homeostasis and protein folding machinery, identifying multiple synergistic targets beyond its known effect on heme alkylation. Importantly, multi-omics also aids in toxicity prediction and safety profiling of phytochemicals. By analyzing how non-target tissues respond at the gene, protein, and metabolite levels, potential off-target effects and adverse outcomes can be detected early in the development pipeline. This is particularly valuable given the complex matrices of plant extracts, which may contain hundreds of bioactive compounds with unknown pharmacological and toxicological profiles. Systems toxicology, an emerging branch of systems biology, combines omics data with toxicokinetic modeling to assess the safety of such compounds comprehensively. Despite its immense potential, integrating multi-omics data is not without challenges. Differences in data formats, experimental conditions, and noise levels across omics platforms necessitate robust data normalization, cross-platform harmonization, and machine learning-based integration. Moreover, computational infrastructure, data storage, and statistical expertise remain significant barriers, particularly in low-resource settings. However, the development of cloud-based platforms (e.g., Galaxy, DNAnexus), open-source tools, and standardized pipelines has begun to democratize access to these powerful techniques. In summary, the integration of multi-omics data with systems biology approaches marks a paradigm shift in phytochemical-based drug discovery. It enables a transition from reductionist, single-target drug development to a systems-level, network-informed framework that better reflects the polypharmacological nature of phytochemicals. By linking molecular perturbations across the transcriptome, proteome, and metabolome with observed phenotypes, researchers can uncover new mechanisms of action, identify multi-target therapeutics, and validate traditional medicinal practices with molecular evidence. As computational tools and biological databases continue to evolve, the synergy between multi-omics and systems biology will remain at the forefront of rational phytochemical drug design, driving innovation in precision medicine and natural product therapeutics.

AI in High-Throughput Screening of Natural Compounds

High-throughput screening (HTS) is a cornerstone of modern drug discovery, allowing researchers to evaluate the biological activity of vast numbers of compounds in a rapid, parallelized, and automated manner. However, traditional HTS, which often involves costly experimental assays and requires extensive compound libraries, instrumentation, and labor, can be resource-intensive and time-consuming. In recent years, the integration of artificial intelligence (AI) with virtual high-throughput screening (vHTS) has emerged as a transformative approach, particularly in the screening of natural products and phytochemicals, which are often structurally diverse, chemically rich, and pharmacologically complex. AI-driven HTS enables the rapid prioritization of promising leads from large-scale natural compound databases while significantly reducing the time, cost, and computational overhead associated with early-stage drug discovery. At the core of this revolution is the use of machine learning (ML) and deep learning (DL) algorithms to automate and optimize the virtual screening pipeline. This includes tasks such as compound filtering, molecular docking, scoring, and hit prediction(Patel et al., 2020). By leveraging historical biological activity data, chemical structure descriptors, and protein-ligand interaction patterns, AI models can rapidly evaluate the potential of millions of natural compounds for their likelihood to bind to specific biological targets. Unlike rule-based or heuristic filtering methods, AI can learn complex nonlinear relationships between molecular features and biological responses, allowing for more accurate and scalable predictions. The virtual screening process typically begins with the construction or selection of a compound library, often sourced from natural product databases such as NPASS, ZINC Natural Products, COCONUT, AfroDb, SuperNatural II, and IMPPAT. These databases offer structurally annotated, curated libraries of plant-derived and microbial metabolites, many of which are underexplored in conventional drug development pipelines. Once a suitable target protein (such as a receptor, enzyme, or ion channel) is selected—based on disease relevance or structural availability—AI can assist in optimizing the screening protocol. For instance, models trained on known ligand-protein pairs can predict the binding potential of natural compounds, pre-filtering candidates before they enter more resource-intensive molecular docking simulations.

One of the most time-saving applications of AI in HTS is automated docking and scoring. Traditional docking tools such as AutoDock Vina, Glide, DOCK, and MOE rely on exhaustive search algorithms to explore the conformational space of ligand binding, often at the cost of computational speed. AI can be used to predict docking poses or refine docking scores based on learned interactions, effectively serving as a surrogate to speed up docking evaluations without significantly compromising accuracy. Deep learning frameworks such as DeepDock, GNINA, TANKBind, and DeepBindRG utilize convolutional neural networks and graph-based architectures to evaluate 3D protein-ligand interactions with higher fidelity and reduced computational requirements compared to classical scoring functions. Moreover, AI plays a pivotal role in compound selection and library enrichment. By identifying molecular fingerprints, pharmacophoric features, or ADMET-related properties that correlate with biological efficacy, ML classifiers (e.g., random forests, support vector machines, gradient boosting) can filter out non-promising candidates early in the process. For instance, if a library consists of 500,000 phytochemicals, AI can narrow this down to a few thousand compounds that meet desirable physicochemical and bioactivity criteria before proceeding to docking or simulation phases(Sadybekov & Katritch, 2023). This enrichment process is critical for hit-to-lead identification, especially when dealing with structurally complex natural products that defy Lipinski's Rule of Five but may still be biologically potent. Natural product-specific challenges such as stereochemical diversity, macrocyclic conformations, and glycosylation patterns can also be addressed by AI. Traditional cheminformatics tools often struggle with these complexities, but DL architectures, particularly graph neural networks (GNNs) and transformer-based models, are capable of learning from structural nuances. GNNs, for example, can represent molecular graphs in a way that captures both local atomic environments and long-range dependencies, making them especially suitable for predicting the bioactivity of large, rigid, or multi-ringed natural compounds. These AI models can also be trained on multi-objective optimization tasks, simultaneously evaluating efficacy, toxicity, solubility, and metabolic stability, thus supporting the identification of drug-like phytochemicals.

Such adaptive screening workflows represent a closed-loop system where AI learns continuously, increasing screening accuracy and reducing attrition rates(Sakthivel et al., 2025). Automation and scalability are additional benefits. Platforms like ChemAI, Schrödinger's LiveDesign, IBM RXN, and DeepChem allow the deployment of AI-augmented HTS pipelines that can operate on cloud infrastructure, enabling real-time analysis of vast datasets. These platforms support parallel processing of molecular docking tasks, active site analysis, machine learning model deployment, and interactive visualization of screening outcomes. Coupled with robotic automation and lab-on-a-chip technologies, AI can also be linked with wet-lab HTS setups, forming AI-augmented experimental screening platforms. This integration is particularly useful in academic or pharmaceutical environments pursuing hybrid discovery models.Another investigation used ML models to filter a marine natural product library, resulting in high-potency hits against kinase targets with nanomolar activity, subsequently validated in vitro. Similar approaches have been applied to

Plasmodium falciparum targets such as PfDHFR, PfATP6, and falcipain-2, where AI-guided vHTS has yielded novel scaffolds with antimalarial potential. While AI has made virtual HTS more efficient and intelligent, several challenges remain(Sarkar et al., 2023).

Challenges and Limitations

The lack of standardized representation formats, such as SMILES or InChI, across different databases leads to inconsistencies in molecular fingerprint generation, which in turn affects downstream predictive modeling and similarity searches. In addition, phytochemicals often violate classical drug-likeness filters, such as Lipinski's Rule of Five, rendering many structure–activity relationship (SAR) models less effective. These structural outliers require specialized descriptors and deep learning architectures, which are more demanding in terms of both computational power and training data.This lack of methodological standardization not only impedes reproducibility but also complicates cross-study comparisons and collaborative research(Thirunagalingam & Selvakumar, 2025). Moreover, AI models trained on proprietary or inaccessible datasets limit reproducibility and hinder peer validation. Open-source platforms and data-sharing initiatives are addressing this issue, but the field still lacks widely accepted benchmarks and reporting standards.A related but often underemphasized limitation is the integration of traditional ethnomedicinal knowledge with computational pipelines. Indigenous and traditional medicine systems such as Ayurveda, Traditional Chinese Medicine (TCM), and African ethnopharmacology offer a vast repository of phytochemical leads and therapeutic hypotheses. However, translating this knowledge into computationally actionable formats remains a significant hurdle. Traditional knowledge is often unstructured, qualitative, and context-dependent, recorded in textual narratives, case studies, or oral traditions rather than standardized scientific formats. Moreover, concepts such as "dosha", "hot-cold balance", or "qi" in traditional systems lack direct equivalents in modern pharmacological terminology, making it difficult to encode them into algorithmic frameworks. Even when ethnopharmacological data are digitized, they frequently lack validation through modern pharmacological assays, making their use in supervised learning models problematic(Yin et al., 2023).

Computational resource limitations also pose challenges, especially for academic and small research institutions in developing countries. High-fidelity simulations such as MD or quantum mechanics/molecular mechanics (QM/MM) require substantial computational power, often only accessible through supercomputing facilities or cloud-based platforms, which may not be affordable or available to all researchers (Wang et al., 2022). Similarly, training large deep learning models requires specialized hardware (e.g., GPUs, TPUs) and expertise in data science, which may be beyond the scope of many pharmacognosy or ethnobotany departments. Model validation and experimental follow-up remain critical bottlenecks in computational drug discovery. Even when AI models identify promising leads, the translation from in silico prediction to in vitro or in vivo validation is non-trivial. Natural compounds may suffer from issues like poor solubility, metabolic instability, or off-target effects that are not adequately captured by current computational tools(Varghese, Shringi & Efferth, 2025). Moreover, the cost and complexity of isolating phytochemicals, particularly from rare or endangered species, further delay validation efforts. Thus, the hit-to-lead conversion rate in phytochemical drug discovery remains relatively low compared to synthetic compound pipelines. Lastly, regulatory and cultural factors can limit the adoption of AI-driven methods in natural product research. Regulatory agencies often require detailed mechanistic evidence for drug approval, which AI models may struggle to provide. Furthermore, conservatism within traditional medicine communities or skepticism within pharmacological circles can inhibit the cross-disciplinary collaboration necessary for integrating computational and ethnopharmacological approaches.

CONCLUSION

In summary, while the application of AI and computational methods holds transformative potential in phytochemical drug discovery, several limitations must be acknowledged and addressed. These include data scarcity and annotation gaps, algorithm interpretability and reproducibility issues, difficulty in integrating traditional medicinal knowledge, regional and epistemic biases, computational resource constraints, and challenges in experimental validation. Tackling these obstacles will require interdisciplinary collaboration, open-access data initiatives, investment in digital infrastructure, and cross-cultural dialogue between modern scientists and traditional knowledge holders. By addressing these barriers thoughtfully and inclusively, the promise of AI-driven phytochemical research can be more equitably and effectively realized in the pursuit of novel therapeutics. Another major challenge lies in the interpretability and reproducibility of AI algorithms. While deep learning models—such as convolutional neural networks (CNNs), graph neural networks (GNNs), and transformers—offer high predictive accuracy, they often operate as "black boxes," offering limited transparency into the decision-making process. This is particularly problematic in drug discovery, where understanding the molecular basis of predictions is essential for hypothesis generation, experimental validation, and regulatory approval. The inability to explain why a particular phytochemical is predicted to interact with a given protein target diminishes user confidence and hinders the integration of AI into medicinal chemistry pipelines. Efforts are being made to incorporate explainable AI (XAI) tools such as SHAP (SHapley Additive exPlanations) and LIME (Local Interpretable Model-agnostic Explanations), but these approaches are still evolving and often lack resolution at the level required for chemical inference. Reproducibility is further challenged by the use of disparate software environments, parameter settings, and preprocessing techniques. For example, differences in molecular docking scoring functions, force fields in molecular dynamics (MD) simulations, or feature selection methods in ML pipelines can yield significantly different outcomes—even when analyzing the same compound-target pair. Despite the immense potential of artificial intelligence (AI) and computational tools in accelerating phytochemical-based drug discovery, several critical challenges and limitations persist that hinder their widespread adoption and full realization. One of the foremost issues is data scarcity, particularly the lack of high-quality, curated, and annotated bioactivity data for many phytochemicals. While large-scale databases such as NPASS, IMPPAT, and AfroDb provide access to structural and ethnobotanical data, they often lack comprehensive pharmacokinetic, pharmacodynamic, and experimental bioactivity information. This deficiency hampers the training and validation of machine learning (ML) models, as predictive algorithms depend heavily on rich datasets that capture diverse biological interactions, dose-response curves, and toxicological profiles. Without robust datasets, models may suffer from overfitting, reduced generalizability, and poor external validation performance, especially when attempting to extrapolate predictions to novel scaffolds commonly found in natural products. Compounding the issue of limited data is the inherent chemical complexity and diversity of phytochemicals. Many plant-derived molecules possess intricate ring systems, chiral centers, and functional group variability that challenge conventional cheminformatics encoding schemes.

REFERENCES

Abbas, S., Rassam, A., Karamshahi, F., Abunora, R., & Abouseada, M. (2024). The role of AI in drug discovery. *ChemBioChem, 3*(14), e202300816. Advance online publication. pubs.acs.org and 3chemistry-europe.onlinelibrary.wiley.com. DOI: 10.1002/cbic.202300816 PMID: 38735845

Amit Kadan, K. Ryczko, E. Lloyd, A. Roitberg, & T. Yamazaki (2024). Guided multi-objective generative AI to enhance structure-based drug design. arXiv. / arXiv.2405.11785 arxiv.orgDOI: 10.48550

Arora, S., Chettri, S., Percha, V., Kumar, D., & Latwal, M. (2024). Artificial intelligence: A virtual chemist for natural product drug discovery. *Journal of Biomolecular Structure & Dynamics, 42*(7), 3826–3835. pmc.ncbi.nlm.nih.gov. DOI: 10.1080/07391102.2023.2216295 PMID: 37232451

Beccari, A., & Vistoli, G. (2022). Exscalate4CoV: innovative high performing computing (HPC) strategies to tackle pandemic crisis. International Journal of Molecular Sciences. ??? (Exact issue pending) en.wikipedia.orgDOI: 10.3390/ijms230

Boldini, D., Ballabio, D., Consonni, V., Todeschini, R., Grisoni, F., & Sieber, S. A. (2024). Effectiveness of molecular fingerprints for exploring the chemical space of natural products. *Journal of Cheminformatics, 16*(1), 35. pmc.ncbi.nlm.nih.gov. DOI: 10.1186/s13321-024-00830-3 PMID: 38528548

Chen, Y., & Kirchmair, J. (2020). Cheminformatics in natural product–based drug discovery. *Molecular Informatics, 39*(12), e2000171. onlinelibrary.wiley.com. DOI: 10.1002/minf.202000171 PMID: 32725781

Chihomvu, P., Ganesan, A., Gibbons, S., Woollard, K., & Hayes, M. A. (2024). Phytochemicals in drug discovery—A confluence of tradition and innovation. International Journal of Molecular Sciences, 25(16), 8792. mdpi.comDOI: 10.3390/ijms25168792

Choudhury, C., Arul Murugan, N., & Priyakumar, U. D. (2022). Structure-based drug repurposing: AI/ML-aided methods. *Drug Discovery Today, 27*(7), 1847–1861. link.springer.com. DOI: 10.1016/j.drudis.2022.03.006 PMID: 35301148

Dara, S., Dhamercherla, S., Jadav, S. S., Babu, C. M., & Ahsan, M. J. (2022). Machine learning in drug discovery: A review. *Artificial Intelligence Review, 55*(3), 1947–1999. link.springer.com. DOI: 10.1007/s10462-021-10058-4 PMID: 34393317

Dou, B., Zhu, Z., Merkurjev, E., et al. (2023). Machine learning methods for small data challenges in molecular science. Chemical Reviews, 123(13), 8736–8780. medium.comDOI: 10.1021/acs.chemrev.3c00189

Fromer, J. C., & Coley, C. W. (2024). An algorithmic framework for synthetic cost-aware decision making in molecular design. Nature Computational Science, 4(6), 440–450. medium.comDOI: 10.1038/s43588-024-00639-y

Gangwal, A., Ansari, A., Ahmad, I., Azad, A. K., Kumarasamy, V., Subramaniyan, V., & Wong, L. S. (2024). Generative artificial intelligence in drug discovery: Basic framework, recent advances, challenges, and opportunities. *Frontiers in Pharmacology, 15*, 1331062. DOI: 10.3389/fphar.2024.1331062 PMID: 38384298

Gangwal, A., Ansari, A., Ahmad, I., Azad, A. K., & Sulaiman, W. M. A. W. (2024). Current strategies to address data scarcity in AI-based drug discovery: A comprehensive review. *Computers in Biology and Medicine*, *179*, 108734. pmc.ncbi.nlm.nih.gov. DOI: 10.1016/j.compbiomed.2024.108734 PMID: 38964243

Gorantla, R., Kubincová, A., Suutari, B., Cossins, B. P., & Mey, A. S. J. S. (2024). Benchmarking active learning protocols for ligand-binding affinity prediction. Journal of Chemical Information and Modeling, 64(6), 1955–1965. DOI: 10.1021/acs.jcim.4c00220

Gu, Y., Wang, Y., Zhu, K., Li, W., Liu, G., & Tang, Y. (2024). DBPP-predictor: Prediction of chemical drug-likeness based on property profiles. *Journal of Cheminformatics*, *16*(1), 4. link.springer.com. DOI: 10.1186/s13321-024-00800-9 PMID: 38183072

Horne, R. I., Andrzejewska, E. A., Alam, P., et al. (2024). Discovery of potent inhibitors of α-synuclein aggregation using structure-based iterative learning. Nature Chemical Biology, 20(5), 634–645. DOI: 10.1038/s41589-024-01580-x

Hubballi, R. B., Selvakumar, P., Seenivasan, R., & Basava Aradhya, S. G., Dinesh, N., & Seelam, P. K. (2025). Overview of Current AI Technologies in Education. In L. Kyei-Blankson & E. Ntuli (Eds.), Transformative AI Practices for Personalized Learning Strategies (pp. 1-26). IGI Global Scientific Publishing. DOI: 10.4018/979-8-3693-8744-3.ch001

Kao, P.-Y., Yang, Y.-C., Chiang, W.-Y., Hsiao, J.-Y., & Cao, Y.. (2022). Exploring the advantages of quantum generative adversarial networks in generative chemistry. ArXiv. https://arxiv.org/abs/2210.16823

Keith, J. A., Vassilev-Galindo, V., Cheng, B., Chmiela, S., Gastegger, M., Müller, K.-R., & Tkatchenko, A. (2021). Combining machine learning and computational chemistry for predictive insights into chemical systems. ArXiv. https://arxiv.org/abs/2102.06321 arxiv.org

Kotte, K. R., Attaluri, V., & Selvakumar, P. (2025). Revolutionising Retail Banking with AI and Virtual Technologies AI-Driven Financial Training. In Nair, A. J., Manohar, S., Limbu, Y. B., & Huhmann, B. A. (Eds.), *Intersecting Natural Language Processing and FinTech Innovations in Service Marketing* (pp. 421–440). IGI Global Scientific Publishing., DOI: 10.4018/979-8-3693-9944-6.ch020

Maheswaran, K., Selvakumar, P., Shaikh, M., Shashank, G., Gupta, S., & Manjunath, T. C. (2025). The Evolution of Smart Urban Mobility With Emerging Technologies. In Ponnusamy, S., Assaf, M., Youssef, B., Jeon, G., & Kalyanaraman, S. (Eds.), *Leveraging VANETs and Blockchain Technology for Urban Mobility* (pp. 1–28). IGI Global Scientific Publishing., DOI: 10.4018/979-8-3373-0265-2.ch001

Min, Y., Wei, Y., Wang, P., Wang, X., Li, H., Wu, N., Bauer, S., Zheng, S., Shi, Y., Wang, Y., Wu, J., Zhao, D., & Zeng, J. (2024). From static to dynamic structures: Improving binding affinity prediction with graph-based deep learning. *Advancement of Science*, *11*(40), 2405404. ouci.dntb.gov.ua. DOI: 10.1002/advs.202405404 PMID: 39206846

Moshawih, S., Goh, H. P., Kifli, N., Idris, A. C., Yassin, H., Kotra, V., Goh, K. W., Liew, K. B., & Ming, L. C. (2022). Synergy between machine learning and natural products cheminformatics: Application to anthraquinone derivatives. *Chemical Biology & Drug Design*, *100*(2), 185–217. onlinelibrary.wiley.com. DOI: 10.1111/cbdd.14062 PMID: 35490393

Nahal, Y., Menke, J., Martinelli, J., ... (2024). Human-in-the-loop active learning for goal-oriented molecule generation. Journal of Cheminformatics, 16(1), 138. pubs.acs.org+2medium.com+2pubs.acs.org+2DOI: 10.1186/s13321-024-00924-y

Odin Zhang, H. Lin, H. Zhang, H. Zhao, Y. Huang, Y. Huang, D. Jiang, C.-Y. Hsieh, P. Pan, & T. Hou (2024). Deep lead optimization: leveraging generative AI for structural modification. arXiv. /arXiv.2404.19230 arxiv.orgDOI: 10.48550

Oliveira, T., Silva, M., Maia, E., Silva, A., & Taranto, A. (2023). Virtual screening algorithms in drug discovery: Machine and deep learning methods. *Drugs and Drug Candidates*, *2*(2), 311–334. link.springer.com. DOI: 10.3390/ddc2020017

Paliwal, A., Jain, S., Kumar, S., Wal, P., Khandai, M., & Khandige, P. S. (2024). Predictive modelling in pharmacokinetics: from in-silico simulations to personalized medicine. Expert Opinion on Drug Metabolism & Toxicology, 20(4), 181–195. premierscience.comDOI: 10.1080/17425255.2024.2330666

Patel, L., Shukla, T., Huang, X., Ussery, D. W., & Wang, S. (2020). Machine learning methods in drug discovery. Molecules, 25(22), 5277. mdpi.comDOI: 10.3390/molecules25225277

Sadybekov, A. V., & Katritch, V. (2023). Computational approaches streamlining drug discovery. Nature, 616, 673–685. frontiersin.orgDOI: 10.1038/s41586-023-05905-z

Sakthivel, M., Jaganathan, A., Mohanraj, M., & Selvakumar, P. Mohit, & Manjunath, T. (2025). Brand Loyalty through AI and Personalisation AI-Generated Content for Financial Marketing. In A. J Nair, S. Manohar, Y. B. Limbu, & B. A. Huhmann (Eds.), Intersecting Natural Language Processing and FinTech Innovations in Service Marketing (pp. 77-96). IGI Global Scientific Publishing. DOI: 10.4018/979-8-3693-9944-6.ch006

Sarkar, C., Das, B., Rawat, V. S., Wahlang, J. B., Nongpiur, A., Tiewsoh, I., & et al. (2023). Artificial intelligence and machine learning technology driven modern drug discovery and development. International Journal of Molecular Sciences, 24(3), 2026. frontiersin.orgDOI: 10.3390/ijms24032026

Thirunagalingam, A., & Selvakumar, P. (2025). Application of Automation and Robotics in the Oil and Gas Industry. In Abdullayev, V., & Khang, A. (Eds.), *Revolutionizing AI and Robotics in the Oil and Gas Industry* (pp. 229–244). IGI Global Scientific Publishing., DOI: 10.4018/979-8-3693-8156-4.ch011

Varghese, R., Shringi, H., & Efferth, T. (2025). Artificial intelligence driven approaches in phytochemical research: trends and prospects. Phytochemistry Reviews, February 27, 1–21. mdpi.com+9link.springer.com+9pmc.ncbi.nlm.nih.gov+9DOI: 10.1007/s11101-025-10096-8

Wang, K., Huang, Y., Wang, Y., You, Q., & Wang, L. (2024). Recent advances from computer-aided drug design to artificial intelligence drug design. *RSC Medicinal Chemistry*, *15*(12), 3978–4000. pubs.acs.orgpubs.rsc.org. DOI: 10.1039/D4MD00522H PMID: 39493228

Wang, Y., Michael, S., Yang, S. M., Huang, R., Cruz-Gutierrez, K., Zhang, Y., et al. (2022). Retro drug design: from target properties to molecular structures. Journal of Chemical Information and Modeling, 62(11), 2659–2669. premierscience.comDOI: 10.1021/acs.jcim.2c00123

Yin, T., Panapitiya, G., Coda, E. D., & Saldanha, E. G. (2023). Evaluating uncertainty-based active learning for accelerating the generalization of molecular property prediction. Journal of Cheminformatics, 15(1), 105. medium.comDOI: 10.1186/s13321-023-00753-5

Compilation of References

Abaza, S. (2024). Recent advances in identification of potential drug targets and development of novel drugs in parasitic diseases: Part V: The value of natural products in drug discovery: Helminths. *Parasitologists United Journal, 17*(2), 57–73. DOI: 10.21608/puj.2024.292672.1250

Abbas, S., Rassam, A., Karamshahi, F., Abunora, R., & Abouseada, M. (2024). The role of AI in drug discovery. *ChemBioChem, 3*(14), e202300816. Advance online publication. pubs.acs.org and 3chemistry-europe.onlinelibrary.wiley.com. DOI: 10.1002/cbic.202300816 PMID: 38735845

Abebe, W., Ashagre, A., Misganaw, T., Dejazmach, Z., Kumie, G., Nigatie, M., Jemal, A., Asmare, Z., Kassahun, W., Gedfie, S., Getachew, E., Gashaw, M., Ayana, S., Gashaw, Y., Sisay, A., Tadesse, S., Eshetu, T., awoke, M., Kassanew, B., & Reta, M. A. (2025). Prevalence of antimalaria drug resistance-conferring mutations associated with sulphadoxine-pyrimethamineine-resistant Plasmodium falciparum in East Africa: A systematic review and meta-analysis. *Annals of Clinical Microbiology and Antimicrobials, 24*(1), 25. DOI: 10.1186/s12941-025-00795-7 PMID: 40241183

Abera, T., Ashebir, R., Basha, H., Debebe, E., Abebe, A., Meresa, A., & Woldekidan, S. (2019). Phytochemical-constituents, safety and efficacy of commonly used medicinal plants for the treatment of malaria in Ethiopia-a review. *Pharmacy & Pharmacology International Journal, 7*(6), 284–295. DOI: 10.15406/ppij.2019.07.00266

Abouelfetouh, M., metwaly., Ali., Marwan., Khan, I., & Shaker, E. (2024). Phytochemical analysis, antimalarial and antioxidant activities of Musa paradisiaca rhizome. Journal of Advanced Pharmacy Research, 8(4), 188 ?"197. doi:10.21608/aprh.2024.291519.1272DOI: 10.21608/aprh.2024.291519.1272

Abu Khalaf, R., Alhusban, A. A., Al-Shalabi, E., Al-Sheikh, I., & Sabbah, D. A. (2019). Chapter 10—Isolation and structure elucidation of bioactive polyphenols. In Atta-ur-Rahman (Ed.), *Studies in Natural Products Chemistry* (Vol. 63, pp. 267–337). Elsevier. DOI: 10.1016/B978-0-12-817901-7.00010-1

Abubakar, A. R., & Haque, M. (2020). Preparation of Medicinal Plants: Basic Extraction and Fractionation Procedures for Experimental Purposes. *Journal of Pharmacy & Bioallied Sciences*, *12*(1), 1–10. DOI: 10.4103/jpbs.JPBS_175_19 PMID: 32801594

Achan, J., Talisuna, A. O., Erhart, A., Yeka, A., Tibenderana, J. K., Baliraine, F. N., Rosenthal, P. J., & D'Alessandro, U. (2011). Quinine, an old anti-malarial drug in a modern world: Role in the treatment of malaria. *Malaria Journal*, *10*(1), 144. DOI: 10.1186/1475-2875-10-144 PMID: 21609473

Addissouky, T. A., El Sayed, I. E. T., Ali, M. M., Alubiady, M. H. S., & Wang, Y. (2024). Schisandra chinensis in liver disease: Exploring the mechanisms and therapeutic promise of an ancient Chinese botanical. *Archives of Pharmacology and Therapeutics*, *6*(1), 27–33. DOI: 10.33696/Pharmacol.6.052

Adebayo, J. O., & Krettli, A. U. (2011). Potential antimalarials from Nigerian plants: A review. Journal of Ethnopharmacology, 133(2), 289 ?"302. doi:10.1016/j.jep.2010.11.024 PubMedDOI: 10.1016/j.jep.2010.11.024 PMID: 21093570

Afakwu-Adimoha, H. C., & Ogidi, O. I., (2025). Health care financing and achieving universal health care in Bayelsa: Changing the narrative through health insurance. *World Journal of Biology Pharmacy and Health Sciences*, *21*(3), 361–373. DOI: 10.30574/wjbphs.2025.21.3.0383

Afzal, I., Habiba, U., & Yasmeen, H. (2023). Review on therapeutic potential of phytochemicals from medicinal plants. *Journal of Bioresource Management*, *10*(4), 7.

Agarwal, G., Blanco, C. P. J., Addo, E. M., & Kinghorn, A. D. (2020). Current status and contemporary approaches to the discovery of antitumor agents from higher plants. *Biotechnology Advances*, *38*, 107337. DOI: 10.1016/j.biotechadv.2019.01.004 PMID: 30633954

Agbodeka, K., Gbekley, H. E., Karou, S. D., Anani, K., Agbonon, A., Tchacondo, T., Batawila, K., Simpore, J., & Gbeassor, M. (2016). Ethnobotanical Study of Medicinal Plants Used for the Treatment of Malaria in the Plateau Region, Togo. Pharmacognosy Research, 8(5, Suppl 1), S12 ?"S18. doi:10.4103/0974-8490.178646 PubMedDOI: 10.4103/0974-8490.178646 PMID: 27114686

Aghili, Z. S., Magnani, M., Ghatrehsamani, M., Nourian Dehkordi, A., Mirzaei, S. A., & Banitalebi Dehkordi, M. (2024). Intelligent berberine-loaded erythrocytes attenuated inflammatory cytokine productions in macrophages. *Scientific Reports*, *14*(1), 9381. DOI: 10.1038/s41598-024-60103-9 PMID: 38654085

Ahmad, F., & Nadeem, H. (2022). *Mass Spectroscopy as an Analytical Tool to Harness the Production of Secondary Plant Metabolites: The Way Forward for Drug Discovery*. DOI: 10.1007/978-1-0716-2716-7_5

Ain, Q. T., Saleem, N., Munawar, N., Nawaz, R., Naseer, F., & Ahmed, S. (2024). Quest for malaria management using natural remedies. *Frontiers in Pharmacology, 15*, 1359890. DOI: 10.3389/fphar.2024.1359890 PMID: 39011507

Ajayi, O., Balogun, O., Fakola, E., Olawuni, I., October, N., & Adewole, A. (2024). Evaluation of Antioxidant & Antidiabetic Activities of Iridoid glycoside Isolated from Stachytarpheta cayennensis (Rich) Vahl Leaf Extract: In vitro combined with molecular docking approach. South African Journal of Botany, 176, 184 ?"196. doi:10.1016/j.sajb.2024.11.008DOI: 10.1016/j.sajb.2024.11.008

Ajibesin, K. K., Ekpo, B. A., Bala, D. N., Essien, E. E., & Adesanya, S. A. (2008). Ethnobotanical survey of Akwa Ibom State, Nigeria. Journal of Ethnopharmacology, 115(3), 387 ?"408. doi:10.1016/j.jep.2007.10.021 PubMedDOI: 10.1016/j.jep.2007.10.021 PMID: 18053664

Akharaiyi, F. C., Ezeanya-Bakpa, C. C., & Otumala, S. O. (2021). Inhibition of methicillin resistant *Staphylococcus aureus* (MRSA) with underutilized medicinal plants extracts. *International Medical Journal, 28*(6), 4953–4964.

Akobundu, I. O., Ekeleme, F., Agyakwa, C. W., & Ogazie, C. A. (2016). A handbook of West African weeds (3rd ed.). International Institute of Tropical Agriculture. Nigeria, OfKAR Publishing Company Limited. Pp 381

Akwaji, P. I., Eyam, E. O., & Bassey, R. A. (2017). Ethnobotanical survey of medicinal plants in Northern Cross River State, Nigeria. World Scientific News, 70(2), 140 ?"157.

Al-Faqeeh, L. A. S. (2023). A comprehensive review of natural products from microbial sources and their applications. *PSM Microbiology, 8*(2), 30–47.

Ali, A. H., Sudi, S., Shi-Jing, N., Hassan, W. R. M., Basir, R., Agustar, H. K., Embi, N., Sidek, H. M., & Latip, J. (2021). Dual anti-malarial and GSK3β-mediated cytokine-modulating activities of quercetin are requisite of its potential as a plant-derived therapeutic in malaria. *Pharmaceuticals (Basel, Switzerland), 14*(3), 248. DOI: 10.3390/ph14030248 PMID: 33803419

Almadiy, A. A., Al-Ghamdi, M. S., Abd Al Galil, F. M., & Dar, S. A. (2025). Azadirachtin from Neem (Azadirachta indica): Efficacy and Mechanisms Against Insects and Diseases. In *Natural Pesticides and Allelochemicals* (pp. 261-278). CRC Press.

Altemimi, A., Lakhssassi, N., Baharlouei, A., Watson, D. G., & Lightfoot, D. A. (2017). Phytochemicals: Extraction, isolation, and identification of bioactive compounds from plant extracts. *Plants*, *6*(4), 42. DOI: 10.3390/plants6040042 PMID: 28937585

Alum, E. U. (2024). Phytochemicals in malaria treatment: Mechanisms of action and clinical efficacy. *KIU J. Health Sci*, *4*(2), 71–84. DOI: 10.59568/KJHS-2024-4-2-06

Alum, E. U. (2024). The role of indigenous knowledge in advancing the therapeutic use of medicinal plants: Challenges and opportunities. *Plant Signaling & Behavior*, *19*(1), 2439255. DOI: 10.1080/15592324.2024.2439255 PMID: 39652401

Alum, E. U. (2025). Sustainable harvesting of medicinal plants: Balancing therapeutic benefits with environmental conservation. *Agroecology and Sustainable Food Systems*, *49*(3), 380–385. DOI: 10.1080/21683565.2024.2421948

Amado, P. S. M., Jesus, A. J. L., Paixão, J. A., Fausto, R., & Cristiano, M. L. S. (2022). Unravelling the Structure of Peroxides with Antiparasitic Activity: The Relative Impact of a Trioxolane or a Tetraoxane Pharmacophore on the Overall Molecular Structure. *ChemPlusChem*, *87*(8), e202200207. DOI: 10.1002/cplu.202200207 PMID: 36000152

Amambua-Ngwa, A., Tetteh, K. K. A., Manske, M., Gomez-Escobar, N., Stewart, L. B., Deerhake, M. E., & Conway, D. J. (2019). Population genomic scan for candidate signatures of balancing selection to guide antigen characterization in malaria parasites. *PLOS Genetics*, *15*(9), e1008535. PMID: 23133397

Amang, A. P., Mezui, C., Siwe, G. T., Emakoua, J., & Tan, P. V. (2017). Healing and antisecretory effects of aqueous extract of Eremomastax speciosa (Acanthaceae) on unhealed gastric ulcers. Evidence-Based Complementary and Alternative Medicine : eCAM, 2017(1), 1924320. doi:10.1155/2017/1924320 PubMedDOI: 10.1155/2017/1924320 PMID: 29234676

Amaral, P. S. T., Klauss, K. S. G., Suárez-Mutis, M. C., Coelho, R. R., Galardo, A. K., Murta, F., Moresco, G. G., Siqueira, A. M., & Gurgel-Gonçalves, R. (2024). Malaria in areas under mining activity in the Amazon: A review. *Revista da Sociedade Brasileira de Medicina Tropical*, *57*, e00200–e02024. DOI: 10.1590/0037-8682-0551-2023 PMID: 38922216

Ambrosino, L., Tangherlini, M., Colantuono, C., Esposito, A., Sangiovanni, M., Miralto, M., Sansone, C., & Chiusano, M. L. (2019). Bioinformatics for marine products: An overview of resources, bottlenecks, and perspectives. *Marine Drugs*, *17*(10), 576. DOI: 10.3390/md17100576 PMID: 31614509

Ameer, S. F., Mohamed, M. Y., Elzubair, Q. A., Sharif, E. A. M., & Ibrahim, W. N. (2024). Curcumin as a novel therapeutic candidate for cancer: Can this natural compound revolutionize cancer treatment? *Frontiers in Oncology*, *14*, 1438040. Advance online publication. DOI: 10.3389/fonc.2024.1438040 PMID: 39507759

Amit Kadan, K. Ryczko, E. Lloyd, A. Roitberg, & T. Yamazaki (2024). Guided multi-objective generative AI to enhance structure-based drug design. arXiv. / arXiv.2405.11785 arxiv.orgDOI: 10.48550

Anchimowicz, J., Zielonka, P., & Jakiela, S. (2025). Plant Secondary Metabolites as Modulators of Mitochondrial Health: An Overview of Their Anti-Oxidant, Anti-Apoptotic, and Mitophagic Mechanisms. *International Journal of Molecular Sciences*, *26*(1), 380. DOI: 10.3390/ijms26010380 PMID: 39796234

Andrade, M. A., Barbosa, C. H., Cerqueira, M. A., Azevedo, A. G., Barros, C., Machado, A. V., Coelho, A., Furtado, R., Correia, C. B., Saraiva, M., Vilarinho, F., Silva, A. S., & Ramos, F. (2023). PLA films loaded with green tea and rosemary polyphenolic extracts as an active packaging for almond and beef. *Food Packaging and Shelf Life*, *36*, 101041. DOI: 10.1016/j.fpsl.2023.101041

Andrade, M. V., Noronha, K., Diniz, B. P., Guedes, G., Carvalho, L. R., Silva, V. A., Calazans, J. A., Santos, A. S., Silva, D. N., & Castro, M. C. (2022). The economic burden of malaria: A systematic review. *Malaria Journal*, *21*(1), 283. DOI: 10.1186/s12936-022-04303-6 PMID: 36199078

Ansari, P., Akther, S., Hannan, J. M. A., Seidel, V., Nujat, N. J., & Abdel-Wahab, Y. H. (2022). Pharmacologically active phytomolecules isolated from traditional antidiabetic plants and their therapeutic role for the management of diabetes mellitus. Molecules (Basel, Switzerland), 27(13), 4278. doi:10.3390/molecules27134278 PubMedDOI: 10.3390/molecules27134278 PMID: 35807526

Antony, A., & Farid, M. (2022). Effect of Temperatures on Polyphenols during Extraction. *Applied Sciences (Basel, Switzerland)*, *12*(4), 2107. DOI: 10.3390/app12042107

Apsari, P. I. B., Suryana, I. K., Satriyasa, B. K., Laksmi, D. A. A. S., Wati, D. K., & Wirasuta, I. M. A. G. (2025). Towards Andrographolide as Antimalarial: A Systematic Review. *Biomedical & Pharmacology Journal*, *18*(1), 499–515. DOI: 10.13005/bpj/3103

Arisco, N. J., Peterka, C., Diniz, C., Singer, B. H., & Castro, M. C. (2024). Ecological change increases malaria risk in the Brazilian Amazon. *Proceedings of the National Academy of Sciences of the United States of America*, *121*(44), e2409583121. DOI: 10.1073/pnas.2409583121 PMID: 39432796

Arora, S., Chettri, S., Percha, V., Kumar, D., & Latwal, M. (2024). Artificial intelligence: A virtual chemist for natural product drug discovery. *Journal of Biomolecular Structure & Dynamics*, *42*(7), 3826–3835. pmc.ncbi.nlm.nih.gov. DOI: 10.1080/07391102.2023.2216295 PMID: 37232451

Asanga, E. E., Noah, K. U., Okokon, J. E., Ekeleme, C. M., Udoh, I. E., Bassey, A., Anagboso, M. O., & Inyang, A. N. (2025). Integrative investigation on Hippocratea africana root: Insights from cardio-protective, antioxidative stress activities, isolation, GC/MS, and pharmacological significance profiling. BMC Complementary Medicine and Therapies, 25(1), 200. doi:10.1186/s12906-025-04941-8 PubMedDOI: 10.1186/s12906-025-04941-8 PMID: 40468373

Ashawat, M. S., Saraf Shailendra, S. S., & Saraf Swarnlata, S. S. (2007). In vitro antioxidant activity of ethanolic extracts of Centella asiatica, Punica granatum, Glycyrrhiza glabra and Areca catechu.

Ashley, E. A., Dhorda, M., Fairhurst, R. M., Amaratunga, C., Lim, P., Suon, S., & Dondorp, A. M. (2018). Spread of artemisinin resistance in *Plasmodium falciparum* malaria. *The New England Journal of Medicine*, *371*(5), 411–423. DOI: 10.1056/NEJMoa1314981 PMID: 25075834

Asigbaase, M., Adusu, D., Anaba, L., Abugre, S., Kang-Milung, S., Acheamfour, S. A., Adamu, I., & Ackah, D. K. (2023). Conservation and economic benefits of medicinal plants: Insights from forest-fringe communities of Southwestern Ghana. Trees, Forests and People, 14, 100462. doi:10.1016/j.tfp.2023.100462DOI: 10.1016/j.tfp.2023.100462

Atanasov, A. G., Waltenberger, B., Pferschy-Wenzig, E. M., Linder, T., Wawrosch, C., Uhrin, P., Temml, V., Wang, L., Schwaiger, S., Heiss, E. H., Rollinger, J. M., Schuster, D., Breuss, J. M., Bochkov, V., Mihovilovic, M. D., Kopp, B., Bauer, R., Dirsch, V. M., & Stuppner, H. (2015). Discovery and resupply of pharmacologically active plant-derived natural products: A review. *Biotechnology Advances*, *33*(8), 1582–1614. DOI: 10.1016/j.biotechadv.2015.08.001 PMID: 26281720

Atanasov, A. G., Zotchev, S. B., Dirsch, V. M., & Supuran, C. T. (2021). Natural products in drug discovery: Advances and opportunities. *Nature Reviews. Drug Discovery*, *20*(3), 200–216. DOI: 10.1038/s41573-020-00114-z PMID: 33510482

Atun, R., & Kazatchkine, M. (2010). The Global Fund's strategic shift: The challenge of integrating HIV, tuberculosis, and malaria programs into health systems. *Health Policy and Planning*, *25*(1), i1–i3. DOI: 10.1093/heapol/czp053 PMID: 19959485

Atwijukire, W., Ayogu, E. E., & Onohuean, H. (2025). Immunomodulatory potentials of Andrographis paniculata and Allium sativum in managing plasmodium infections. *Discover Applied Sciences, 7*(7), 661. DOI: 10.1007/s42452-025-07010-4

Aziz, S. M. A., Ahmed, O. M., El-Twab, S. M. A., Al-Muzafar, H. M., Amin, K. A., & Abdel-Gabbar, M. (2020). Antihyperglycemic Effects and Mode of Actions of Musa paradisiaca Leaf and Fruit Peel Hydroethanolic Extracts in Nicotinamide/Streptozotocin ??Induced Diabetic Rats. Evidence-based Complementary and Alternative Medicine, 2020(1). https://doi.org/doi:10.1155/2020/9276343DOI: 10.1155/2020/9276343

Bajpai, V. K., Majumder, R., & Park, J. G. (2016). Isolation and purification of plant secondary metabolites using column-chromatographic technique. *Bangladesh Journal of Pharmacology, 11*(4), 844–848. DOI: 10.3329/bjp.v11i4.28185

Balaji, S. N., Deshmukh, R., & Trivedi, V. (2020). Severe malaria: Biology, clinical manifestation, pathogenesis and consequences. *Journal of Vector Borne Diseases, 57*(1), 1–13. DOI: 10.4103/0972-9062.308793 PMID: 33818449

Balandrin, M. F., Kinghorn, A. D., & Farnsworth, N. R. (1993). *Plant-derived natural products in drug discovery and development: An overview*. In American Chemical Society., DOI: 10.1021/bk-1993-0534.ch001

Balikagala, B., Fukuda, N., Ikeda, M., Katuro, O. T., Tachibana, S. I., Yamauchi, M., & Tsuboi, T. (2021). Evidence of artemisinin-resistant malaria in Africa. *The New England Journal of Medicine, 385*(13), 1163–1171. DOI: 10.1056/NEJMoa2101746 PMID: 34551228

Banjari, I., Misir, A., Savikin, K., Jokic, S., Molnar, M., & Waisundara, V. Y. (2017). Antidiabetic effects of Aronia melanocarpa and its other therapeutic properties. *Frontiers in Nutrition, 4*, 53. DOI: 10.3389/fnut.2017.00053 PMID: 29164127

Bankole, A. E., Adekunle, A. A., Sowemimo, A. A., Umebese, C. E., Abiodun, O., & Gbotosho, G. O. (2016). Phytochemical screening and in vivo antimalarial activity of extracts from three medicinal plants used in malaria treatment in Nigeria. *Parasitology Research, 115*(1), 299–305. DOI: 10.1007/s00436-015-4747-x PMID: 26391173

Banu, K. S., & Cathrine, D. L. (2015). *General Techniques Involved in Phytochemical Analysis*.

Barman, P., & Biswas, A. (2025). *The Contribution of Traditionally Used Medicinal Plants to Modern Medicine: An Update on the Successful Journey of Medicinal Plants of North East Africa*. Bentham Science Publishers. https://www.benthamdirect.com/content/books/9789815313178.chapter-6

Barreto, J. R., Rocha, R., Barlow, J., & Loyola, R. (2025). Indigenous territories safeguard human health in the Brazilian Amazon. *Communications Earth & Environment*, *6*(1), 1–9. DOI: 10.1038/s43247-025-02620-7 PMID: 39830897

Bassey, N. O., Eteng, O. E., Nelson, V. A., Essien, N. M., Udo, E. P., Ogar, B. A., & Udosen, E. O. (2022). Proximate And Phytochemical Screening: Evaluation of Minerals And Vitamin Composition Of (Hypoestes rosea) Plant Harvested In Calabar, Cross River State, Nigeria. FUDMA Journal of Sciences, 5(4), 229 ?"234. doi:10.33003/fjs-2021-0504-809DOI: 10.33003/fjs-2021-0504-809

Beat Malaria. (2024). *2024 World Malaria Report: What you need to know*. Retrieved from https://beatmalaria.org

Beccari, A., & Vistoli, G. (2022). Exscalate4CoV: innovative high performing computing (HPC) strategies to tackle pandemic crisis. International Journal of Molecular Sciences. ??? (Exact issue pending) en.wikipedia.orgDOI: 10.3390/ijms230

Bedri, S., Khalil, E. A., Khalid, S. A., Alzohairy, M. A., Mohieldein, A., Aldebasi, Y. H., Etet, P. F. S., & Farahna, M. (2013). Azadirachta indica ethanolic extract protects neurons from apoptosis and mitigates brain swelling in experimental cerebral malaria. Malaria Journal, 12(1), 298. doi:10.1186/1475-2875-12-298 PubMedDOI: 10.1186/1475-2875-12-298 PMID: 23984986

Behl, T., Kumar, K., Brisc, C., Rus, M., Nistor-Cseppento, D. C., Bustea, C., Aron, R. A. C., Pantis, C., Zengin, G., Sehgal, A., Kaur, R., Kumar, A., Arora, S., Setia, D., Chandel, D., & Bungau, S. (2021). Exploring the multifocal role of phytochemicals as immunomodulators. Biomedicine and Pharmacotherapy, 133, 110959. doi:10.1016/j.biopha.2020.110959 PubMedDOI: 10.1016/j.biopha.2020.110959 PMID: 33197758

Bekono, B. D., Ntie-Kang, F., Onguéné, P. A., Lifongo, L. L., Sippl, W., Fester, K., & Owono, L. C. (2020). The potential of anti-malarial compounds derived from African medicinal plants: A review of pharmacological evaluations from 2013 to 2019. *Malaria Journal*, *19*(1), 183. DOI: 10.1186/s12936-020-03231-7 PMID: 32423415

Belete, T. M. (2020). Recent progress in the development of new antimalarial drugs with novel targets. *Drug Design, Development and Therapy*, *14*, 3875–3889. DOI: 10.2147/DDDT.S265602 PMID: 33061294

Bency Baby, T., & Suriyaprakash, T. N. K. (2022). Intellectual Property Rights: Bioprospecting, Biopiracy. *Intellectual Property*, 25.

Beniwal, P., Joshi, J., & Kaur, S. (2025). A comprehensive review of cerebral malaria. *Journal of Parasitic Diseases : Official Organ of the Indian Society for Parasitology*, *49*(2), 257–272. DOI: 10.1007/s12639-024-01758-z PMID: 40458503

Berlowitz, I., Cuya-Velásquez, L., Brabec de Mori, B., & Rozin, A. (2025). Towards culturally inclusive healthcare in Peru: Epistemic concepts in Indigenous-Amazonian medicine. *Journal of Ethnobiology and Ethnomedicine*, *21*(1), 1–18. PMID: 39794744

Berlowitz, I., Pesantes, M. A., Cárdenas Palacios, C., Martin-Soelch, C., Wolf, U., & Maake, C. (2025). Towards culturally inclusive healthcare in Peru: Mapping epistemic concepts in contemporary Indigenous Amazonian medicine—Traditional healers' perspectives. *PLOS Global Public Health*, *5*(1), e0003912. DOI: 10.1371/journal.pgph.0003912 PMID: 39823398

Bezerra, J. J. L., Pinheiro, A. A. V., & Dourado, D. (2023). *Antimalarial potential of* Moringa oleifera *Lam. (Moringaceae): A review of the ethnomedicinal, pharmacological, toxicological, and phytochemical evidence*. https://doi.org/DOI: 10.1590/1678-9199-JVATITD-2022-0079

Bhambhani, S., Kondhare, K. R., & Giri, A. P. (2021). Diversity in Chemical Structures and Biological Properties of Plant Alkaloids. *Molecules (Basel, Switzerland)*, *26*(11), 3374. DOI: 10.3390/molecules26113374 PMID: 34204857

Bhatnagar, A. (2023). Chemical constituents of Andrographis paniculata (Burm. F) Nees: A review. International Journal of Pharmaceutical Sciences and Research, 14(7), 3238 ?"3245.

Bhatt, S., Weiss, D. J., Cameron, E., Bisanzio, D., Mappin, B., Dalrymple, U., Battle, K. E., Moyes, C. L., Henry, A., Eckhoff, P. A., Wenger, E. A., Briët, O., Penny, M. A., Smith, T. A., Bennett, A., Yukich, J., Eisele, T. P., Griffin, J. T., Fergus, C. A., & Gething, P. W. (2015). The effect of malaria control on *Plasmodium falciparum* in Africa between 2000 and 2015. *Nature*, *526*(7572), 207–211. DOI: 10.1038/nature15535 PMID: 26375008

Bitwell, C., Indra, S. S., Luke, C., & Kakoma, M. K. (2023). A review of modern and conventional extraction techniques and their applications for extracting phytochemicals from plants. *Scientific African*, *19*, e01585. DOI: 10.1016/j.sciaf.2023.e01585

Bloom, D. E., Sachs, J. D., Collier, P., & Udry, C. (1998). Geography, demography, and economic growth in Africa. *Brookings Papers on Economic Activity*, *1998*(2), 207–273. DOI: 10.2307/2534695 PMID: 12295931

Blunt, J. W., Carroll, A. R., Copp, B. R., Davis, R. A., Keyzers, R. A., & Prinsep, M. R. (2018). Marine natural products. *Natural Product Reports*, *35*(1), 8–53. DOI: 10.1039/C7NP00052A PMID: 29335692

Bochkov, D. V., Sysolyatin, S. V., Kalashnikov, A. I., & Surmacheva, I. A. (2012). Shikimic acid: Review of its analytical, isolation, and purification techniques from plant and microbial sources. *Journal of Chemical Biology*, *5*(1), 5–17. DOI: 10.1007/s12154-011-0064-8 PMID: 22826715

Boldini, D., Ballabio, D., Consonni, V., Todeschini, R., Grisoni, F., & Sieber, S. A. (2024). Effectiveness of molecular fingerprints for exploring the chemical space of natural products. *Journal of Cheminformatics*, *16*(1), 35. pmc.ncbi.nlm.nih.gov. DOI: 10.1186/s13321-024-00830-3 PMID: 38528548

Boulet, C., Doerig, C. D., & Carvalho, T. G. (2018). Manipulating eryptosis of human red blood cells: A novel antimalarial strategy? *Frontiers in Cellular and Infection Microbiology*, *8*, 419. DOI: 10.3389/fcimb.2018.00419 PMID: 30560094

Boye, G. L., & Ampofo, O. (2018). Cryptolepine hydrochloride: An alkaloid from *Cryptolepis sanguinolenta. Journal of Ethnopharmacology*, *213*, 36–45.

Brackney, D. E., LaReau, J. C., & Smith, R. C. (2021). Frequency matters: How successive feeding episodes by blood-feeding insect vectors influences disease transmission. *PLoS Pathogens*, *17*(6), e1009590. DOI: 10.1371/journal.ppat.1009590 PMID: 34111228

Bregman, H., Simard, J. R., Andrews, K. L., Ayube, S., Chen, H., Gunaydin, H., & Huang, X. (2017). The discovery and hit-to-lead optimization of tricyclic sulfonamides as potent and efficacious potentiators of glycine receptors. *Journal of Medicinal Chemistry*, *60*(3), 1105–1125. DOI: 10.1021/acs.jmedchem.6b01496 PMID: 28001399

Bučević Popović, V., Karahmet Farhat, E., Banjari, I., Jeličić Kadić, A., & Puljak, L. (2024). Bioavailability of oral curcumin in systematic reviews: A methodological study. *Pharmaceuticals (Basel, Switzerland)*, *17*(2), 164. DOI: 10.3390/ph17020164 PMID: 38399379

Bülbül, E. F., Bode, H. B., Schmitt, S., & Bozhüyük, K. A. J. (2025). Engineering the future of medicine: Natural products, synthetic biology and artificial intelligence for next-generation therapeutics. *Clinical and Translational Medicine*, *15*(2), e70146. DOI: 10.1002/ctm2.70146 PMID: 39856487

Burkot, T. R., & Graves, P. M. (2000). Malaria, babesiosis, theileriosis and related diseases. In *Medical Entomology: A Textbook on Public Health and Veterinary Problems Caused by Arthropods* (pp. 187–230). Springer Netherlands. DOI: 10.1007/978-94-011-6472-6_7

Burrows, J. N., van Huijsduijnen, R. H., Mohrle, J. J., Oeuvray, C., & Wells, T. N. (2017). Designing the next generation of medicines for malaria control and eradication. *Malaria Journal, 16*(1), 187. DOI: 10.1186/1475-2875-12-187 PMID: 23742293

Bussmann, R. W., & Sharon, D. (2022). Ethnobotany in the Andes and the Amazon in a changing world. *Canadian Journal of Botany, 100*(6), 431–444. DOI: 10.1139/cjb-2021-0062

Butler, M. S., & Newman, D. J. (2008). Mother Nature's gifts to diseases of mankind: The impact of natural products on anti-infective drug discovery. *Annals of the New York Academy of Sciences, 1213*(1), 136–156.

Bykerk, V. P., Keystone, E. C., Kuriya, B., Larché, M., Thorne, J. C., & Haraoui, B. (2013). Achieving remission in clinical practice: Lessons from clinical trial data. *Clinical and Experimental Rheumatology, 31*(4), 621–632. PMID: 23622099

Caminade, C., Kovats, S., Rocklov, J., Tompkins, A. M., Morse, A. P., Colón-González, F. J., Stenlund, H., Martens, P., & Lloyd, S. J. (2014). Impact of climate change on global malaria distribution. *Proceedings of the National Academy of Sciences of the United States of America, 111*(9), 3286–3291. DOI: 10.1073/pnas.1302089111 PMID: 24596427

Candini, O., Grisendi, G., Foppiani, E. M., Brogli, M., Aramini, B., Masciale, V., Spano, C., Petrachi, T., Veronesi, E., Conte, P., Mari, G., & Dominici, M. (2019). A novel 3D in-vitro platform for pre-clinical investigations in drug testing, gene therapy, and immuno-oncology. *Scientific Reports, 9*(1), 7154. DOI: 10.1038/s41598-019-43613-9 PMID: 31073193

Cao, Y., Wu, H., Zhang, Y., Wu, X., Li, J., Chen, H., & Gao, W. (2025). Time trends in malaria incidence from 1992 to 2021 in high-risk regions: An age-period-cohort analysis based on the Global Burden of Disease study 2021. *International Journal of Infectious Diseases, 153*, 107770. DOI: 10.1016/j.ijid.2024.107770 PMID: 39736331

Carrara, V. I., Lwin, K. M., Ashley, E., Price, R. N., & Nosten, F. (2013). Malaria burden and artemisinin resistance in mobile populations on the Thai–Myanmar border. *Malaria Journal, 12*(1), 1–9.

Carvalho, M. T., AraA jo-Filho, H. G., Barreto, A. S., Quintans-JA nior, L. J., Quintans, J. S., & Barreto, R. S. (2021). Wound healing properties of flavonoids: A systematic review highlighting the mechanisms of action. Phytomedicine, 90, 153636. doi:10.1016/j.phymed.2021.153636 PubMedDOI: 10.1016/j.phymed.2021.153636 PMID: 34333340

Celik, O. F., Kilicaslan, M., Akcaoglu, S., & Ozturk, Y. (2023). Improving the antioxidant activity of yogurt through black and green tea supplementation. *International Journal of Food Science & Technology*, *58*(11), 6121–6130. DOI: 10.1111/ijfs.16722

Centers for Disease Control and Prevention. (2024). *Malaria: Biology*. https://www.cdc.gov/malaria/

Ceravolo, I. P., Aguiar, A. C., Adebayo, J. O., & Krettli, A. U. (2021). Studies on activities and chemical characterization of medicinal plants in search for new Antimalarials: A ten year review on Ethnopharmacology. *Frontiers in Pharmacology*, *12*, 734263. DOI: 10.3389/fphar.2021.734263 PMID: 34630109

Ceravolo, I. P., Arcas, R. D. C. C., & Ursine, A. (2024). Plants from South America: A Systematic Review of Their Antiplasmodial and Antimalarial Activities Based on Ethnopharmacological Use. *Journal of Biomedical Research & Environmental Sciences*, *2766*(8), 2276. DOI: 10.37871/jbres1972

Chaachouay, N., Azeroual, A., Bencharki, B., Douira, A., & Zidane, L. (2022c). Ethnoveterinary medicines plants for animal therapy in the Rif, North of Morocco. *South African Journal of Botany*, *147*, 176–191. DOI: 10.1016/j.sajb.2021.12.037

Chaachouay, N., Azeroual, A., Douira, A., & Zidane, L. (2022b). Ethnoveterinary practices of medicinal plants among the Zemmour and Zayane tribes, Middle Atlas, Morocco. *South African Journal of Botany*, *151*, 826–840. DOI: 10.1016/j.sajb.2022.11.009

Chaachouay, N., Benkhnigue, O., Fadli, M., El Ayadi, R., & Zidane, L. (2019b). Ethnobotanical study of medicinal plants used to treat osteoarticular diseases in the Moroccan Rif, Morocco. *Journal of Pharmacy & Pharmacognosy Research*, *7*(6), 454–470. DOI: 10.56499/jppres19.644_7.6.454

Chaachouay, N., Benkhnigue, O., Fadli, M., El Ibaoui, H., El Ayadi, R., & Zidane, L. (2019a). Ethnobotanical and ethnopharmacological study of medicinal and aromatic plants used in the treatment of respiratory system disorders in the Moroccan Rif. *Ethnobotany Research and Applications*, *18*, 1–16. DOI: 10.32859/era.18.22.1-17

Chaachouay, N., Douira, A., & Zidane, L. (2022a). Herbal medicine used in the treatment of human diseases in the Rif, Northern Morocco. *Arabian Journal for Science and Engineering*, *47*(1), 131–153. DOI: 10.1007/s13369-021-05501-1 PMID: 33842189

Chang, J., Kim, Y., & Kwon, H. J. (2016). Advances in identification and validation of protein targets of natural products without chemical modification. *Natural Product Reports*, *33*(5), 719–730. DOI: 10.1039/C5NP00107B PMID: 26964663

Chao, W. W., & Lin, B. F. (2010). Isolation and identification of bioactive compounds in Andrographis paniculata (Chuanxinlian). Chinese Medicine, 5(1), 17. doi:10.1186/1749-8546-5-17 PubMedDOI: 10.1186/1749-8546-5-17 PMID: 20465823

Chen, J., Tian, X., Guo, D., Gu, H., Duan, Y., & Li, D. (2025). Global trends and burdens of neglected tropical diseases and malaria from 1990 to 2021: A systematic analysis of the Global Burden of Disease Study 2021. *BMC Public Health*, *25*(1), 1307. DOI: 10.1186/s12889-025-22477-x PMID: 40197173

Chen, Y., & Kirchmair, J. (2020). Cheminformatics in natural product-based drug discovery. *Molecular Informatics*, *39*(12), 2000171. DOI: 10.1002/minf.202000171 PMID: 32725781

Chihomvu, P., Ganesan, A., Gibbons, S., Woollard, K., & Hayes, M. A. (2024). Phytochemicals in Drug Discovery—A Confluence of Tradition and Innovation. *International Journal of Molecular Sciences*, *25*(16), 8792. DOI: 10.3390/ijms25168792 PMID: 39201478

Chima, R. I., Goodman, C. A., & Mills, A. (2003). The economic impact of malaria in Africa: A critical review of the evidence. *Health Policy (Amsterdam)*, *63*(1), 17–36. DOI: 10.1016/S0168-8510(02)00036-2 PMID: 12468115

Chinsembu, K. C. (2016). Plants as antimalarial agents in Sub-Saharan Africa. *Acta Tropica*, *152*, 32–48. DOI: 10.1016/j.actatropica.2015.08.009 PMID: 26297798

Chirangi, R. B., Pandey, D. K., Kumar, N., & Mishra, S. (2018). Phytochemicals of traditional medicinal plants with potential antimalarial activity: An updated review. *Journal of Ethnopharmacology*, *225*, 352–381.

Choudhary, R., Kaushik, R., Akhtar, A., Manna, S., Sharma, J., & Bains, A. (2025). Nutritional, Phytochemical, and Antimicrobial Properties of Carica papaya Leaves: Implications for Health Benefits and Food Applications. Foods, 14(2), 154. doi:10.3390/foods14020154 PubMedDOI: 10.3390/foods14020154 PMID: 39856820

Choudhury, A. (2022). Potential role of bioactive phytochemicals in combination therapies against antimicrobial activity. *Journal of Pharmacopuncture*, *25*(2), 79–87. DOI: 10.3831/KPI.2022.25.2.79 PMID: 35837140

Choudhury, C., Arul Murugan, N., & Priyakumar, U. D. (2022). Structure-based drug repurposing: AI/ML-aided methods. *Drug Discovery Today*, *27*(7), 1847–1861. link.springer.com. DOI: 10.1016/j.drudis.2022.03.006 PMID: 35301148

Clark, A. M. (1996). Natural products as a resource for new drugs. *Pharmaceutical Research*, *13*(8), 1133–1141. DOI: 10.1023/A:1016091631721 PMID: 8865302

Colella, J. P. (2023). Engaging with the Nagoya Protocol on Access and Benefit-Sharing: Implications for noncommercial research. *Journal of Mammalogy*, *104*(3), 430–440. DOI: 10.1093/jmammal/gyac122

Colonia, C. B., Vásquez-Rodríguez, A. B., Alexander, N., & de la Hoz Restrepo, F. (2024). Malaria, relationship with climatic variables and deforestation in Colombia, Latin America and the Caribbean from 2000 to 2020: A systematic review. *Malaria Journal*, *23*(1), 347. DOI: 10.1186/s12936-024-05140-5 PMID: 39558332

Combrinck, J. M., Mabotha, T. E., Ncokazi, K. K., Ambele, M. A., Taylor, D., Smith, P. J., Hoppe, H. C., & Egan, T. J. (2013). Insights into the Role of Heme in the Mechanism of Action of Antimalarials. *ACS Chemical Biology*, *8*(1), 133–137. DOI: 10.1021/cb300454t PMID: 23043646

Convention on Biological Diversity. (2014). *Nagoya Protocol on Access and Benefit-Sharing*. CBD.

Convention on Biological Diversity. (2018). Decision 3/13 on a global multilateral benefit-sharing mechanism (Article 10) (CBD/NP/MOP/DEC/3/13). https://www.cbd.int/doc/decisions/np-mop-03/np-mop-03-dec-13-en.pdf

Cortez-Maya, S., Moreno-Herrera, A., Palos, I., & Rivera, G. (2020). Old antiprotozoal drugs: Are they still viable options for parasitic infections or new options for other diseases? *Current Medicinal Chemistry*, *27*(32), 5403–5428. DOI: 10.2174/0929867326666190628163633 PMID: 31264538

Couillaud, J., Leydet, L., Duquesne, K., & Iacazio, G. (2021). The Terpene Mini-Path, a New Promising Alternative for Terpenoids Bio-Production. *Genes*, *12*(12), 1974. DOI: 10.3390/genes12121974 PMID: 34946923

Cowell, A. N., & Winzeler, E. A. (2019). Exploration of the Plasmodium falciparum kinome for targets of established chemotherapeutic agents. *Nature Reviews. Microbiology*, *17*(1), 33–46.

Cragg, G. M., & Newman, D. J. (2013). Natural products: A continuing source of novel drug leads.

Daher, A., Pereira, D., Lacerda, M. V., Alexandre, M. A., Nascimento, C. T., Alves de Lima e Silva, J. C., Tada, M., Ruffato, R., Maia, I., dos Santos, T. C., Marchesini, P., Santelli, A. C., & Lalloo, D. G. (2018). Efficacy and safety of artemisinin-based combination therapy and chloroquine with concomitant primaquine to treat Plasmodium vivax malaria in Brazil: An open label randomized clinical trial. *Malaria Journal, 17*(1), 45. DOI: 10.1186/s12936-018-2192-x PMID: 29361939

Dara, S., Dhamercherla, S., Jadav, S. S., Babu, C. M., & Ahsan, M. J. (2022). Machine learning in drug discovery: A review. *Artificial Intelligence Review, 55*(3), 1947–1999. link.springer.com. DOI: 10.1007/s10462-021-10058-4 PMID: 34393317

Das, G., Shin, H.-S., & Patra, J. K. (2024). The Antiviral and Antimalarial Prodrug Artemisinin from the Artemisia Species: A Review. *Current Issues in Molecular Biology, 46*(11), 12099–12118. DOI: 10.3390/cimb46110718 PMID: 39590312

Datoo, M. S., Natama, H. M., Somé, A., Traoré, O., Rouamba, T., Bellamy, D., Yameogo, P., Valia, D., Tegneri, M., Ouedraogo, F., Soma, R., Sawadogo, S., Sorgho, F., Derra, K., Rouamba, E., Orindi, B., Ramos Lopez, F., Flaxman, A., Cappuccini, F., & Tinto, H. (2021). Efficacy of a low-dose candidate malaria vaccine, R21/Matrix-M, with seasonal administration to children in Burkina Faso: A randomized controlled trial. *Lancet, 397*(10287), 1809–1818. DOI: 10.1016/S0140-6736(21)00943-0 PMID: 33964223

David, P. E., Luis, B. S. G., Alma, D. E. A., Martha, P. N. H., & Mariadel, C. V. M. (2017). HIV-1 Infection Inhibition by Neem (Azadirachta indica A. Juss.) leaf extracts and azadirachtin. Indian Journal of Traditional Knowledge, 16, 437 ?"441.

Davis, K., Guimarães, M., Davis, G., & Amarante, L. (2021). Ethnobotanical study of anti-malarial plants among riverine communities, Portel, Pará, Brazil. *Revista Fitos, 15*(4), 498–511. DOI: 10.32712/2446-4775.2021.1156

de Lima, E. P., Laurindo, L. F., Catharin, V. C. S., Direito, R., Tanaka, M., Jasmin Santos German, I., Lamas, C. B., Guiguer, E. L., Araújo, A. C., Fiorini, A. M. R., & Barbalho, S. M. (2025). Polyphenols, Alkaloids, and Terpenoids Against Neurodegeneration: Evaluating the Neuroprotective Effects of Phytocompounds Through a Comprehensive Review of the Current Evidence. *Metabolites, 15*(2), 124. DOI: 10.3390/metabo15020124 PMID: 39997749

de Páscoa Júnior, J. G., & Luna de Souza, I. L. (2021). *Medicinal plants used in the Amazon region: A systematic review.* Research. *Social Development, 10*(14), e163101419965.

De Salazar, P. M., Parra-Salazar, A., Niles-Robin, R., Valz, O., James, K., Buckee, C. O., & Cox, H. (2025). Malaria spillover in Indigenous Guyanese communities following a crackdown on illegal gold mining in Brazil. *Lancet Regional Health. Americas*, *42*, 42. DOI: 10.1016/j.lana.2024.100969 PMID: 39830894

De Smet, P. A. G. M. (1983). A multidisciplinary overview of intoxicating enema rituals in the Western Hemisphere. Journal of Ethnopharmacology, 9(2-3), 129 ?"166. doi:10.1016/0378-8741(83)90031-4 PubMedDOI: 10.1016/0378-8741(83)90031-4 PMID: 6677814

de Sousa, D. P., Damasceno, R. O. S., Amorati, R., Elshabrawy, H. A., de Castro, R. D., Bezerra, D. P., Nunes, V. R. V., Gomes, R. C., & Lima, T. C. (2023). Essential Oils: Chemistry and Pharmacological Activities. *Biomolecules*, *13*(7), 1144. DOI: 10.3390/biom13071144 PMID: 37509180

de Swiet, M. (2023). Cinchona: The source of quinine and quinidine. In *Modern Medicines from Plants* (pp. 93-102). CRC Press.

de Villiers, K. A., & Egan, T. J. (2021). Heme Detoxification in the Malaria Parasite: A Target for Antimalarial Drug Development. *Accounts of Chemical Research*, *54*(11), 2649–2659. DOI: 10.1021/acs.accounts.1c00154 PMID: 33982570

Del Prado-Audelo, M. L., Cortés, H., Caballero-Florán, I. H., González-Torres, M., Escutia-Guadarrama, L., Bernal-Chávez, S. A., Giraldo-Gomez, D. M., Magaña, J. J., & Leyva-Gómez, G. (2021). Therapeutic Applications of Terpenes on Inflammatory Diseases. *Frontiers in Pharmacology*, *12*, 704197. Advance online publication. DOI: 10.3389/fphar.2021.704197 PMID: 34483907

Deressa, T., Mekonnen, Y., & Animut, A. (2010). In-vivo antimalarial activities of Clerodendrum myricoides, Dodonea angustifolia, and Aloe debrana against Plasmodium berghei. The Ethiopian Journal of Health Development, 24(1), 25 ?"29. doi:10.4314/ejhd.v24i1.62941DOI: 10.4314/ejhd.v24i1.62941

Dev, M., & Mukadam, M. (2025). *Functional group profiling of medicinal plants using FTIR spectroscopy*. World Journal of Biology Pharmacy and Health Sciences., DOI: 10.30574/wjbphs.2025.21.1.0039

Dewees, J. (2023). Bittersweet Empire: Clements Robert Markham, Cinchona, and Botanical Exploitation. *PhD diss., Wesleyan University*.

Dey, P., Kundu, A., Kumar, A., Gupta, M., Lee, B. M., Bhakta, T., Dash, S., & Kim, H. S. (2020). Analysis of alkaloids (indole alkaloids, isoquinoline alkaloids, tropane alkaloids). *Recent Advances in Natural Products Analysis*, 505–567. DOI: 10.1016/B978-0-12-816455-6.00015-9

Diala, C. C., Pennas, T., Marin, C., & Belay, K. A. (2013). Perceptions of intermittent preventive treatment of malaria in pregnancy (IPTp) and barriers to adherence in Nasarawa and Cross River States in Nigeria. Malaria Journal, 12(1), 342. doi:10.1186/1475-2875-12-342 PubMedDOI: 10.1186/1475-2875-12-342 PMID: 24059757

Dias, M. C., Pinto, D. C. G. A., & Silva, A. M. S. (2021). Plant Flavonoids: Chemical Characteristics and Biological Activity. *Molecules (Basel, Switzerland)*, *26*(17), 5377. DOI: 10.3390/molecules26175377 PMID: 34500810

Dimitrova, Z. (1999). The history of pharmacy. *Sofija: St Clement of Ohrid*, 13-26.

Djokic, V., Rocha, S. C., & Parveen, N. (2021). Lessons learned for pathogenesis, immunology, and disease of erythrocytic parasites: Plasmodium and Babesia. *Frontiers in Cellular and Infection Microbiology*, *11*, 685239. DOI: 10.3389/fcimb.2021.685239 PMID: 34414129

Domingo-Fernández, D., Gadiya, Y., Preto, A. J., Krettler, C. A., Mubeen, S., Allen, A., Healey, D., & Colluru, V. (2024). Natural Products Have Increased Rates of Clinical Trial Success throughout the Drug Development Process. *Journal of Natural Products*, *87*(7), 1844–1851. DOI: 10.1021/acs.jnatprod.4c00581 PMID: 38970498

Dondorp, A. M., Fairhurst, R. M., Slutsker, L., MacArthur, J. R., Breman, J. G., Guerin, P. J., & Ringwald, P. (2009). The threat of artemisinin-resistant malaria. *The New England Journal of Medicine*, *361*(5), 455–457. DOI: 10.1056/NEJMoa0808859 PMID: 19641202

Dou, B., Zhu, Z., Merkurjev, E., et al. (2023). Machine learning methods for small data challenges in molecular science. Chemical Reviews, 123(13), 8736–8780. medium.comDOI: 10.1021/acs.chemrev.3c00189

Drabu, S., Khatri, S., & Babu, S. (2012). Neem: Healer of all ailments. Research Journal of Pharmaceutical, Biological and Chemical Sciences, 3, 120 ?"126.

Duda-Madej, A., Viscardi, S., Niezgódka, P., Szewczyk, W., & Wińska, K. (2025). The Impact of Plant-Derived Polyphenols on Combating Efflux-Mediated Antibiotic Resistance. *International Journal of Molecular Sciences*, *26*(9), 4030. DOI: 10.3390/ijms26094030 PMID: 40362268

Dunn, J. P., Krige, J. E. J., Wood, R., Bornman, P. C., & Terblanche, J. (1991). Colonic complications after toxic tribal enemas. British Journal of Surgery, 78(5), 545 ?"548. doi:10.1002/bjs.1800780510 PubMedDOI: 10.1002/bjs.1800780510 PMID: 2059802

Duval, R., & Duplais, C. (2017). Fluorescent natural products as probes and tracers in biology. *Natural Product Reports*, *34*(2), 161–193. DOI: 10.1039/C6NP00111D PMID: 28125109

Dwivedi, G. R., Tripathi, P., & Mishra, S. K. (2013). Repurposing quercetin as a potential anti-malarial: In vitro and in silico studies. Journal of Biomolecular Structure & Dynamics, 31(4), 400 ?"410.

Dwivedi, M. K., Mishra, S., Sonter, S., & Singh, P. K. (2021). Diterpenoids as potential anti-malarial compounds from Andrographis panculata. *Beni-Suef University Journal of Basic and Applied Sciences*, *10*(1), 7. Advance online publication. DOI: 10.1186/s43088-021-00098-8

Ebenyi, L. N., Yongabi, K. A., Ali, F. U., Ominyi, M. C., Anyanwu, C. B., Benjamin, E., & Ogbanshi, M. E. (2021). Effect of aqueous leaf extract of Jatropha tanjorensis on parasitaemia and haematological parameters in mice infected with Plasmodium berghei. Nigerian Journal of Biotechnology, 38(1), 146 ?"153. doi:10.4314/njb.v38i1.17DOI: 10.4314/njb.v38i1.17

Ediriweera, M. K., Tennekoon, K. H., & Samarakoon, S. R. (2017). A review on ethnopharmacological applications, pharmacological activities, and bioactive compounds of Mangifera indica (Mango). Evidence-Based Complementary and Alternative Medicine : eCAM, 6949835(1), 6949835. Advance online publication. doi:10.1155/2017/6949835 PubMedDOI: 10.1155/2017/6949835 PMID: 29456572

Ekasari, W., Widya Pratiwi, D., Amanda, Z., Suciati, Widyawaruyanti, A. & Arwati H. (2019). Various Parts of *Helianthus annuus* Plants as New Sources of Antimalarial Drugs. *Evidence-Based Complement Alternative Medicine*, .DOI: 10.1155/2019/7390385

Elebiyo, T. C., Oluba, O. M., & Adeyemi, O. S. (2023). Anti-malarial and haematological evaluation of the ethanolic, ethyl acetate, and aqueous fractions of Chromolaena odorata. BMC Complementary Medicine and Therapies, 23(1), 402. Advance online publication. doi:10.1186/s12906-023-04200-8 PubMedDOI: 10.1186/s12906-023-04200-8 PMID: 37946127

Emeribe, A. U., Anyanwu, S. O., Isong, I. K., Bassey, U. R., Inyang, I. J., Ibeneme, E. O., Asemota, E. A., Okhormhe, Z., Icha, B., & Abdullahi, I. N. (2021). Phytochemical analysis and toxicological evaluation of the ethanolic Leaves extract of Hypoestes rosea on the morphology and biochemical indices of the Kidneys of albino Wistar Rats. Saudi Journal of Biological Sciences, 28(12), 6748 ?"6755. doi:10.1016/j.sjbs.2021.07.045 PubMedDOI: 10.1016/j.sjbs.2021.07.045 PMID: 34866973

Enenebeaku, C. K., Ogukwe, C. E., Nweke, C. O., Anyado-Nwadike, S. O., Obi, M., Duru, I. A., Enenebeaku, U. E., & Ogidi, O. I. (2022a). Antiplasmodial and *in vitro* antioxidant potentials of crude aqueous and methanol extracts of *Chasmanthera dependens* (Hochst). *Bulletin of the National Research Center*, *46*(33), 1–12. DOI: 10.1186/s42269-022-00721-3

Enenebeaku, U. E., Duru, C. E., Okotcha, E. N., Ogidi, O. I., Mgbemena, I. C., Nwigwe, H. C., & Enenebeaku, C. K. (2022b). Phytochemical analysis and antioxidant evaluation of crude extracts from the roots, stem and leaves of *Dictyandra arborescens* (Welw.). *Tropical Journal of Natural Product Research*, *6*(1), 62–70. DOI: 10.26538/tjnpr/v6i1.12

Enenebeaku, U. E., Ukwandu, N. C., Mgbemena, I. C., Nwigwe, H. C., Enenebeaku, C. K., Duru, C. E., & Ogidi, O. I. (2021). Oral acute toxicity and antimalarial potentials of aqueous and methanolic extracts of roots, leaves and stem of *Dictyandra arborescens* (Welw.) on *Plasmodium berghei* infected mice. *Bulletin of the National Research Center*, *45*(75), 1–12. DOI: 10.1186/s42269-021-00530-0

Erinoso, S. M., & Aworinde, D. O. (2018). Current outlook and future promise of ethnobotany in Nigeria: A review and personal observation. African Journal of Plant Science, 12(4), 73-80. ? https://doi.org/doi:10.5897/AJPS2017.1571DOI: 10.5897/AJPS2017.1571

Ernst, M., Grace, O. M., Saslis-Lagoudakis, C. H., Nilsson, N., Simonsen, H. T., & Ronsted, N. (2015). Global medicinal uses of Euphorbia L. (Euphorbiaceae). *Journal of Ethnopharmacology*, *176*, 90–101. DOI: 10.1016/j.jep.2015.10.025 PMID: 26485050

Ettling, M. B., McFarland, D. A., Schultz, L. J., & Chitsulo, L. (1994). Economic impact of malaria in Malawian households. *Tropical Medicine and Parasitology*, *45*(1), 74–79. PMID: 8066390

European Medicines Agency (2020). Guidelines on Quality of Medicinal Products Derived from Biological Sources.

Ewart, L., Dehne, E. M., Fabre, K., Gibbs, S., Hickman, J., Hornberg, E., & Swanson, B. (2018). Application of microphysiological systems to enhance safety assessment in drug discovery. *Annual Review of Pharmacology and Toxicology*, *58*(1), 65–82. DOI: 10.1146/annurev-pharmtox-010617-052722 PMID: 29029591

Ezeanya-Bakpa, C. C., Inobeme, A., & Adekoya, M. A. (2022). Hospital laundries and their effect on medical textiles. In: Medical Textiles from Natural Resources, Elsevier, United Kingdom, Pp, 767-792. DOI: DOI: 10.1016/B978-0-323-90479-7.00004-X

Ezeanya-Bakpa, C. C., & Adams, A. A. (2024). *In vitro* susceptibility of drug-resistant fungi and urinary bacteria to *Psidium guajava* L. leaf extract. *Nigerian Journal of Biotechnology*, *41*(1), 157–164. DOI: 10.4314/njb.v41i1.17

Ezeanya-Bakpa, C. C., Adetunji, C. O., Enosabata, I. A., & Olori, E. (2021). Lycopene for wound infection: In vitro susceptibility of drug-resistant clinical pathogens. *Tropical Journal of Natural Product Research*, *5*(1), 49–52. DOI: 10.26538/tjnpr/v5i1.4

Ezeanya-Bakpa, C. C., Agbakoba, N. R., Enweani, I. B., & Oguejiofor, C. B. (2019). Predominance of cervicitis agents with minimal testing rate within the student population in Benin City, Nigeria. *Journal of Obstetrics & Gynaecology*, *39*(6), 840–844. DOI: 10.1080/01443615.2019.1584888 PMID: 31007108

Ezeanya-Bakpa, C. C., Agbakoba, N. R., Enweani-Nwokelo, I. B., & Oguejiofor, C. B. (2022). Phylogeny-based identification of *Mycoplasma genitalium* in a Nigerian population of apparently healthy sexually active female students. *The Pan African Medical Journal*, *41*, 71–76. PMID: 35382058

Ezeanya-Bakpa, C. C., Akinola, K., Adebayo, O. P., & Akharaiyi, F. C. (2023). Antibacterial combination effect of allicin, lycopene and quercetin on antibiotic-resistant bacteria. *Microbes and Infectious Diseases*, *5*(1), 0. Advance online publication. DOI: 10.21608/mid.2023.253557.1701

Ezeigbo, O., Awomukwu, D., & Ezeigbo, I. (2016). The Antimicrobial and Phytochemical Analysis of the Leaves of Aspilia africana on Clinical Isolates. European Journal of Medicinal Plants, 15(2), 1 ?"6. doi:10.9734/EJMP/2016/26481DOI: 10.9734/EJMP/2016/26481

Ezema, C. A., Okagu, I. U., & Ezeorba, T. P. C. (2023). Escaping the enemy's bullets: An update on how malaria parasites evade host immune response. *Parasitology Research*, *122*(8), 1715–1731. DOI: 10.1007/s00436-023-07868-6 PMID: 37219610

Feachem, R. G., Chen, I., Akbari, O., Bertozzi-Villa, A., Bhatt, S., Binka, F., & Weiss, D. J. (2019). Malaria eradication within a generation: Ambitious, achievable, and necessary. *Lancet*, *394*(10203), 1056–1112. DOI: 10.1016/S0140-6736(19)31139-0 PMID: 31511196

Ferreira, M. U., Gamboa, D., Torres, K., Rodriguez-Ferrucci, H., Soto-Calle, V. E., Pardo, K., Fontoura, P. S., Tomko, S. S., Gazzinelli, R. T., Conn, J. E., Castro, M. C., Llanos-Cuentas, A., & Vinetz, J. M. (2022). Evidence-based malaria control and elimination in the Amazon: Input from the International Center of excellence in malaria research network in Peru and Brazil. *The American Journal of Tropical Medicine and Hygiene*, *107*(4, Suppl), 160–167. DOI: 10.4269/ajtmh.21-1272 PMID: 36228907

Ferreira, T. S., Moreira, C. Z., Cária, N. Z., Victoriano, G., Silva, W. F.Jr, & Magalhães, J. C. (2014). Phytotherapy: An introduction to its history, use and application. *Revista Brasileira de Plantas Medicinais*, *16*(2), 290–298. DOI: 10.1590/S1516-05722014000200019

Filli, M. S., Ibrahim, A. A., Kesse, S., Aquib, M., Boakye-Yiadom, K. O., Farooq, M. A., Raza, F., Zhang, Y., & Wang, B. (2022). Synthetic berberine derivatives as potential new drugs. *Brazilian Journal of Pharmaceutical Sciences*, *58*, e18835. DOI: 10.1590/s2175-97902020000318835

Fix, J. H. (2013). Fixing a broken drug development process. *Journal of Commercial Biotechnology*, *19*, 5–8.

Fletcher, I. K., Grillet, M. E., Moreno, J. E., Drakeley, C., Hernández-Villena, J., Jones, K. E., & Lowe, R. (2022). Synergies between environmental degradation and climate variation on malaria re-emergence in southern Venezuela: A spatiotemporal modelling study. *The Lancet. Planetary Health*, *6*(9), e739–e748. DOI: 10.1016/S2542-5196(22)00192-9 PMID: 36087604

Fokou, P. V. T., Tali, M. B. T., Mbouna, C. D. J., Yamthe, L. R. T., Sharifi-Rad, J., Calina, D., Radha, , Kumar, M., Tchouankeu, J. C., & Boyom, F. F. (2025). Natural products as transmission-blocking agents against malaria: A comprehensive review of bioactive compounds and their therapeutic potential. *Malaria Journal*, *24*(1), 164. DOI: 10.1186/s12936-025-05395-6 PMID: 40420292

Folawewo, A. D., Madu, A. N., Agbaje-Daniels, F. V., Faboyede, A. O., & Coker, A. R. (2017). Phytochemical screening and antibacterial activities of the root bark extracts of Hippocratea africana (Willd.) Locs. cx Engl. European Journal of Medicinal Plants, 19(1), 1 ?"8. doi:10.9734/EJMP/2017/32765DOI: 10.9734/EJMP/2017/32765

Frolova, N., Orlova, A., Popova, V., Bilova, T., & Frolov, A. (2025). *GC-MS-based metabolomics – Part 1 Gas chromatography-mass spectrometry (GC-MS) and its place in the plant metabolomics toolbox*. Chemistry. DOI: 10.26434/chemrxiv-2025-5kgvt

Fromer, J. C., & Coley, C. W. (2024). An algorithmic framework for synthetic cost-aware decision making in molecular design. Nature Computational Science, 4(6), 440–450. medium.comDOI: 10.1038/s43588-024-00639-y

Gallup, J. L., & Sachs, J. D. (2001). The economic burden of malaria. *The American Journal of Tropical Medicine and Hygiene*, *64*(1–2), 85–96. DOI: 10.4269/ajtmh.2001.64.85 PMID: 11425181

Gangwal, A., Ansari, A., Ahmad, I., Azad, A. K., Kumarasamy, V., Subramaniyan, V., & Wong, L. S. (2024). Generative artificial intelligence in drug discovery: Basic framework, recent advances, challenges, and opportunities. *Frontiers in Pharmacology, 15*, 1331062. DOI: 10.3389/fphar.2024.1331062 PMID: 38384298

Gangwal, A., Ansari, A., Ahmad, I., Azad, A. K., & Sulaiman, W. M. A. W. (2024). Current strategies to address data scarcity in AI-based drug discovery: A comprehensive review. *Computers in Biology and Medicine*, *179*, 108734. pmc.ncbi.nlm.nih.gov. DOI: 10.1016/j.compbiomed.2024.108734 PMID: 38964243

Garcia, C. G. R., Ribeiro, B. C., Souza, A. S., Lima, L. J. P., Póvoa, M. M., Laporta, G. Z., & Cunha, M. G. (2025). Assessing the spatial influence of deforestation on malaria incidence in Pará State, Amazon region, Brazil, 2008-2019. *Memorias do Instituto Oswaldo Cruz, 120*, e240143. DOI: 10.1590/0074-02760240143 PMID: 40531672

García, M., Magi, M. S., & García, M. C. (2025). Harnessing Phytonanotechnology to Tackle Neglected Parasitic Diseases: Focus on Chagas Disease and Malaria. *Pharmaceutics*, *17*(8), 1043. DOI: 10.3390/pharmaceutics17081043 PMID: 40871066

Gautam, P. K., Prajapati, B., & Sujatha, R. (2020). Chapter-5 Life Cycle, Pathogenesis and Laboratory Diagnosis of Malaria Parasite. *Chief Editor Dr. Durgadas Govind Naik*, *105*, 105.

Gavi. (2024). *Rolling out vaccines to beat malaria together: Time to harness the power of immunisation for a malaria-free future*. https://www.gavi.org/news-resources/resources/knowledge-products/rolling-out-vaccines-beat-malaria-together-time-harness-power-immunisation-malaria-free-future

Gebara, M. F., Ramcilovic-Suominen, S., & Schmidlehner, M. F. (2023). Indigenous Knowledge in the Amazon's Bioeconomy: Unveiling Bioepistemicide through the case of Kambo Medicine. *Forest Policy and Economics*, *154*, 103012. DOI: 10.1016/j.forpol.2023.103012

Gerheart, W. A., Edward, E. K., Mohammed, A., Prince, N. A., Jeremiah, A. S., & Boansi, A. A. (2024). Comparative analysis of phytochemical constituents in different parts of Aspilia africana: A potential medicinal plant for therapeutic applications. Phytomedicine Plus : International Journal of Phytotherapy and Phytopharmacology, 4(4), 100656. Advance online publication. doi:10.1016/j.phyplu.2024.100656DOI: 10.1016/j.phyplu.2024.100656

Gil, M. I., Tomás-Barberán, F. A., Hess-Pierce, B., & Kader, A. A. (2002). Antioxidant capacities, phenolic compounds, carotenoids, and vitamin C contents of nectarine, peach, and plum cultivars from California. *Journal of Agricultural and Food Chemistry, 50*(17), 4976–4982. DOI: 10.1021/jf020136b PMID: 12166993

Gleave, K., Lissenden, N., Richardson, M., Choi, L., & Ranson, H. (2018). Piperonyl butoxide (PBO) combined with pyrethroids in insecticide-treated nets to prevent malaria in Africa. *Cochrane Database of Systematic Reviews, 2018*(11). Advance online publication. DOI: 10.1002/14651858.CD012776.pub2 PMID: 30488945

Global Fund. (2023). *Malaria: Global Fund results report 2023.* Retrieved from https://www.theglobalfund.org

Gomes, A. R., Albuquerque, K. C., Brígido, H. P., Correa-Barbosa, J., Dolabela, M. F., & Percário, S. (2021). Development of Antimalarial and Antileishmanial Drugs from Amazonian Biodiversity. [Bentham Science Publishers.]. *Frontiers in Clinical Drug Research-Anti-Infectives, 7*, 127–172. DOI: 10.2174/9789814998093121070007

Gorantla, R., Kubincová, A., Suutari, B., Cossins, B. P., & Mey, A. S. J. S. (2024). Benchmarking active learning protocols for ligand-binding affinity prediction. Journal of Chemical Information and Modeling, 64(6), 1955–1965. DOI: 10.1021/acs.jcim.4c00220

Gozubuyuk, G. S., Aktas, E., & Yigit, N. (2014). An ancient plant Lawsonia inermis (henna): Determination of in vitro antifungal activity against dermatophytes species. *Journal de Mycologie Médicale, 24*(4), 313–318. DOI: 10.1016/j.mycmed.2014.07.002 PMID: 25442917

Grant, W. F. (1994). The present status of higher plant bioassays for the detection of environmental mutagens. *Mutation Research, 310*(2), 175–185. DOI: 10.1016/0027-5107(94)90112-0 PMID: 7523890

Graziose, R., Lila, M. A., & Raskin, I. (2010). Merging traditional Chinese medicine with modern drug discovery technologies to find novel drugs and functional foods. *Current Drug Discovery Technologies, 7*(1), 2–12. DOI: 10.2174/157016310791162767 PMID: 20156139

Grigalunas, M., Brakmann, S., & Waldmann, H. (2022). Chemical evolution of natural product structure. *Journal of the American Chemical Society, 144*(8), 3314–3329. DOI: 10.1021/jacs.1c11270 PMID: 35188375

Gunaseelan, R. J., Raj, A., Nagarajan, P., Perumal, S., Kumar, J., & Patil, S. J. (2025). Biotechnological Phytochemical Synthesis: Innovations, Challenges, Advantages, Implications. In *Biotechnology and Phytochemical Prospects in Drug Discovery* (pp. 83–101). Springer., DOI: 10.1007/978-981-96-2790-5_3

Gupta, M., Kumar, S., Kumar, R., Kumar, A., Verma, R., Darokar, M. P., Rout, P., & Pal, A. (2021). Inhibition of heme detoxification pathway in malaria parasite by 3-hydroxy-11-keto-β-boswellic acid isolated from Boswellia serrata. *Biomedicine and Pharmacotherapy*, *144*, 112302. DOI: 10.1016/j.biopha.2021.112302 PMID: 34678731

Gupta, S. C., Patchva, S., Koh, W., & Aggarwal, B. B. (2012). Discovery of curcumin, a component of the golden spice, and its miraculous biological activities. *Clinical and Experimental Pharmacology & Physiology*, *39*(3), 283–299. DOI: 10.1111/j.1440-1681.2011.05648.x PMID: 22118895

Gutiérrez-Grijalva, E. P., López-Martínez, L. X., Contreras-Angulo, L. A., Elizalde-Romero, C. A., & Heredia, J. B. (2020). Plant Alkaloids: Structures and Bioactive Properties. In Swamy, M. K. (Ed.), *Plant-derived Bioactives* (pp. 85–117). Springer Singapore., DOI: 10.1007/978-981-15-2361-8_5

Gu, Y., Wang, Y., Zhu, K., Li, W., Liu, G., & Tang, Y. (2024). DBPP-predictor: Prediction of chemical drug-likeness based on property profiles. *Journal of Cheminformatics*, *16*(1), 4. link.springer.com. DOI: 10.1186/s13321-024-00800-9 PMID: 38183072

Hagazy, K., Sibhat, G. G., Karim, A., Tekulu, G. H., Periasamy, G., & Hiben, M. (2020). Antimalarial activity of Meriandra dianthera leaf extracts in Plasmodium berghei-infected mice. Evidence-Based Complementary and Alternative Medicine : eCAM, 12(1), 8980212. doi:10.1155/2020/8980212 PubMedDOI: 10.1155/2020/8980212 PMID: 32104197

Hailu, A., Lindtjørn, B., Deressa, W., Gari, T., & Loha, E. (2009). Economic burden of malaria and predictors of cost variability to rural households in south-central Ethiopia. *Malaria Journal*, *8*(1), 214.

Haines, A., Sanders, D., Lehmann, U., Rowe, A. K., Lawn, J. E., Jan, S., Walker, D. G., & Bhutta, Z. (2007). Achieving child survival goals: Potential contribution of community health workers. *Lancet*, *369*(9579), 2121–2131. DOI: 10.1016/S0140-6736(07)60325-0 PMID: 17586307

Haines, D. D., & Tosaki, A. (2020). Heme degradation in pathophysiology of and countermeasures to inflammation-associated disease. *International Journal of Molecular Sciences*, *21*(24), 9698. DOI: 10.3390/ijms21249698 PMID: 33353225

Hamilton, A. C. (2004). Medicinal plants, conservation and livelihoods. *Biodiversity and Conservation, 13*(8), 1477–1517. DOI: 10.1023/B:BIOC.0000021333.23413.42

Harrison, C. (2014). Patenting natural products just got harder. *Nature Biotechnology, 32*(5), 403–404. DOI: 10.1038/nbt0514-403a PMID: 24811496

Harshberger, J. W. (1896). The purposes of ethno-botany. Botanical Gazette (Chicago, Ill.), 21(3), 146 ?"154. doi:10.1086/327316DOI: 10.1086/327316

Harvey, A. L., Edrada-Ebel, R., & Quinn, R. J. (2015). The re-emergence of natural products for drug discovery in the genomics era. *Nature Reviews. Drug Discovery, 14*(2), 111–129. DOI: 10.1038/nrd4510 PMID: 25614221

Hawadak, J., Dongang Nana, R. R., & Singh, V. (2021). Global trend of Plasmodium malariae and Plasmodium ovale spp. malaria infections in the last two decades (2000–2020): A systematic review and meta-analysis. *Parasites & Vectors, 14*(1), 297. DOI: 10.1186/s13071-021-04797-0 PMID: 34082791

Hawkins, J., Baker, C., Cherry, L., & Dunne, E. (2019). Black elderberry (Sambucus nigra) supplementation effectively treats upper respiratory symptoms: A meta-analysis of randomized, controlled clinical trials. *Complementary Therapies in Medicine, 42*, 361–365. DOI: 10.1016/j.ctim.2018.12.004 PMID: 30670267

Heinrich, M. (2020). Access and Benefit-Sharing under the Nagoya Protocol: Opportunities and challenges in Latin America. *Frontiers in Pharmacology / PMC.* https://www.ncbi.nlm.nih.gov/pmc/articles/PMC7294742/

Heinrich, M. (2010). Galanthamine from *Galanthus* and other Amaryllidaceae—Chemistry and biology based on traditional use. *The Alkaloids. Chemistry and Biology, 68*, 157–165. DOI: 10.1016/S1099-4831(10)06804-5 PMID: 20334038

Heinrich, M., Scotti, F., Andrade-Cetto, A., Berger-Gonzalez, M., Echeverría, J., Friso, F., Garcia-Cardona, F., Hesketh, A., Hitziger, M., Maake, C., Politi, M., Spadafora, C., & Spadafora, R. (2020). Access and benefit sharing under the Nagoya protocol—Quo Vadis? Six Latin American case studies assessing opportunities and risk. *Frontiers in Pharmacology, 11*, 765. DOI: 10.3389/fphar.2020.00765 PMID: 32581783

Hemingway, J., Ranson, H., Magill, A., Kolaczinski, J., Fornadel, C., Gimnig, J., & Gething, P. W. (2016). Averting a malaria disaster: Will insecticide resistance derail malaria control? *Lancet, 387*(10029), 1785–1788. DOI: 10.1016/S0140-6736(15)00417-1 PMID: 26880124

Hermanto, F., Haq, F. A., & Khasanah, R. (2024). The effect of resveratrol on the relationship of antioxidant activity and beta-hematin inhibition as an antimalarial action target. *Journal of Advanced Pharmaceutical Technology & Research, 15*(4), 359–363. DOI: 10.4103/JAPTR.JAPTR_144_24

Hogan, K. M., Gilmore, M., McCarron, G. P., Griffiths, B. M., Koehler, J. W., García, G. A., & von Fricken, M. E. (2024). Knowledge, attitudes, and practices regarding malaria transmission and prevention in an indigenous Maijuna community: A qualitative study in the Peruvian Amazon. *Malaria Journal*, *23*(1), 314. DOI: 10.1186/s12936-024-05121-8 PMID: 39425050

Holding, P. A., & Snow, R. W. (2001). Impact of *Plasmodium falciparum* malaria on performance and learning: Review of the evidence. *The American Journal of Tropical Medicine and Hygiene*, *64*(1–2), 68–75. DOI: 10.4269/ajtmh.2001.64.68 PMID: 11425179

Hooda, P., Malik, R., Bhatia, S., Al-Harrasi, A., Najmi, A., Zoghebi, K., Halawi, M. A., Makeen, H. A., & Mohan, S. (2024). Phytoimmunomodulators: A review of natural modulators for complex immune system. *Heliyon*, *10*(1), e23790. DOI: 10.1016/j.heliyon.2023.e23790 PMID: 38205318

Horackova, J., Chuspe Zans, M. E., Kokoska, L., Sulaiman, N., & Clavo Peralta, Z. M. (2023). Ethnobotanical inventory of medicinal plants used by Cashinahua herbalists in the Peruvian Amazon. *Journal of Ethnobiology and Ethnomedicine*, *19*(16). Advance online publication. DOI: 10.1186/s13002-023-00586-4 PMID: 37170108

Horne, R. I., Andrzejewska, E. A., Alam, P., et al. (2024). Discovery of potent inhibitors of α-synuclein aggregation using structure-based iterative learning. Nature Chemical Biology, 20(5), 634–645. DOI: 10.1038/s41589-024-01580-x

Hossain, M. S., Wazed, M. A., Asha, S., Amin, M. R., & Shimul, I. M. (2025). Dietary phytochemicals in health and disease: Mechanisms, clinical evidence, and applications a comprehensive review. *Food Science & Nutrition*, *13*(3), e70101. DOI: 10.1002/fsn3.70101 PMID: 40115248

Hosseinzadeh, S., Jafarikukhdan, A., Hosseini, A., & Armand, R. (2015). The application of medicinal plants in traditional and modern medicine: A review of Thymus vulgaris. International Journal of Clinical Medicine, 6(9), 635 ?"642. doi:10.4236/ijcm.2015.69084DOI: 10.4236/ijcm.2015.69084

Hotwani, K., Baliga, S., & Sharma, K. (2014). Phytodentistry: Use of medicinal plants. *Journal of Complementary & Integrative Medicine*, *11*(2), 233–251. DOI: 10.1515/jcim-2013-0015 PMID: 25153610

Huang, Y., Xiao, D., Burton-Freeman, B. M., & Edirisinghe, I. (2016). Chemical changes of bioactive phytochemicals during thermal processing

Huang, J., Zaynab, M., Sharif, Y., Khan, J., Al-Yahyai, R., Sadder, M., Ali, M., Alarab, S. R., & Li, S. (2024). Tannins as antimicrobial agents: Understanding toxic effects on pathogens. *Toxicon, 247*, 107812. DOI: 10.1016/j.toxicon.2024.107812 PMID: 38908527

Huang, W., Wang, Y., Tian, W., Cui, X., Tu, P., Li, J., Shi, S., & Liu, X. (2022). Biosynthesis Investigations of Terpenoid, Alkaloid, and Flavonoid Antimicrobial Agents Derived from Medicinal Plants. *Antibiotics (Basel, Switzerland), 11*(10), 1380. DOI: 10.3390/antibiotics11101380 PMID: 36290037

Huang, Y., Wang, S., Cai, Q., & Jin, H. (2021). Effective methods for isolation and purification of extracellular vesicles from plants. *Journal of Integrative Plant Biology, 63*(9), 2020–2030. DOI: 10.1111/jipb.13181 PMID: 34668639

Hubballi, R. B., Selvakumar, P., Seenivasan, R., & Basava Aradhya, S. G., Dinesh, N., & Seelam, P. K. (2025). Overview of Current AI Technologies in Education. In L. Kyei-Blankson & E. Ntuli (Eds.), Transformative AI Practices for Personalized Learning Strategies (pp. 1-26). IGI Global Scientific Publishing. DOI: 10.4018/979-8-3693-8744-3.ch001

Hutchinson, J., & Dalziel, J. M. (1973). Flora of West Tropical Africa (2nd ed., Vol. 1, Pt. 2. Crown Agents for Overseas Governments and Administrations.

Hu, W., Yu, A., Wang, S., Bai, Q., Tang, H., Yang, B., Wang, M., & Kuang, H. (2023). Extraction, purification, structural characteristics, biological activities, and applications of the polysaccharides from Zingiber officinale Roscoe (Ginger): A review. *Molecules (Basel, Switzerland), 28*(11), 4477. DOI: 10.3390/molecules28093855 PMID: 37175266

Hu, Y., Guo, N., Yang, T., Yan, J., Wang, W., & Li, X. (2022). The Potential Mechanisms by which Artemisinin and Its Derivatives Induce Ferroptosis in the Treatment of Cancer. *Oxidative Medicine and Cellular Longevity, 2022*(1), 1458143. DOI: 10.1155/2022/1458143 PMID: 35028002

Ibok, M. G., Odeja, O. O., Okpala, E. O., Eghwubare, J. E., & Anifalaje, E. O. (2023). Eremomastax speciosa (Hochst.): GC/MS profiling, antioxidant and antimicrobial activities of stem essential oil. Future Journal of Pharmaceutical Sciences, 9(1), 51. doi:10.1186/s43094-023-00501-4DOI: 10.1186/s43094-023-00501-4

Ibrahim, N. I., Wong, S. K., Mohamed, I. N., Mohamed, N., Chin, K. Y., Ima-Nirwana, S., & Shuid, A. N. (2018). Wound healing properties of selected natural products. International Journal of Environmental Research and Public Health, 15(11), 2360. doi:10.3390/ijerph15112360 PubMedDOI: 10.3390/ijerph15112360 PMID: 30366427

Iftikhar, A., Saleem, M., Raza, S. A., Achuthan, A., Luwor, R., Muhammad, T., & Majeed, U. (2025). Immunomodulatory properties of a methanolic extract of Ficus lyrata mitigate inflammation in Complete Freund's Adjuvant-induced arthritis. *Inflammopharmacology*, *33*(4), 1–14. DOI: 10.1007/s10787-025-01700-6 PMID: 40140117

Ikot, M., Mbong, E., Akpabio, K., & Uyoh, V. (2025). Morpho-statistical variation and taxonomic characterization of Andrographis paniculata (Burm. F.) Nees population obtained from selected locations within Southern Nigeria. Dutse Journal of Pure and Applied Sciences, 10(4c), 14 ?"23. doi:10.4314/dujopas.v10i4c.2DOI: 10.4314/dujopas.v10i4c.2

Imam, M. Z., & Akter, S. (2011). Musa paradisiaca L. and Musa sapientum L.: A phytochemical and pharmacological review. Journal of Applied Pharmaceutical Science, 1(5), 14 ?"20.

Imran, M., Arshad, M. S., Butt, M. S., Kwon, J. H., Arshad, M. U., & Sultan, M. T. (2017). Mangiferin: A natural miracle bioactive compound against lifestyle-related disorders. Lipids in Health and Disease, 16(1), 1 ?"17. doi:10.1186/s12944-017-0449-y PubMedDOI: 10.1186/s12944-017-0449-y PMID: 28464819

Ippolito, M. M., Moser, K. A., Kabuya, J. B. B., Cunningham, C., & Juliano, J. J. (2021). Antimalarial drug resistance and implications for the WHO global technical strategy. *Current Epidemiology Reports*, *8*(2), 46–62. DOI: 10.1007/s40471-021-00266-5 PMID: 33747712

Iqbal, T., Altaf, S., Fatima, M., Rasheed, R., Laraib, K., Azam, M., & Usman, S. (2024). A narrative review on effective use of medicinal plants for the treatment of parasitic foodborne diseases. Agrobiological Records 16: 79-92. *Agric Res J*, *16*, 79–92.

Ishola, A. A., Adewole, K. E., Adebayo, J. O., & Balogun, E. A. (2023). Potentials of Terpenoids as Inhibitors of Multiple Plasmodium falciparum Protein Drug Targets. *Acta Parasitologica*, *68*(4), 793–806. DOI: 10.1007/s11686-023-00711-z PMID: 37603126

Iwu, I. C., Onu, U. L., Ukaoma, A. A., & Oze, R. N. (2018). Phytochemical, antimicrobial, and Gc/Ms analysis of the root of Stachytarpheta cayennensis (L. Vahl) grown in Eastern Nigeria. International Research Journal of Natural Sciences., 6(2), 1 ?"14. 10.37745/irjns.13

Jaiswal, Y., Liang, Z., & Zhao, Z. (2016). Botanical drugs in Ayurveda and Traditional Chinese Medicine. Journal of Ethnopharmacology, 194, 245 ?"259. doi:10.1016/j.jep.2016.06.052 PubMedDOI: 10.1016/j.jep.2016.06.052 PMID: 27394388

Jamil, S. N. H., Ali, A. H., Feroz, S. R., Lam, S. D., Agustar, H. K., Mohd Abd Razak, M. R., & Latip, J. (2023). Curcumin and Its Derivatives as Potential Antimalarial and Anti-Inflammatory Agents: A Review on Structure–Activity Relationship and Mechanism of Action. *Pharmaceuticals (Basel, Switzerland)*, *16*(4), 609. DOI: 10.3390/ph16040609 PMID: 37111366

Jamil, S. N. H., Bakar, K. A., Ali, A. H., Marzuki, N. F. N., Shahid, F., Mahmud, F., Feroz, S. R., Lam, S. D., Oka, N., Zakaria, Y., Muhajir, M. I., Maharani, R., Supratman, U., & Latip, J. (2025). *Promising bioactivity of curcumin derivatives against malaria: In silico, in vitro and ITC studies. Research Square*. DOI: 10.21203/rs.3.rs-7148737/v1

Jan, R., Asaf, S., Numan, M., Lubna, , & Kim, K.-M. (2021). Plant secondary metabolite biosynthesis and transcriptional regulation in response to biotic and abiotic stress conditions. *Agronomy (Basel)*, *11*(5), 968. DOI: 10.3390/agronomy11050968

Javanmardi, J., Stushnoff, C., Locke, E., & Vivanco, J. M. (2003). Antioxidant activity and total phenolic content of Iranian Ocimum accessions. *Food Chemistry*, *83*(4), 547–550. DOI: 10.1016/S0308-8146(03)00151-1

Jayakumar, T., Hsieh, C. Y., Lee, J. J., & Sheu, J. R. (2013). Experimental and Clinical Pharmacology of Andrographis paniculata and Its Major Bioactive Phytoconstituent Andrographolide. Evidence-Based Complementary and Alternative Medicine : eCAM, 846740, 1 ?"16. Advance online publication. doi:10.1155/2013/846740 PubMedDOI: 10.1155/2013/846740 PMID: 23634174

Jensen, A. R., Adams, Y., & Hviid, L. (2020). Cerebral Plasmodium falciparum malaria: The role of PfEMP1 in its pathogenesis and immunity, and PfEMP1-based vaccines to prevent it. *Immunological Reviews*, *293*(1), 230–252. DOI: 10.1111/imr.12807 PMID: 31562653

Kaiser, A. (2019). Druggable targets in cyclic nucleotide signaling pathways in apicomplexan parasites and kinetoplastids against disabling protozoan diseases in humans. *International Journal of Molecular Sciences*, *20*(1), 138. DOI: 10.3390/ijms20010138 PMID: 30609697

Kamaraj, C., Ragavendran, C., Prem, P., Naveen Kumar, S., Ali, A., Kazmi, A., Ullah, A., Chandra Satish Kumar, R., Khan, S. U., Luna-Arias, J. P., Mashwani, Z.-U.-R., Balasubramani, G., & Rehman, S. U. (2023). Exploring the therapeutic potential of traditional antimalarial and antidengue plants: A mechanistic perspective. *The Canadian Journal of Infectious Diseases & Medical Microbiology*, *2023*(1), 1860084. DOI: 10.1155/2023/1860084 PMID: 37927532

Kangwanrangsan, N., Niramolyanun, G., Praikongkatham, C., Chantree, P., Martviset, P., & Pankao, V. (2025). Growth Inhibition and Additive Effect to Antimalarial Drugs of Brucea javanica Extracts on Asexual Blood-Stage Plasmodium falciparum. *Pathogens (Basel, Switzerland)*, *14*(7), 646. DOI: 10.3390/pathogens14070646 PMID: 40732696

Kao, P.-Y., Yang, Y.-C., Chiang, W.-Y., Hsiao, J.-Y., & Cao, Y.. (2022). Exploring the advantages of quantum generative adversarial networks in generative chemistry. ArXiv. https://arxiv.org/abs/2210.16823

Karunamoorthi, K., Jegajeevanram, K., Vijayalakshmi, J., & Mengistie, E. (2013). Traditional medicinal plants: A source of phytotherapeutic modality in resource-constrained health care settings. *Journal of Evidence-Based Complementary & Alternative Medicine*, *18*(1), 67–74. DOI: 10.1177/2156587212460241

Kato, L. S., Lelis, C. A., da Silva, B. D., Galvan, D., & Conte-Junior, C. A. (2023). Micro-and nanoencapsulation of natural phytochemicals: Challenges and recent perspectives for the food and nutraceuticals industry applications. *Advances in Food and Nutrition Research*, *104*, 77–137. DOI: 10.1016/bs.afnr.2022.10.003 PMID: 37236735

Kayamba, F., Faya, M., Pooe, O. J., Kushwaha, B., Kushwaha, N. D., Obakachi, V. A., Nyamori, V. O., & Karpoormath, R. (2021). Lactate dehydrogenase and malate dehydrogenase: Potential antiparasitic targets for drug development studies. *Bioorganic & Medicinal Chemistry*, *50*, 116458. DOI: 10.1016/j.bmc.2021.116458 PMID: 34687983

Kayani, S., Ahmad, M., Zafar, M., Sultana, S., Khan, M. P. Z., Ashraf, M. A., Hussain, J., & Yaseen, G. (2014). Ethnobotanical uses of medicinal plants for respiratory disorders among the inhabitants of Gallies ?"Abbottabad, Northern Pakistan. Journal of Ethnopharmacology, 156, 47 ?"60. doi:10.1016/j.jep.2014.08.005 PubMedDOI: 10.1016/j.jep.2014.08.005 PMID: 25153021

Keiser, J., Singer, B. H., & Utzinger, J. (2005). Reducing the burden of malaria in different eco-epidemiological settings with environmental management: A systematic review. *The Lancet. Infectious Diseases*, *5*(11), 695–708. DOI: 10.1016/S1473-3099(05)70268-1 PMID: 16253887

Keith, J. A., Vassilev-Galindo, V., Cheng, B., Chmiela, S., Gastegger, M., Müller, K.-R., & Tkatchenko, A. (2021). Combining machine learning and computational chemistry for predictive insights into chemical systems. ArXiv. https://arxiv.org/abs/2102.06321 arxiv.org

Kesarwani, K., & Gupta, R. (2013). Bioavailability enhancers of herbal origin: An overview. *Asian Pacific Journal of Tropical Biomedicine*, *3*(4), 253–266. DOI: 10.1016/S2221-1691(13)60060-X PMID: 23620848

Khosropour, E., Ahangari, S., & Hakimi, L. (2024). Antimalarial Response, Traditional and Other Potential Uses of Cinchona Genera. In *Antimalarial Medicinal Plants* (pp. 174–187). CRC Press. DOI: 10.1201/9781003378396-11

Kim, H. W., Wang, M., Leber, C. A., Nothias, L. F., Reher, R., Kang, K. B., van der Hooft, J. J. J., Dorrestein, P. C., Gerwick, W. H., & Cottrell, G. W. (2021). NP Classifier: A deep neural network-based structural classification tool for natural products. *Journal of Natural Products*, *84*(11), 2795–2807. DOI: 10.1021/acs.jnatprod.1c00399 PMID: 34662515

Kimura, L. T., Andrade, E. R., Nobre, I., Nobre, C. A., De Medeiros, B. A., Riaño-Pachón, D. M., Shiraishi, F. K., Carvalho, T. C. M. B., & Simplicio, M. A.Jr. (2023). Amazon Biobank: A collaborative genetic database for bioeconomy development. *Functional & Integrative Genomics*, *23*(2), 101. DOI: 10.1007/s10142-023-01015-1 PMID: 36964864

Klemow, K. M., Bartlow, A., Crawford, J., Kocher, N., Shah, J., & Ritsick, M. (2011). Medical attributes of St. John's Wort (*Hypericum perforatum*). In *Herbal Medicine* (2nd ed.). Biomolecular and Clinical Aspects. DOI: 10.1201/b10787-12

Kohnen-Johannsen, K. L., & Kayser, O. (2019). Tropane Alkaloids: Chemistry, Pharmacology, Biosynthesis and Production. *Molecules (Basel, Switzerland)*, *24*(4), 796. DOI: 10.3390/molecules24040796 PMID: 30813289

Kolawole, E., Ayeni, E., Abolade, S., Ugwu, S., Awoyinka, T., Ofeh, A., & Okolo, B. (2023). Malaria endemicity in sub-Saharan Africa: Past and present issues in public health. Microbes and Infectious Diseases, 4(1), 242-251. https://doi.org/10.21608/mid.. 2022.150194.1346

Komolafe, C. J., Adetoyinbo, I. I., Alao, F. O., & Ogunsola, J. F. (2024). Phytochemical Analyses and Antibacterial Activities of Jatropha tanjorensis J. L. Ellis and Saroja leaves extract against clinical pathogens. Asian Journal of Applied Chemistry Research, 15(4), 79 ?"93. doi:10.9734/ajacr/2024/v15i5298DOI: 10.9734/ajacr/2024/v15i5298

Kong, Y. R., Jong, Y. X., Balakrishnan, M., Bok, Z. K., Weng, J. K. K., Tay, K. C., Goh, B. H., Ong, Y. S., Chan, K. G., Lee, L. H., & Khaw, K. Y. (2021). Beneficial Role of Carica papaya Extracts and Phytochemicals on Oxidative Stress and Related Diseases: A Mini Review. Biology (Basel), 10(4), 287. doi:10.3390/biology10040287 PubMedDOI: 10.3390/biology10040287 PMID: 33916114

Kotte, K. R., Attaluri, V., & Selvakumar, P. (2025). Revolutionising Retail Banking with AI and Virtual Technologies AI-Driven Financial Training. In Nair, A. J., Manohar, S., Limbu, Y. B., & Huhmann, B. A. (Eds.), *Intersecting Natural Language Processing and FinTech Innovations in Service Marketing* (pp. 421–440). IGI Global Scientific Publishing., DOI: 10.4018/979-8-3693-9944-6.ch020

Kuiate, J. R., Amvam-Zollo, P. H., Lamaty, G., Menut, C., & Bessiere, J. M. (1999). Composition of the Essential Oils from the Leaves of two varieties of Aspilia africana (Pers). C.D. Adams from Cameroon. Flavour and Fragrance Journal, 14(3), 167 ?"169. doi:10.1002/(SICI)1099-1026(199905/06)14:3<167::AID-FFJ802>3.0.CO;2-ODOI: 10.1002/(SICI)1099-1026(199905/06)14:3<167::AID-FFJ802>3.0.CO;2-O

Kumar, R., Pal, O. P., Kamboj, N., & Jaiswal, A. (2025). Phytonutrients in Neuroprotection and Neurodegenerative Disorders. *Current Research in Nutrition and Food Science Journal, 13*(Special Issue Phytonutrients June 2025).

Kumar, S., Singh, B., & Bajpai, V. (2021). Andrographis paniculata (Burm.f.) Nees: Traditional uses, phytochemistry, pharmacological properties, and quality control/quality assurance. Journal of Ethnopharmacology, 275, 114054. doi:10.1016/j.jep.2021.114054 PubMedDOI: 10.1016/j.jep.2021.114054 PMID: 33831465

Kumar, A., P, N., Kumar, M., Jose, A., Tomer, V., Oz, E., Proestos, C., Zeng, M., Elobeid, T., K, S., & Oz, F. (2023). Major phytochemicals: Recent advances in health benefits and extraction method. *Molecules (Basel, Switzerland), 28*(2), 887. DOI: 10.3390/molecules28020887 PMID: 36677944

Kumaratilake, L. M., Ferrante, A., Robinson, B. S., Jaeger, T., & Poulos, A. (1997). Enhancement of the neutrophil-mediated killing of Plasmodium falciparum asexual blood forms by fatty acids: Importance of fatty acid structure. Infection and Immunity, 65(10), 4152 ?"4157. doi:10.1128/iai.65.10.4152-4157.1997 PubMedDOI: 10.1128/iai.65.10.4152-4157.1997 PMID: 9317021

Kumar, M., Saadaoui, M., & Al Khodor, S. (2022). Infections and pregnancy: Effects on maternal and child health. *Frontiers in Cellular and Infection Microbiology, 12*, 873253. DOI: 10.3389/fcimb.2022.873253 PMID: 35755838

Laajala, T. D., Jumppanen, M., Huhtaniemi, R., Väisanen, M. R., Yetukuri, L., Suni, V., & Aittokallio, T. (2016). Optimized design and analysis of preclinical intervention studies in vivo. *Scientific Reports, 6*(1), 30723. DOI: 10.1038/srep30723 PMID: 27480578

Lacerda, U. V., da Costa, C. V. P., Cardoso, R. R., D'Almeida, C. T. dos S., do Carmo, M. A. V., Lima, A. dos S., Cruz, L. da S., de Souza, A. B., Fernandes, P. O., Maltarollo, V. G., Ferreira, M. S. L., Azevedo, L., Eller, M. R., Corich, V., Giacomini, A., & de Barros, F. A. R. (2025). Antioxidant, Antiproliferative, Antibacterial, and Antimalarial Effects of Phenolic-Rich Green Tea Kombucha. *Beverages, 11*(1), 7. DOI: 10.3390/beverages11010007

Laeliocattleya, R. A., Estiasih, T., Griselda, G., & Muchlisyiyah, J. (2018). The bioactive compounds and antioxidant activity of ethanol and ethyl acetate extracts of CandiBanana (Musa paradisiaca). IOP Conference Series. Earth and Environmental Science, 131, 012013. doi:10.1088/1755-1315/131/1/012013DOI: 10.1088/1755-1315/131/1/012013

Lahlou, M. (2013). The success of natural products in drug discovery. *Pharmacology & Pharmacy, 4*(3, 3A), 17–31. DOI: 10.4236/pp.2013.43A003

Lalita Nargawe, G. Malathi, Vidhya C. S., Lalit Upadhyay. (. (2023). Ethnobotanical Survey of Medicinal Plants Used in Traditional Medicine in Africa. Plant Science Archives, 26-28. Advance online publication. doi:10.51470/PSA.2023.8.4.26DOI: 10.51470/PSA.2023.8.4.26

Larayetan, R., Ololade, Z. S., Ogunmola, O. O., & Ladokun, A. (2019). Phytochemical Constituents, Antioxidant, Cytotoxicity, Antimicrobial, Antitrypanosomal, and Antimalarial Potentials of the Crude Extracts of *Callistemon citrinus. Evidence-Based Complementary and Alternative Medicine : eCAM, 2019*, 1–14. Advance online publication. DOI: 10.1155/2019/5410923 PMID: 31558912

Lautie, E., Russo, O., Ducrot, P., & Boutin, J. A. (2020). Unraveling plant natural chemical diversity for drug discovery purposes. *Frontiers in Pharmacology, 11*, 397. DOI: 10.3389/fphar.2020.00397 PMID: 32317969

Lawal, I. O., Rafiu, B. O., Ale, J. E., Majebi, O. E., & Aremu, A. O. (2022). Ethnobotanical Survey of Local Flora Used for Medicinal Purposes among Indigenous People in Five Areas in Lagos State, Nigeria. Plants, 11(5), 633. doi:10.3390/plants11050633 PubMedDOI: 10.3390/plants11050633 PMID: 35270103

Lawal, L., Buhari, A. O., Jaji, T. A., Alatare, A. S., Adeyemo, A. O., Olumoh, A. O., Yusuff, Y. A., Osborn, G., Mogaji, A. B., Adoto, B. H., Ibrahim, N. G., Saliu, W. O., & Abdul-Rahman, T. (2024). Lingering challenges in malaria elimination efforts in sub-Saharan Africa: Insights and potential solutions. *Health Science Reports*, *7*(6), e2122. DOI: 10.1002/hsr2.2122 PMID: 38831778

Letchuman, S., Madhuranga, H. D. T., Madhurangi, B. L. N. K., Premarathna, A. D., & Saravanan, M. (2025). Alkaloids unveiled: A comprehensive analysis of novel therapeutic properties, mechanisms, and plant-based innovations. *Intelligent Pharmacy*, *3*(4), 268–276. DOI: 10.1016/j.ipha.2024.09.007

Li, F., & Weng, J. (2017). Demystifying traditional herbal medicine with modern approach. Nature Plants, 3(8), 17109. Advance online publication. doi:10.1038/nplants.2017.109 PubMedDOI: 10.1038/nplants.2017.109 PMID: 28758992

Lifongo, L. L., Simoben, C. V., Ntie-Kang, F., Babiaka, S. B., & Judson, P. N. (2014). A bioactivity versus ethnobotanical survey of medicinal plants from Nigeria, West Africa. Natural Products and Bioprospecting, 4(1), 1 ?"19. doi:10.1007/s13659-014-0005-7 PubMedDOI: 10.1007/s13659-014-0005-7 PMID: 24660132

Li, M., Qian, M., Jiang, Q., Tan, B., Yin, Y., & Han, X. (2023). Evidence of Flavonoids on Disease Prevention. *Antioxidants*, *12*(2), 527. DOI: 10.3390/antiox12020527 PMID: 36830086

Lindberg, K., Martvall, A., Lima, M. G. B., & Franca, C. S. (2023). Herbal medicine promotion for a restorative bioeconomy in tropical forests: A reality check on the Brazilian Amazon. *Forest Policy and Economics*, *155*, 103058. DOI: 10.1016/j.forpol.2023.103058

Lins, F. S. V., da Silva, V. F., Tavares, J. F., dos Santos, V. L., & da Silva Alves, H. (2021). Bioguided isolation of alkaloids and pharmacological effects of the total alkaloid fraction from *Aspidosperma pyrifolium* Mart. (Apocynaceae). *Plants*, *10*(11), 2526. DOI: 10.3390/plants10112526 PMID: 34834889

Liu, Q., Lawrence, A. J., & Liang, J. H. (2011). Traditional Chinese medicine for treatment of

Liu, Q., Jing, W., Kang, L., Liu, J., & Liu, M. (2021). Trends of the global, regional and national incidence of malaria in 204 countries from 1990 to 2019 and implications for malaria prevention. *Journal of Travel Medicine*, *28*(5), taab046. DOI: 10.1093/jtm/taab046 PMID: 33763689

Liu, Q., Lawrence, A. J., & Liang, J.-H. (2011, January). alcoholism: From ancient to modern. *The American Journal of Chinese Medicine*, *39*(1), 1–13. DOI: 10.1142/S0192415X11008609 PMID: 21213394

M'bondoukwé, N. P., Moutongo, R., Gbédandé, K., Ndong Ngomo, J. M., Hountohotegbé, T., Adamou, R., Koumba Lengongo, J. V., Pambou Bello, K., Mawili-Mboumba, D. P., Luty, A. J. F., & Bouyou-Akotet, M. K. (2022). Circulating IL-6, IL-10, and TNF-alpha and IL-10/IL-6 and IL-10/TNF-alpha ratio profiles of polyparasitized individuals in rural and urban areas of gabon. *PLoS Neglected Tropical Diseases*, *16*(4), e0010308. DOI: 10.1371/journal.pntd.0010308 PMID: 35421083

Maafoh, C., & Onyedibe, K. (2024). Alternative first-line malaria treatment. Annals of African Medicine, 23(1), 5 ?"12. doi:10.4103/aam.aam_35_23 PubMedDOI: 10.4103/aam.aam_35_23 PMID: 38358164

Mabuza, M. J. (2022). *Antiplasmodial properties of extracts from Pappea capensis Eckl. & Zeyh.* Sapindaceae.

Machado, B. A. S., Pereira, C. G., Nunes, S. B., Padilha, F. F., & Umsza-Guez, M. A. (2013). Supercritical fluid extraction using CO_2: Main applications and future perspectives. *Separation Science and Technology*, *48*(17), 2741–2760. DOI: 10.1080/01496395.2013.811422

Magozwi, D. K., Dinala, M., Mokwana, N., Siwe-Noundou, X., Krause, R. W. M., Sonopo, M., McGaw, L. J., Augustyn, W. A., & Tembu, V. J. (2021). Flavonoids from the Genus Euphorbia: Isolation, Structure, Pharmacological Activities and Structure–Activity Relationships. *Pharmaceuticals (Basel, Switzerland)*, *14*(5), 428. DOI: 10.3390/ph14050428 PMID: 34063311

Maheswaran, K., Selvakumar, P., Shaikh, M., Shashank, G., Gupta, S., & Manjunath, T. C. (2025). The Evolution of Smart Urban Mobility With Emerging Technologies. In Ponnusamy, S., Assaf, M., Youssef, B., Jeon, G., & Kalyanaraman, S. (Eds.), *Leveraging VANETs and Blockchain Technology for Urban Mobility* (pp. 1–28). IGI Global Scientific Publishing., DOI: 10.4018/979-8-3373-0265-2.ch001

Mallo, N., Lamas, J., Sueiro, R. A., & Leiro, J. M. (2020). Molecular targets implicated in the antiparasitic and anti-inflammatory activity of the phytochemical curcumin in Trichomoniasis. *Molecules (Basel, Switzerland)*, *25*(22), 5321. DOI: 10.3390/molecules25225321 PMID: 33202696

Mamede, C. C., & Cristina, L. (2024). *Metabolomic Investigation of Natural Antiplasmodial Agents*. https://orbi.uliege.be/handle/2268/311229

Manisha, M., Babu, R., Begam, A. M., Shakya Chahal, K., & Ashok Harale, A. (2025). Medicinal Plants and Traditional Uses and Modern Applications. *Journal of Neonatal Surgery*, *14*(3), 162–175. DOI: 10.52783/jns.v14.2210

Mannangatti, P., & Naidu, K. N. (2016). Indian herbs for the treatment of neurodegenerative disease. *Advances in Neurobiology*, *12*, 323–336. DOI: 10.1007/978-3-319-28383-8_17 PMID: 27651261

Marchev, A. S., Vasileva, L. V., Amirova, K. M., Savova, M. S., Balcheva-Sivenova, Z. P., & Georgiev, M. I. (2021). Metabolomics and health: From nutritional crops and plant-based pharmaceuticals to profiling of human biofluids. *Cellular and Molecular Life Sciences : CMLS*, *78*(15), 6487–6503. DOI: 10.1007/s00018-021-03918-3 PMID: 34410445

Martens, P., & Hall, L. (2000). Malaria on the move: Human population movement and malaria transmission. *Emerging Infectious Diseases*, *6*(2), 103–109. DOI: 10.3201/eid0602.000202 PMID: 10756143

Martins, A., Vieira, H., Gaspar, H., & Santos, S. (2019). Marketed marine natural products in the pharmaceutical and cosmeceutical industries: Tips for success. *Marine Drugs*, *17*(3), 145. PMID: 30832207

Matte, E. H. C., Luciano, F. B., & Evangelista, A. G. (2023). Essential oils and essential oil compounds in animal production as antimicrobials and anthelmintics: An updated review. *Animal Health Research Reviews*, *24*(1), 1–11. DOI: 10.1017/S1466252322000093 PMID: 37401263

McCarthy, M. W. (2019). Teixobactin: A novel anti-infective agent. *Expert Review of Anti-Infective Therapy*, *17*(1), 1–3. DOI: 10.1080/14787210.2019.1550357 PMID: 30449226

Medicines for Malaria Venture. (2023). *Annual report 2023: Advancing the fight against malaria*. MMV.

Memariani, H., Memariani, M., & Ghasemian, A. (2024). Quercetin as a promising antiprotozoan phytochemical: Current knowledge and future research avenues. *BioMed Research International*, *2024*(1), 7632408. DOI: 10.1155/2024/7632408 PMID: 38456097

Mensah, J. K., Okoli, R. I., Ohagu-Obodo, J. O., & Lifediyi, K. (2008). Phytochemical, nutritional, and medicinal properties of some leafy Vegetables consumed by the Edo people of Nigeria. African Journal of Biotechnology, 7(3), 2304 ?"2309. 10.4314/ajb.v7i14.58988

Mezieobi, K. C., Alum, E. U., Ugwu, O. P. C., Uti, D. E., Alum, B. N., Egba, S. I., & Michael, E. C. (2025). Economic burden of malaria on developing countries: A mini review. *Parasite Epidemiology and Control*, *30*, 00435. DOI: 10.1016/j.parepi.2025.e00435 PMID: 40519859

Middleton, T. (2024). *Quinine's Remains: Empire's Medicine and the Life Thereafter*. University of California Press.

Milliken, W., Walker, B. E., Howes, M. J. R., Forest, F., & Nic Lughadha, E. (2021). Plants used traditionally as antimalarials in Latin America: Mining the tree of life for potential new medicines. *Journal of Ethnopharmacology*, *279*, 114221. DOI: 10.1016/j.jep.2021.114221 PMID: 34029639

Min, Y., Wei, Y., Wang, P., Wang, X., Li, H., Wu, N., Bauer, S., Zheng, S., Shi, Y., Wang, Y., Wu, J., Zhao, D., & Zeng, J. (2024). From static to dynamic structures: Improving binding affinity prediction with graph-based deep learning. *Advancement of Science*, *11*(40), 2405404. ouci.dntb.gov.ua. DOI: 10.1002/advs.202405404 PMID: 39206846

Mishra, K., Dash, A. P., Swain, B. K., & Dey, N. (2009). Anti-malarial activities of Andrographis paniculata and Hedyotis corymbosa extracts and their combination with curcumin. Malaria Journal, 8(1), 26. Advance online publication. doi:10.1186/1475-2875-8-26 PubMedDOI: 10.1186/1475-2875-8-26 PMID: 19216765

Mishra, A., Shaik, H. A., Sinha, R. K., & Shah, B. R. (2021). Andrographolide: A herbal-chemosynthetic approach for enhancing immunity, combating viral infections, and its implication on human health. *Molecules (Basel, Switzerland)*, *26*(22), 7036. DOI: 10.3390/molecules26227036 PMID: 34834128

Mishra, R., Xavier, J. da C., Kumar, N., Krishna, G., Dhakad, P. K., Santos, H. S., dos, , Bandeira, P. N., Rodrigues, T. H. S., Gondim, D. R., Ribeiro, W. H. F., Silva, D. S., da, , Teixeira, A. M. R., Pereira, W. F., & Marinho, E. S. (2025). Exploring Quinoline Derivatives: Their Antimalarial Efficacy and Structural Features. *Medicinal Chemistry (Shariqah, United Arab Emirates)*, *21*(2), 96–121. DOI: 10.2174/0115734064318361240827072124 PMID: 40007183

Mohammadi, S., Jafari, B., Asgharian, P., Martorell, M., & Sharifi-Rad, J. (2020). Medicinal plants used in the treatment of Malaria: A key emphasis to Artemisia, Cinchona, Cryptolepis, and Tabebuia genera. *Phytotherapy Research*, *34*(7), 1556–1569. DOI: 10.1002/ptr.6628 PMID: 32022345

Mohammed, A. E., Abdul-Hameed, Z. H., Alotaibi, M. O., Bawakid, N. O., Sobahi, T. R., Abdel-Lateff, A., & Alarif, W. M. (2021). Chemical Diversity and Bioactivities of Monoterpene Indole Alkaloids (MIAs) from Six Apocynaceae Genera. *Molecules (Basel, Switzerland), 26*(2), 488. DOI: 10.3390/molecules26020488 PMID: 33477682

Mohanraj, K., Karthikeyan, B. S., Vivek-Ananth, R. P., Chand, R. B., Aparna, S. R., Mangalapandi, P., & Samal, A. (2018). IMPPAT: A curated database of Indian Medicinal P lants, Phytochemistry And Therapeutics. *Scientific Reports, 8*(1), 4329.

Molina-Franky, J., Patarroyo, M. E., Kalkum, M., & Patarroyo, M. A. (2022). The cellular and molecular interaction between erythrocytes and Plasmodium falciparum merozoites. *Frontiers in Cellular and Infection Microbiology, 12*, 816574. DOI: 10.3389/fcimb.2022.816574 PMID: 35433504

Moon, K. B., Park, J. S., Park, Y. I., Song, I. J., Lee, H. J., Cho, H. S., Jeon, J. H., & Kim, H. S. (2019). Development of systems for the production of plant-derived biopharmaceuticals. *Plants, 9*(1), 30. DOI: 10.3390/plants9010030 PMID: 31878277

Moshawih, S., Goh, H. P., Kifli, N., Idris, A. C., Yassin, H., Kotra, V., Goh, K. W., Liew, K. B., & Ming, L. C. (2022). Synergy between machine learning and natural products cheminformatics: Application to anthraquinone derivatives. *Chemical Biology & Drug Design, 100*(2), 185–217. onlinelibrary.wiley.com. DOI: 10.1111/cbdd.14062 PMID: 35490393

Mosquera, M. E. G., Jiménez, G., Tabernero, V., Vinueza-Vaca, J., García-Estrada, C., Kosalková, K., Sola-Landa, A., Monje, B., Acosta, C., Alonso, R., & Valera, M. Á. (2021). Terpenes and Terpenoids: Building Blocks to Produce Biopolymers. *Sustainable Chemistry, 2*(3), 467–492. DOI: 10.3390/suschem2030026

Muhammad, R. H., Sanusi, F. S., & Safiyanu, M. (2025). In-vitro Anti-Plasmodial Activity of Mangifera indica Leaves Against Plasmodium falciparum. Bima Journal of Science and Technology Gombe, 9(2B), 295 ?"301. doi:10.64290/bima.v9i2B.1300DOI: 10.64290/bima.v9i2B.1300

Mukherjee, S., Mukherjee, N., Gayen, P., Roy, P., Sinha, P., & Babu, S. (2016). Metabolic inhibitors as antiparasitic drugs: Pharmacological, biochemical and molecular perspectives. *Current Drug Metabolism, 17*(10), 937–970. DOI: 10.2174/1389200217666161004143152 PMID: 27719626

Mutai, B. K., & Waitumbi, J. N. (2010). Apoptosis stalks Plasmodium falciparum maintained in continuous culture condition. *Malaria Journal, 9*(S3, Suppl 3), S6. DOI: 10.1186/1475-2875-9-S3-S6 PMID: 21144086

Mutha, R. E., Kalaskar, M., & Khan, Z. G. (2025). *Modern Analytical Techniques for Quality Control and Chemical Identification of Phytochemicals*. Retrieved September 28, 2025, from https://onlinelibrary.wiley.com/doi/10.1002/9781394203680.ch09

Nagai, K., & Goto, Y. (2022). Parasitomimetics: Can we utilize parasite-derived immunomodulatory molecules for interventions to immunological disorders? *Frontiers in Immunology, 13*, 824695. DOI: 10.3389/fimmu.2022.824695 PMID: 35386686

Nahal, Y., Menke, J., Martinelli, J., ... (2024). Human-in-the-loop active learning for goal-oriented molecule generation. Journal of Cheminformatics, 16(1), 138. pubs.acs.org+2medium.com+2pubs.acs.org+2DOI: 10.1186/s13321-024-00924-y

Nandi, S., Ahmed, S., & Saxena, A. K. (2022). Exploring the role of antioxidants to combat oxidative stress in malaria Parasites. *Current Topics in Medicinal Chemistry, 22*(24), 2029–2044. DOI: 10.2174/1568026622666220405121643 PMID: 35382719

Narzary, D., & Boro, I. (2025). Plants in Bodo Folklore and Ritual Practices: An Ethnobotanical Perspective. International Journal for Multidisciplinary Research, 7(4), 53553. Advance online publication. doi:10.36948/ijfmr.2025.v07i04.53553DOI: 10.36948/ijfmr.2025.v07i04.53553

Nascimento Brandão, D. L., Martins, M. T., Silva, A. O., Almeida, A. D., Aguiar Gomes, A. T., Vasconcelos, F., & Dolabela, M. F. (2020). Anti-malarial activity and toxicity of *Aspidosperma nitidum* Benth: A plant used in traditional medicine in the Brazilian Amazon. *Research. Social Development, 9*(10), e5059108817.

Naser, R. H., Rajaii, T., Farash, B. R. H., Seyyedtabaei, S., Hajali, V., Sadabadi, F., & Saburi, E. (2024). Hematological changes due to malaria–An update. *Molecular and Biochemical Parasitology, 259*, 111635. DOI: 10.1016/j.molbiopara.2024.111635 PMID: 38857772

Natolino, A., Passaghe, P., Brugnera, G., & Comuzzo, P. (2024). Intensification of grape marc (*Vitis vinifera*) exploitation by subcritical water-ethanol extraction: Effect on polyphenol bioactivities and kinetic modelling. *Journal of Food Engineering, 381*, 112185. DOI: 10.1016/j.jfoodeng.2024.112185

Nayak, C., Oberai, P., Varanasi, R., Baig, H. Ch. R., & Reddy, G. R. (2013). A prospective multi-centric open clinical trial of homeopathy in diabetic distal symmetric polyneuropathy. *Homeopathy, 102*(2), 130–138. DOI: 10.1016/j.homp.2013.02.004 PMID: 23622263

Ndem, J. I., Eteng, M. U., & Uwah, A. F. (2014). Effect of Hippocratea Africana Root Bark Extract on Lipid Profile of Female and Male Albino Wistar Rats. Journal of Scientific Research and Reports, 3(19), 2574 ?"2583. doi:10.9734/JSRR/2014/12491DOI: 10.9734/JSRR/2014/12491

Ndem, J., Uwah, A., Effiong, B., Bassey, U., Umanah, B., & Chukwudike, C. (2020). Ethanol leaf extract of Jatropha tanjorensis ameliorates hepatorenal toxicity of Plasmodium berghi-berghi infected mice treated with Hippocratea africana root bark extract. The Journal of Phytopharmacology, 9(5), 374 ?"377. doi:10.31254/phyto.2020.9515DOI: 10.31254/phyto.2020.9515

Newman, D. J., & Cragg, G. M. (2016). Natural Products as Sources of New Drugs over the 30 Years from 1981 to 2010. *Journal of Natural Products*, *79*(3), 629–661. DOI: 10.1021/acs.jnatprod.5b01055 PMID: 26852623

Newman, D. J., & Cragg, G. M. (2020). Natural products as sources of new drugs over the nearly four decades from 01/1981 to 09/2019. *Journal of Natural Products*, *83*(3), 770–803. DOI: 10.1021/acs.jnatprod.9b01285 PMID: 32162523

Ng, X., Venkatanarayanan, N., & Ho, C. Y. (2017). Clinical use of Hypericum perforatum (St John's wort) in depression: A meta-analysis. *Journal of Affective Disorders*, *210*, 211–221. DOI: 10.1016/j.jad.2016.12.048 PMID: 28064110

Nikolovski, B. (1995). Essays on the history of health culture in Macedonia. *Skopje: Macedonian pharmaceutical association*, 17-27.

Nirmala, C., & Sridevi, M. (2021). Ethnobotanical, phytochemistry, and pharmacological property of Waltheria Indica Linn. *Future Journal of Pharmaceutical Sciences*, *7*(1), 14. DOI: 10.1186/s43094-020-00174-3

Njama-Meya, D., Clark, T. D., Nzarubara, B., Staedke, S. G., Kamya, M. R., Dorsey, G., & Rosenthal, P. J. (2017). Treatment of malaria restricted to laboratory-confirmed cases: A prospective cohort study in Ugandan children. *Malaria Journal*, *16*(1), 1–8. PMID: 28049519

Nosten, F., Richard-Lenoble, D., & Danis, M. (2022). A brief history of malaria. *La Presse Medicale*, *51*(3), 104130. DOI: 10.1016/j.lpm.2022.104130 PMID: 35667599

Nureye, D., & Assefa, S. (2020). Old and recent advances in life cycle, pathogenesis, diagnosis, prevention, and treatment of malaria including perspectives in Ethiopia. *TheScientificWorldJournal*, *2020*(1), 1295381. DOI: 10.1155/2020/1295381

Nwaka, S., Ilunga, T. B., Da Silva, J. S., Rial Verde, E., Hackley, D., De Vré, R., & Ridley, R. G. (2010). Developing ANDI: A novel approach to health product R&D in Africa. *Nature Reviews. Drug Discovery*, *9*(6), 437–443. PMID: 20613865

Nworgu, C. O., Elele, K., & Adikwu, E. (2022). Toxicity and antiplasmodial assessments of Chromolaena odorata leaf extract on Plasmodium berghei-infected mice. Journal of Infectious Diseases and Epidemiology, 8(8), 276. doi:10.23937/2474-3658/1510276DOI: 10.23937/2474-3658/1510276

O'Shaughnessy, D. M., & Berlowitz, I. (2021). Amazonian medicine and the psychedelic revival: Considering the "Dieta". *Frontiers in Pharmacology, 12*, 639124. DOI: 10.3389/fphar.2021.639124 PMID: 34149407

Obeagu, E. I. (2024). Role of cytokines in immunomodulation during malaria clearance. *Annals of Medicine and Surgery (London), 86*(5), 2873–2882. DOI: 10.1097/MS9.0000000000002019 PMID: 38694310

Obinna, A., Onyedikachi, U., Alaebo, P., Odo, C., Okechukwu, G., & Omodamiro, O. (2021). Methanol leaf extract of Jatropha tanjorensis Ellis and Saroja possesses phytoconstituents with free radical scavenging activity. FUDMA Journal of Sciences, 5(3), 286 ?"293. doi:10.33003/fjs-2021-0503-660DOI: 10.33003/fjs-2021-0503-660

Odugbemi, T. O., Akinsulire, O. R., Aibinu, I. E., & Fabeku, P. O. (2006). Medicinal plants useful for malaria therapy in Okeigbo, Ondo State, Southwest Nigeria. African Journal of Traditional, Complementary, and Alternative Medicines : AJTCAM, 4(2), 191 ?"198. doi:10.4314/ajtcam.v4i2.31207 PubMedDOI: 10.4314/ajtcam.v4i2.31207 PMID: 20162091

Ogidi, O. I. (2020). A review on the use of herbal remedies and clinical therapeutics for the management of COVID-19 pandemic. *ASIO Journal of Pharmaceutical & Herbal Medicines Research, 6*(2), 68–77. http://doi.org/doilink/10.2020.85722646

Ogidi, O. I. (2022). Omicron (B.1.1.529): Variant of concern—A mini review. *Biomedical Journal of Scientific & Technical Research, 41*(5), 33106–33112. DOI: 10.26717/BJSTR.2022.41.006672

Ogidi, O. I., Afakwu-Adimoha, H. C., & Indiamaowei, D. L. (2023). E-health care system in Nigeria: The current status, issues and future prospective. *World Journal of Advanced Healthcare Research*, 7(4), 75–83.

Ogidi, O. I., Aye, T., & Felagha, I. (2025b). Antiviral therapeutics for emerging viruses. In Aslam, M., Yingngam, B., Javed, T., & Riaz, S. (Eds.), *Global perspectives on antiviral drug development* (pp. 217–260). IGI Global., DOI: 10.4018/979-8-3693-9276-8.ch006

Ogidi, O. I., Berefagha, W. L., & Okara, E. (2021). COVID-19 vaccination: The pros and cons. *World Journal of Biology Pharmacy and Health Sciences*, 7(1), 15–22. DOI: 10.30574/wjbphs.2021.7.1.0072

Ogidi, O. I., Ebong, C. U., & Ikimi, C. G. (2025c). Lifespan-extending natural compounds. In Chen, J. (Ed.), *Drug discovery and antiaging approaches for human longevity* (pp. 351–390). IGI Global., DOI: 10.4018/979-8-3693-9730-5.ch010

Ogidi, O. I., Ogoun, T. R., & Tobia, P. S. (2025a). Antimalarial activities and lipid profile of ethanolic extract of *Ficus sur* Forssk (described by Peter Forsskål) in *Plasmodium berghei* infected albino rats. *Journal of Ethnopharmacology, 348*, 119901. DOI: 10.1016/j.jep.2025.119901 PMID: 40306496

Ogorzewska, Z. (2022). Intercultural health in the Peruvian Amazon: Problems and potentials. *Anuario Latinoamericano, 10*(1), 93–111. DOI: 10.17951/al.2022.10.93-111

Okello, D., Lee, J., & Kang, Y. (2020). Ethnopharmacological Potential of Aspilia africana for the Treatment of Inflammatory Diseases. Evidence-Based Complementary and Alternative Medicine : eCAM, 2020(1), 1 ?"11. doi:10.1155/2020/8091047 PubMedDOI: 10.1155/2020/8091047 PMID: 32733588

Okoh, M. P., Egua, M. O., Alli, L. A., Dalu, D., Gundamaraju, R., Singla, R. K., & Shen, B. (2025). Unveiling the Potential of Natural Resources-Derived Therapeutics for Improved Malaria Management: Computational to Experimental Studies. *Advanced Biology, 9*(2), 2400282. DOI: 10.1002/adbi.202400282 PMID: 39703011

Okokon, J. E., Akpan, H. D., Umoh, E. E., & Ekaidem, I. S. (2011). Antidiarrhoeal and antiulcer activities of Hippocratea africana root extract. Pakistan Journal of Pharmaceutical Sciences, 24(2), 201 ?"205. PubMed PMID: 21454170

Okokon, J. E., Antia, B. S., Umoh, E. E., & Etim, E. I. (2010). Antidiabetic, cardioprotective, and hypolipidaemic activities of Hippocratea africana. International Journal of Drug Development Research, 2, 501 ?"506.

Okokon, J. E., Chinyere, P. C., Amaechi, P., Bassey, A. L., & Thomas, P. S. (2022). Antioxidant, antidiabetic, and hypolipidemic activities of ethanol root extract and fractions of Hippocratea africana. Tropical Journal of Natural Product Research, 6(3), 446 ?"453.

Okokon, J. E., Dar, A., & Choudhary, M. I. (2013b). Immunomodulatory, cytotoxic, and antileishmanial activities of Hippocratea africana. Journal of Natural Pharmaceuticals, 4(2), 81 ?"85.

Okokon, J. E., Ettebong, E., & Antia, B. S. (2008). In vivo antimalarial activity of ethanolic leaf extract of Stachytarpheta cayennensis. Indian Journal of Pharmacology, 40(3), 111 ?"113. doi:10.4103/0253-7613.42303 PubMedDOI: 10.4103/0253-7613.42303 PMID: 20040937

Okokon, J. E., Ita, B. N., & Udokpoh, A. E. (2006). The In Vivo Antimalarial Activities of Uvariae chamae and Hippocratea africana. Annals of Tropical Medicine and Parasitology, 100(9), 585 ?"590. doi:10.1179/136485906X118512 PubMedDOI: 10.1179/136485906X118512 PMID: 16989684

Okokon, J. E., Nwafor, P. A., Charles, U., Dar, A., & Choudhary, M. I. (2013a). The antioxidative burst and hepatoprotective effects of ethanolic root extract of Hippocratea africana against paracetamol-induced liver injury. Pharmaceutical Biology, 51(7), 872 ?"880. doi:10.3109/13880209.2013.768273 PubMedDOI: 10.3109/13880209.2013.768273 PMID: 23530960

Okokon, J. E., Okokon, P. J., & Sahal, D. (2017). In vitro antiplasmodial activity of some Nigerian medicinal plants. International Journal of Herbal Medicine, 5(5), 102 ?"109.

Okoli, C., Akah, P. A., Nwafor, S. V., Anisiobi, A. I., Ibegbunam, I. N., & Erojikwe, O. (2006). Anti-inflammatory activity of hexane leaf extract of Aspilia africana C.D. Adams. Journal of Ethnopharmacology, 109(2), 219 ?"225. doi:10.1016/j.jep.2006.07.037 PubMedDOI: 10.1016/j.jep.2006.07.037 PMID: 16950582

Okombo, J., & Fidock, D. A. (2025). Towards next-generation treatment options to combat Plasmodium falciparum malaria. *Nature Reviews. Microbiology*, *23*(3), 178–191. DOI: 10.1038/s41579-024-01099-x PMID: 39367132

Oksana, S. (2012). Plant phenolic compounds for food, pharmaceutical and cosmetics production. *Journal of Medicinal Plants Research*, *6*(13). Advance online publication. DOI: 10.5897/JMPR11.1695

Olas, B., Urbańska, K., & Bryś, M. (2020). Saponins as modulators of the blood coagulation system and perspectives regarding their use in the prevention of venous thromboembolic incidents. *Molecules (Basel, Switzerland)*, *25*(21), 5171. DOI: 10.3390/molecules25215171 PMID: 33172028

Oleinikov, A. V. (2022). Malaria parasite Plasmodium falciparum proteins on the surface of infected erythrocytes as targets for novel drug discovery. *Biochemistry (Moscow)*, *87*(S1, Suppl 1), S192–S202. DOI: 10.1134/S0006297922140152 PMID: 35501996

Oliveira-Ferreira, J., Lacerda, M. V. G., Brasil, P., Ladislau, J. L. B., Tauil, P. L., & Daniel-Ribeiro, C. T. (2010). Malaria in Brazil: An overview. *Malaria Journal*, *9*(1), 115. DOI: 10.1186/1475-2875-9-115 PMID: 20433744

Oliveira, T., Silva, M., Maia, E., Silva, A., & Taranto, A. (2023). Virtual screening algorithms in drug discovery: Machine and deep learning methods. *Drugs and Drug Candidates*, *2*(2), 311–334. link.springer.com. DOI: 10.3390/ddc2020017

Omar, F., Tareq, A. M., Alqahtani, A. M., Dhama, K., Sayeed, M. A., Emran, T. B., & Simal-Gandara, J. (2021). Plant-Based Indole Alkaloids: A Comprehensive Overview from a Pharmacological Perspective. *Molecules (Basel, Switzerland)*, *26*(8), 2297. DOI: 10.3390/molecules26082297 PMID: 33921093

Onyesom, I., Elu, C. O., Acha, J. O., Ojugbeli, E. T., Ochonogor, E. P., & Udumebraye, L. O. (2022). Evaluation of Antiplasmodial Activity and Inhibitions of Lipid Peroxidation and Parasite Haem Polymerization Activity by Medicinal Phytochemicals of Phyllanthus amarus. *Nigerian Journal of Parasitology*, *43*(2), 293–302. DOI: 10.4314/njpar.v43i2.12

Oseghale, I. D., Ikokwu, G. M., Ralph-Okhiria, O. H., Odunvbun, P., & Adedotun, A. M. (2025). Comprehensive ethnomedicinal and phytopharmacological review of Jatropha tanjorensis. Asian Journal of Research in Biochemistry, 15(4), 62 ?"76. doi:10.9734/ajrb/2025/v15i4407DOI: 10.9734/ajrb/2025/v15i4407

Ottinger, M. A., & Geiselman, C. (2023). *One Health meets the exposome: Human, wildlife, and ecosystem health*. Elsevier.

Oxborough, R. M. (2016). Trends in US President's Malaria Initiative–supported indoor residual spray coverage and insecticide choice in sub-Saharan Africa (2008–2015): Implications for future vector control. *Malaria Journal*, *15*(1), 146. DOI: 10.1186/s12936-016-1201-1 PMID: 26957210

Paddon, C. J., & Keasling, J. D. (2014). Semi-synthetic artemisinin: A model for the use of synthetic biology in pharmaceutical development. *Nature Reviews. Microbiology*, *12*(5), 355–367. DOI: 10.1038/nrmicro3240 PMID: 24686413

Paddon, C. J., Westfall, P. J., Pitera, D. J., Benjamin, K., Fisher, K., McPhee, D., Leavell, M. D., Tai, A., Main, A., Eng, D., Polichuk, D. R., Teoh, K. H., Reed, D. W., Treynor, T., Lenihan, J., Jiang, H., Fleck, M., Bajad, S., Dang, G., & Newman, J. D. (2013). High-level semi-synthetic production of the potent antimalarial artemisinin. *Nature*, *496*(7446), 528–532. DOI: 10.1038/nature12051 PMID: 23575629

Paliwal, A., Jain, S., Kumar, S., Wal, P., Khandai, M., & Khandige, P. S. (2024). Predictive modelling in pharmacokinetics: from in-silico simulations to personalized medicine. Expert Opinion on Drug Metabolism & Toxicology, 20(4), 181–195. premierscience.comDOI: 10.1080/17425255.2024.2330666

Panieri, E., & Saso, L. (2021). Inhibition of the NRF2/KEAP1 axis: A promising therapeutic strategy to alter redox balance of cancer cells. *Antioxidants & Redox Signaling*, *34*(18), 1428–1483. DOI: 10.1089/ars.2020.8146 PMID: 33403898

Patel, L., Shukla, T., Huang, X., Ussery, D. W., & Wang, S. (2020). Machine learning methods in drug discovery. Molecules, 25(22), 5277. mdpi.comDOI: 10.3390/molecules25225277

Patil, P. R, A. R., Sivakumar, B., Bora, N. R., V, V., D, S. S., A, M. V., Rajaram, R., Prathyusha, K., Datta, P. L., & Nath, I. (2024). *A Comprehensive Review on Sustainable Cultivation Practices of Medicinal Plants | International Journal of Plant & Soil Science*. Retrieved September 28, 2025, from https://journalijpss.com/index.php/IJPSS/article/view/5002

Patouillard, E., Griffin, J., Bhatt, S., Ghani, A. C., Cibulskis, R., & Eckert, E. (2017). Global investment targets for malaria control and elimination between 2016 and 2030. *BMJ Global Health*, *2*(2), e000176. DOI: 10.1136/bmjgh-2016-000176 PMID: 29242750

Paudel, S., Mishra, N., & Agarwal, R. (2023). Phytochemicals as immunomodulatory molecules in cancer therapeutics. *Pharmaceuticals (Basel, Switzerland)*, *16*(12), 1652. DOI: 10.3390/ph16121652 PMID: 38139779

Pawłowska, M., Mila-Kierzenkowska, C., Szczegielniak, J., & Woźniak, A. (2023). Oxidative stress in parasitic diseases—Reactive oxygen species as mediators of interactions between the host and the parasites. *Antioxidants*, *13*(1), 38. DOI: 10.3390/antiox13010038 PMID: 38247462

Payne, D. (1987). Spread of chloroquine resistance in Plasmodium falciparum. *Parasitology Today (Personal Ed.)*, *3*(8), 241–246. DOI: 10.1016/0169-4758(87)90147-5 PMID: 15462966

Pell, C., MeA aca, A., Afrah, N. A., Manda-Taylor, L., Chatio, S., Were, F., Abraham Hodgson, A., Hamel, M. J., Kalilani, L., Tagbor, H., & Pool, R. (2013). Prevention and management of malaria during pregnancy: Findings from a comparative qualitative study in Ghana, Kenya, and Malawi. Malaria Journal, 12(1), 427. doi:10.1186/1475-2875-12-427 PubMedDOI: 10.1186/1475-2875-12-427 PMID: 24257105

Penido, C., Costa, K., Futuro, D., Paiva, S., Kaplan, M., Figueiredo, M. R., & Henriques, M. G. M. O. (2005). Anti-inflammatory and anti-ulcerogenic properties of Stachytarpheta cayennensis (L.C. Rich) Vahl. Journal of Ethnopharmacology, 104(1 ?"2), 225 ?"233. doi:10.1016/j.jep.2005.09.006 PubMedDOI: 10.1016/j.jep.2005.09.006 PMID: 16219439

Periferakis, A.-T., Periferakis, A., Periferakis, K., Caruntu, A., Badarau, I. A., Savulescu-Fiedler, I., Scheau, C., & Caruntu, C. (2023). Antimicrobial Properties of Capsaicin: Available Data and Future Research Perspectives. *Nutrients*, *15*(19), 4097. DOI: 10.3390/nu15194097 PMID: 37836381

Piechowiak, T., & Skóra, B. (2023). Edible coating enriched with cinnamon oil reduces the oxidative stress and improves the quality of strawberry fruit stored at room temperature. *Journal of the Science of Food and Agriculture*, *103*(5), 2389–2400. DOI: 10.1002/jsfa.12463 PMID: 36683377

Pons, D. G. (2024). Roles of phytochemicals in cancer prevention and therapeutics. *International Journal of Molecular Sciences*, *25*(10), 5450. DOI: 10.3390/ijms25105450 PMID: 38791488

Porwal, O., Ozdemir, M., Kala, D., & Anwer, E. T. (2021). A review on medicinal plants as potential sources of natural immunomodulatory action. *Journal of Drug Delivery and Therapeutics*, *11*(6), 324–331. DOI: 10.22270/jddt.v11i6.5125

Price, R. N., Commons, R. J., Battle, K. E., Thriemer, K., & Mendis, K. (2020). Plasmodium vivax in the era of the shrinking P. falciparum map. *Trends in Parasitology*, *36*(6), 560–570. DOI: 10.1016/j.pt.2020.03.009 PMID: 32407682

Pulford, J., Hetzel, M. W., Bryant, M., Siba, P. M., & Mueller, I. (2011). Reported reasons for not using a mosquito net when one is available: A review of the published literature. *Malaria Journal*, *10*(1), 83. DOI: 10.1186/1475-2875-10-83 PMID: 21477376

Quintana, S. E., Salas, S., & GarcA-a Zapateiro, L. A. (2021). Bioactive compounds of mango (Mangifera indica): A review of extraction technologies and chemical constituents. Journal of the Science of Food and Agriculture, 101(15), 6186 ?"6192. doi:10.1002/jsfa.11455 PubMedDOI: 10.1002/jsfa.11455 PMID: 34324201

Rahaman, S. T., & Mondal, S. (2020). Flavonoids: A vital resource in healthcare and medicine. *Pharmacy & Pharmacology International Journal*, *8*(2), 91–104. DOI: 10.15406/ppij.2020.08.00285

Ramos, D. P. (2022). Indigenous leadership, anthropology and intercultural initiatives in the Upper Rio Negro, Brazilian Amazon. *Anthropology in Action : Newsletter of the British Association for Social Anthropology in Policy and Practice (BASAPP)*, *29*(1), 59–65. DOI: 10.3167/aia.2022.290105

Ranson, H., & Lissenden, N. (2016). Insecticide resistance in African *Anopheles* mosquitoes: A worsening situation that needs urgent action to maintain malaria control. *Trends in Parasitology*, *32*(3), 187–196. DOI: 10.1016/j.pt.2015.11.010 PMID: 26826784

Rasmussen, C., Alonso, P., & Ringwald, P. (2022). Current and emerging strategies to combat antimalarial resistance. *Expert Review of Anti-Infective Therapy*, *20*(3), 353–372. DOI: 10.1080/14787210.2021.1962291 PMID: 34348573

Rasoulian, B., & Kheirandish, F. (2017). Herbal medicines: From traditional medicine to modern experimental approaches. *Herbal Medicine Journal*, *2*, 1–2.

Rauf, A., Abu-Izneid, T., Khalil, A. A., Imran, M., Shah, Z. A., Emran, T. B., Mitra, S., Khan, Z., Alhumaydhi, F. A., Aljohani, A. S. M., Khan, I., Rahman, M. M., Jeandet, P., & Gondal, T. A. (2021). Berberine as a potential anticancer agent: A comprehensive review. *Molecules (Basel, Switzerland)*, *26*(23), 7368. DOI: 10.3390/molecules26237368 PMID: 34885950

Reddy, V., Weiss, D. J., Rozier, J., Ter Kuile, F. O., & Dellicour, S. (2023). Global estimates of the number of pregnancies at risk of malaria from 2007 to 2020: A demographic study. *The Lancet. Global Health*, *11*(1), e40–e47. DOI: 10.1016/S2214-109X(22)00431-4 PMID: 36521951

Remigante, A., Spinelli, S., Straface, E., Gambardella, L., Caruso, D., Falliti, G., Dossena, S., Marino, A., & Morabito, R. (2022). Antioxidant Activity of Quercetin in a H2O2-Induced Oxidative Stress Model in Red Blood Cells: Functional Role of Band 3 Protein. *International Journal of Molecular Sciences*, *23*(19), 10991. DOI: 10.3390/ijms231910991 PMID: 36232293

Reyes-López, M., Aguirre-Armenta, B., Piña-Vázquez, C., De la Garza, M., & Serrano-Luna, J. (2023). Hemoglobin uptake and utilization by human protozoan parasites: A review. *Frontiers in Cellular and Infection Microbiology*, *13*, 1150054. DOI: 10.3389/fcimb.2023.1150054 PMID: 37360530

Ribbiso, K. A., Heller, L. E., Taye, A., Julian, E., Willems, A. V., & Roepe, P. D. (2021). Artemisinin-Based Drugs Target the Plasmodium falciparum Heme Detoxification Pathway. *Antimicrobial Agents and Chemotherapy*, *65*(4), . https://doi.org/DOI: 10.1128/AAC.02137-20

Ribeiro, G. D. J. G., Rei Yan, S. L., Palmisano, G., & Wrenger, C. (2023). Plant extracts as a source of natural products with potential antimalarial effects: An update from 2018 to 2022. *Pharmaceutics*, *15*(6), 1638. DOI: 10.3390/pharmaceutics15061638 PMID: 37376086

Riss, T., Niles, A., Moravec, R., Karassina, N., & Vidugiriene, J. (2019). *Cytotoxicity assays: In-vitro methods to measure dead cells*. Eli Lilly & Company and the National Center for Advancing Translational Sciences.

Roll Back Malaria Partnership. (2020). *The RBM Partnership to End Malaria: Annual Report*. Retrieved from https://endmalaria.org

Rowe, A. K., Rowe, S. Y., Snow, R. W., Korenromp, E. L., Schellenberg, J. R., Stein, C., & Bryce, J. (2009). The burden of malaria mortality among African children in the year 2000. *International Journal of Epidemiology*, *38*(3), 791–801. PMID: 19351697

Rudrapal, M., & Chetia, D. (2021). Malaria and recent developments in antimalarial drugs. *Neglected tropical diseases and phytochemicals in drug discovery*, 499-542.

Rupasinghe, H. P. V. (2020). Special Issue "Flavonoids and Their Disease Prevention and Treatment Potential": Recent Advances and Future Perspectives. *Molecules (Basel, Switzerland)*, *25*(20), 4746. DOI: 10.3390/molecules25204746 PMID: 33081132

Ryan, S. J., Carlson, C. J., Mordecai, E. A., & Johnson, L. R. (2020). Global expansion and redistribution of Aedes-borne virus transmission risk with climate change. *PLoS Neglected Tropical Diseases*, *14*(3), e0007213. DOI: 10.1371/journal.pntd.0007213 PMID: 30921321

Sachs, J., & Malaney, P. (2002). The economic and social burden of malaria. *Nature*, *415*(6872), 680–685. DOI: 10.1038/415680a PMID: 11832956

Sadybekov, A. V., & Katritch, V. (2023). Computational approaches streamlining drug discovery. Nature, 616, 673–685. frontiersin.orgDOI: 10.1038/s41586-023-05905-z

Saini, A., Kumar, R., & Devi, R. (2025). Natural products in modern drug discovery: Challenges, advances, and emerging opportunities. *International Journal of Pharma Sciences*, *3*(1), 1187–1199. DOI: 10.5281/zenodo.14652293

Sakthivel, M., Jaganathan, A., Mohanraj, M., & Selvakumar, P. Mohit, & Manjunath, T. (2025). Brand Loyalty through AI and Personalisation AI-Generated Content for Financial Marketing. In A. J Nair, S. Manohar, Y. B. Limbu, & B. A. Huhmann (Eds.), Intersecting Natural Language Processing and FinTech Innovations in Service Marketing (pp. 77-96). IGI Global Scientific Publishing. DOI: 10.4018/979-8-3693-9944-6.ch006

Sakyi, P. O., Twumasi, E. B., Twumasi, M. A., Akolgo, G. A., Amewu, R. K., & Osei-Safo, D. (2025). Therapeutic Potential of Natural Products as Innovative and New Frontiers for Combating Parasitic Diseases. *Parasitologia*, *5*(3), 49. DOI: 10.3390/parasitologia5030049

Salagre, K. D., Sahay, R. N., Pazare, A. R., Dubey, A., & Marathe, K. K. (2017). A study of clinical profile of patients presenting with complications of acute febrile illnesses during monsoon. *The Journal of the Association of Physicians of India, 65*(9), 37–42. PMID: 29313575

Samtiya, M., Aluko, R. E., Dhewa, T., & Moreno-Rojas, J. M. (2021). Potential Health Benefits of Plant Food-Derived Bioactive Components: An Overview. *Foods, 10*(4), 839. DOI: 10.3390/foods10040839 PMID: 33921351

Sandhir, R., Khurana, M., & Singhal, N. K. (2021). Potential benefits of phytochemicals from Azadirachta indica against neurological disorders. Neurochemistry International, 146, 105023. doi:10.1016/j.neuint.2021.105023 PubMedDOI: 10.1016/j.neuint.2021.105023 PMID: 33753160

Sarkar, C., Das, B., Rawat, V. S., Wahlang, J. B., Nongpiur, A., Tiewsoh, I., & et al. (2023). Artificial intelligence and machine learning technology driven modern drug discovery and development. International Journal of Molecular Sciences, 24(3), 2026. frontiersin.orgDOI: 10.3390/ijms24032026

Sarkar, A., Basak, S., Ghosh, S., Mahalanobish, S., & Sil, P. C. (2021). Insights into the relation between oxidative stress and malaria: A mechanistic and therapeutic approach. *Reactive Oxygen Species (Apex, N.C.), 11*, m26–m41. DOI: 10.20455/ros.2021.m.805

Sawerus, M. G., Kamel, H. H., Ahmed, W. M., Ata, E. B., El Amir, D., Mahdi, E. A., Ibrahim, M. A., & Shehata, O. (2025). Antitrypanosomal potential of Salvia officinalis terpenoids-rich fraction in Trypanosoma evansi-infected rat model. *BMC Veterinary Research, 21*(1), 410. DOI: 10.1186/s12917-025-04861-2 PMID: 40571943

Schultes, R. E. (1960). Tapping our heritage of ethnobotanical lore. Economic Botany, 14(4), 257 ?"262. https://www.jstor.org/stable/4252190. doi:10.1007/BF02908034DOI: 10.1007/BF02908034

Scott, C. S. (2023). Biopiracy: Using New Laws and Databases to Protect Indigenous Communities. *Rich. JL & Tech., 30*, 434.

Sebghatollahi, Z., Yogesh, R., Mahato, N., Kumar, V., Mohanta, Y. K., Baek, K. H., & Mishra, A. K. (2025). Signaling Pathways in Oxidative Stress-Induced Neurodegenerative Diseases: A Review of Phytochemical Therapeutic Interventions. *Antioxidants, 14*(4), 457. DOI: 10.3390/antiox14040457 PMID: 40298834

Septembre-Malaterre, A., Lalarizo Rakoto, M., Marodon, C., Bedoui, Y., Nakab, J., Simon, E., Hoarau, L., Savriama, S., Strasberg, D., Guiraud, P., Selambarom, J., & Gasque, P. (2020). Artemisia annua, a traditional plant brought to light. *International Journal of Molecular Sciences, 21*(14), 4986. DOI: 10.3390/ijms21144986 PMID: 32679734

Seshadri, K., Abad, A. N. D., Nagasawa, K. K., Yost, K. M., Johnson, C. W., Dror, M. J., & Tang, Y. (2025). Synthetic Biology in Natural Product Biosynthesis. *Chemical Reviews, 125*(7), 3814–3931. DOI: 10.1021/acs.chemrev.4c00567 PMID: 40116601

Shamsudin, N. F., Ahmed, Q. U., Mahmood, S., Shah, S. A. A., Sarian, M. N., Khattak, M. M. A. K., Khatib, A., Sabere, A. S. M., Yusoff, Y. M., & Latip, J. (2022). Flavonoids as Antidiabetic and Anti-Inflammatory Agents: A Review on Structural Activity Relationship-Based Studies and Meta-Analysis. *International Journal of Molecular Sciences, 23*(20), 12605. DOI: 10.3390/ijms232012605 PMID: 36293459

Shariff, N., Sudarshana, M. S., Umesha, S., & Hariprasad, P. (2006). Antimicrobial activity of Rauvolfia tetraphylla and Physalis minima leaf and callus extracts. *African Journal of Biotechnology, 5*(10).

Sharifi-Rad, J., Kobarfard, F., Ata, A., Ayatollahi, S. A., Khosravi-Dehaghi, N., Jugran, A. K., Tomas, M., Capanoglu, E., Matthews, K. R., Popović-Djordjević, J., Kostić, A., Kamiloglu, S., Sharopov, F., Choudhary, M. I., & Martins, N. (2019). Prosopis Plant Chemical Composition and Pharmacological Attributes: Targeting Clinical Studies from Preclinical Evidence. *Biomolecules, 9*(12), 777. DOI: 10.3390/biom9120777 PMID: 31775378

Shegokar, R. (2020). Preclinical testing—understanding the basics first. In Drug Delivery Aspects (pp. 19–32).

Shepard, D. S., Ettling, M. B., Brinkmann, U., & Sauerborn, R. (2013). The economic cost of malaria in Africa. *Tropical Medicine and Parasitology, 45*(1), 74–79. PMID: 1801147

Sherrard-Smith, E., Hogan, A. B., Hamlet, A., Watson, O. J., Whittaker, C., Winskill, P., & Ghani, A. C. (2022). The potential public health consequences of COVID-19 on malaria in Africa. *Nature Medicine, 26*(9), 1411–1416. DOI: 10.1038/s41591-020-1025-y PMID: 32770167

Shibeshi, M. A., Kifle, Z. D., & Atnafie, S. A. (2020). Antimalarial drug resistance and novel targets for antimalarial drug discovery. *Infection and Drug Resistance, 13*, 4047–4060. DOI: 10.2147/IDR.S279433 PMID: 33204122

Shinyuy, L. M., Loe, G. E., Jansen, O., Mamede, L., Ledoux, A., Noukimi, S. F., Abenwie, S. N., Ghogomu, S. M., Souopgui, J., Robert, A., Demeyer, K., & Frederich, M. (2023). Secondary metabolites isolated from Artemisia afra and Artemisia annua and their anti-malarial, anti-inflammatory and Immunomodulating properties—pharmacokinetics and pharmacodynamics: A review. *Metabolites, 13*(5), 613. DOI: 10.3390/metabo13050613 PMID: 37233654

Sifuna, N. (2022). African Traditional Medicine: Its Potential, Limitations and Challenges. J Healthcare, 5(1), 141 ?"150. doi:10.36959/569/475DOI: 10.36959/569/475

Silva, J. C. K., Soliani, R. D., Ferreira-Júnior, G. C., de Abreu Freitas, R. G., & Lobão, M. S. P. (2025). Bioeconomy In The Amazon: Challenges, opportunities, and trends for regional development. *Revista de Gestão Social e Ambiental, 19*(1), 1–16. DOI: 10.24857/rgsa.v19n1-166

Singh, R., & Sharma, B. (2019). *Therapeutic Potential of Plant Based Natural Compounds for Malaria—Recent Advances and Future Perspective.*

Singh, H., & Bharadvaja, N. (2021). Treasuring the computational approach in medicinal plant research. *Progress in Biophysics and Molecular Biology, 164*, 19–32. DOI: 10.1016/j.pbiomolbio.2021.05.004 PMID: 34004233

Singh, N., & Yeh, P. J. (2017). Suppressive drug combinations and their potential to combat antibiotic resistance. *The Journal of Antibiotics, 70*(11), 1033–1042. DOI: 10.1038/ja.2017.102 PMID: 28874848

Singla, R. K., De, R., Efferth, T., Mezzetti, B., Uddin, M. S., & Ntie-Kang, F. (2023). The international natural product sciences Taskforce (INPST) and the power of Twitter networking exemplified through #INPST hashtag analysis. *Phytomedicine, 108*, 154520. DOI: 10.1016/j.phymed.2022.154520 PMID: 36334386

Sinha, S., Batovska, D. I., Medhi, B., Radotra, B. D., Bhalla, A., Markova, N., & Sehgal, R. (2019). In vitro anti-malarial efficacy of chalcones: Cytotoxicity profile, mechanism of action and their effect on erythrocytes. *Malaria Journal, 18*(1), 421. DOI: 10.1186/s12936-019-3060-z PMID: 31842914

Sinka, M. E., Pironon, S., Massey, N. C., Longbottom, J., Hemingway, J., Moyes, C. L., & Hay, S. I. (2020). A new malaria vector in Africa: Predicting the expansion range of Anopheles stephensi and identifying the urban populations at risk. *Proceedings of the National Academy of Sciences of the United States of America, 117*(40), 24900–24908. DOI: 10.1073/pnas.2003976117 PMID: 32929020

Siqueira-Neto, J. L., Wicht, K. J., Chibale, K., Burrows, J. N., Fidock, D. A., & Winzeler, E. A. (2023). Antimalarial drug discovery: Progress and approaches. *Nature Reviews. Drug Discovery*, *22*(10), 807–826. DOI: 10.1038/s41573-023-00772-9 PMID: 37652975

Siraj, A. S., Santos-Vega, M., Bouma, M. J., Yadeta, D., Ruiz Carrascal, D., & Pascual, M. (2014). Altitudinal changes in malaria incidence in highlands of Ethiopia and Colombia. *Science*, *343*(6175), 1154–1158. DOI: 10.1126/science.1244325 PMID: 24604201

Sircar, N. N. (1982). Medicinal plants. *The Eastern Pharmacist*, *29*(291), 49–52.

Slater, L. B. (2009). *War and disease: Biomedical research on malaria in the twentieth century*. Rutgers University Press.

Snow, R. W., Sartorius, B., & Kyalo, D.. (2021). The prevalence of *Plasmodium falciparum* in sub-Saharan Africa since 1900. *Nature*, *601*(7891), 547–553. DOI: 10.1038/s41586-021-04264-3 PMID: 29019978

Sobhani, M., Farzaei, M. H., Kiani, S., & Khodarahmi, R. (2021). Immunomodulatory; anti-inflammatory/antioxidant effects of polyphenols: A comparative review on the parental compounds and their metabolites. *Food Reviews International*, *37*(8), 759–811. DOI: 10.1080/87559129.2020.1717523

Sofowora, A., Ogunbodede, E., & Onayade, A. (2013). The role and place of medicinal plants in the strategies for disease prevention. *African Journal of Traditional, Complementary, and Alternative Medicines : AJTCAM*, *10*(3), 210–229. DOI: 10.4314/ajtcam.v10i5.2 PMID: 24311829

Sojka, D., Jalovecká, M., & Perner, J. (2022). Babesia, Theileria, plasmodium and hemoglobin. *Microorganisms*, *10*(8), 1651. DOI: 10.3390/microorganisms10081651 PMID: 36014069

Sok Yen, F., & Qin, S. (2021). C., Tan Shi Xuan, S., Jia Ying, P., Yi Le, H., Darmarajan, T., Gunasekaran, B., & Salvamani, S. (2021). Hypoglycemic Effects of Plant Flavonoids: A Review. *Evidence-Based Complementary and Alternative Medicine : eCAM*, *2057333*(1), 1–12. DOI: 10.1155/2021/2057333 PMID: 34925525

Sokan-Adeaga, A. A., Sokan-Adeaga, M. A., Sokan-Adeaga, E. D., Oparaji, A. N., Edris, H., Tella, E. O., Balogun, F. A., Aledeh, M., & Amubieya, O. E. (2023). Environmental toxicants and health adversities: A review on interventions of phytochemicals. *Journal of Public Health Research*, *12*(2), 22799036231181226. DOI: 10.1177/22799036231181226 PMID: 37440795

Soni, R., Sharma, D., Rai, P., Sharma, B., & Bhatt, T. K. (2017). Signaling strategies of malaria parasite for its survival, proliferation, and infection during erythrocytic stage. *Frontiers in Immunology*, *8*, 349. DOI: 10.3389/fimmu.2017.00349 PMID: 28400771

Sorkin, B. C., Kuszak, A. J., Bloss, G., Fukagawa, N. K., Hoffman, F. A., Jafari, M., Barrett, B., Brown, P. N., Bushman, F. D., Casper, S. J., Chilton, F. H., Coffey, C. S., Ferruzzi, M. G., Hopp, D. C., Kiely, M., Lakens, D., MacMillan, J. B., Meltzer, D. O., Pahor, M., & Pauli, G. F. (2020). Improving natural product research translation: From source to clinical trial. [FASEB]. *The FASEB Journal*, *34*(1), 41–65. DOI: 10.1096/fj.201902143R PMID: 31914647

Srivastava, R., Jaiswal, N., Kharkwal, H., Dubey, N. K., & Srivastava, R. (2025). Phytomedical Properties of Carica papaya for Boosting Human Immunity Against Viral Infections. Viruses, 17(2), 271. doi:10.3390/v17020271 PubMedDOI: 10.3390/v17020271 PMID: 40007026

Suganya, T., Packiavathy, I. A. S. V., Aseervatham, G. S. B., Carmona, A., Rashmi, V., Mariappan, S., Devi, N. R., & Ananth, D. A. (2022). Tackling multiple-drug-resistant bacteria with conventional and complex phytochemicals. *Frontiers in Cellular and Infection Microbiology*, *12*, 883839. DOI: 10.3389/fcimb.2022.883839 PMID: 35846771

Sun, J., Xufeng, J., Qiu, Z., Gao, Q., Zhu, Z., He, J., Gao, S., & Sui, X. (2025). Artemisiae Annuae Herba: From anti-malarial legacy to emerging anti-cancer potential. *Theranostics*, *15*(15), 7346–7377. DOI: 10.7150/thno.115414 PMID: 40756346

Sun, S., Yu, Y., Jo, Y., Han, J. H., Xue, Y., Cho, M., Bae, S.-J., Ryu, D., Park, W., Ha, K.-T., & Zhuang, S. (2025). Impact of extraction techniques on phytochemical composition and bioactivity of natural product mixtures. *Frontiers in Pharmacology*, *16*, 1615338. Advance online publication. DOI: 10.3389/fphar.2025.1615338 PMID: 40808686

Su, X., Liang, Z., Xue, Q., Liu, J., Hao, X., & Wang, C. (2023). A comprehensive review of azadirachtin: Physicochemical properties, bioactivities, production, and biosynthesis. *Acupuncture and Herbal Medicine*, *3*(4), 256–270. DOI: 10.1097/HM9.0000000000000086

Takken, W., Charlwood, D., & Lindsay, S. W. (2024). The behaviour of adult Anopheles gambiae, sub-Saharan Africa's principal malaria vector, and its relevance to malaria control: A review. *Malaria Journal*, *23*(1), 161. DOI: 10.1186/s12936-024-04982-3 PMID: 38783348

Tansaz, M., & Tajadini, H. (2016). Comparison of leiomyoma of modern medicine and traditional Persian medicine. *Journal of Evidence-Based Complementary & Alternative Medicine*, *21*(2), 160–163. DOI: 10.1177/2156587215595299 PMID: 26177818

Tarkang, P. A., Appiah-Opong, R., Ofori, M. F., Ayong, L. S., & Nyarko, A. K. (2016). Application of multi-target phytotherapeutic concept in malaria drug discovery: A systems biology approach in biomarker identification. *Biomarker Research*, *4*(1), 25. DOI: 10.1186/s40364-016-0077-0 PMID: 27999673

Thakur, A., & Sharma, R. (2018). Health promoting phytochemicals in vegetables: A mini review. *International Journal of Food and Fermentation Technology*, *8*(2), 107–117. DOI: 10.30954/2277-9396.02.2018.1

Thakur, V. (2024). Food Vacuole as a Drug Target. In *Drug Targets for Plasmodium Falciparum: Historic to Future Perspectives* (pp. 183–199). Springer Nature Singapore. DOI: 10.1007/978-981-19-4484-0_10

Thirunagalingam, A., & Selvakumar, P. (2025). Application of Automation and Robotics in the Oil and Gas Industry. In Abdullayev, V., & Khang, A. (Eds.), *Revolutionizing AI and Robotics in the Oil and Gas Industry* (pp. 229–244). IGI Global Scientific Publishing., DOI: 10.4018/979-8-3693-8156-4.ch011

Thomford, N. E., Awortwe, C., Dzobo, K., Adu, F., Chopera, D., Wonkam, A., & Dandara, C. (2016a). Inhibition of CYP2B6 by medicinal plant extracts: Implication for use of efavirenz and nevirapine-based highly active anti-retroviral therapy (HAART) in resource-limited settings. *Molecules (Basel, Switzerland)*, *21*(2), 211. DOI: 10.3390/molecules21020211 PMID: 26891286

Thomford, N. E., Dzobo, K., Chopera, D., Wonkam, A., Skelton, M., Blackhurst, D., & Dandara, C. (2016b). In vitro reversible and time-dependent CYP450 inhibition profiles of medicinal herbal plant extracts Newbouldia laevis and Cassia abbreviata: Implications for herb-drug interactions. *Molecules (Basel, Switzerland)*, *21*(7), 891. DOI: 10.3390/molecules21070891 PMID: 27399660

Thomford, N. E., Dzobo, K., Chopera, D., Wonkam, A., Skelton, M., Blackhurst, D., & Dandara, C. (2016c). Pharmacogenomics implications of using herbal medicinal plants on African populations in health transition. *Pharmaceuticals (Basel, Switzerland)*, *8*(3), 637–663. DOI: 10.3390/ph8030637 PMID: 26402689

Tiamiyu, M., & Okunlade, O. A. (2020). Benefits and detriments of Siam weed (Chromolaena odorata): A review. Biochemistry and Biotechnology Research (Delta), 8(2), 21 ?"28.

Timothy, F. M., & Zininga, T. (2023). Small heat shock proteins as modulators of cell death in Plasmodium falciparum parasites and its human host. *Frontiers in Cell Death*, *2*, 1322780. DOI: 10.3389/fceld.2023.1322780

Tinto, H., Valea, I., Sorgho, H., Rouamba, N., Kaboré, Y., Kazienga, A., & D'Alessandro, U. (2015). Efficacy and safety of the candidate malaria vaccine RTS,S/AS01 administered according to different schedules in African children: A randomised controlled trial. *The Lancet. Infectious Diseases*, *15*(12), 1451–1460.

Tiralongo, E., Wee, S., & Lea, R. (2016, March 24). Elderberry supplementation reduces cold duration and symptoms in air-travellers: A randomized, double-blind placebo-controlled clinical trial. *Nutrients*, *8*(4), 182. DOI: 10.3390/nu8040182 PMID: 27023596

Titanji, V. P. K., Zofou, D., & Ngenenya, M. N. (2008). The antimalarial potential of medicinal plants used for the treatment of malaria in Cameroonian folk medicine. (2008, April 10). PubMed. https://pubmed.ncbi.nlm.nih.gov/20161952/

Tiwari, R., Latheef, S. K., Ahmed, I., Iqbal, H. M., Bule, M. H., Dhama, K., Samad, H. A., Karthik, K., Alagawany, M., El-Hack, M. E. A., Yatoo, M. I., & Farag, M. R. (2018). Herbal immunomodulators-a remedial panacea for designing and developing effective drugs and medicines: Current scenario and future prospects. *Current Drug Metabolism*, *19*(3), 264–301. DOI: 10.2174/1389200219666180129125436 PMID: 29380694

Tucakov, J. (1971). Healing with plants–phytotherapy. *Beograd. Culture (Québec)*, *180*, 90.

Tusting, L. S., Rek, J., Arinaitwe, E., Staedke, S. G., Kamya, M. R., Cano, J., & Lindsay, S. W. (2017). Why is malaria associated with poverty? Findings from a cohort study in rural Uganda. *Infectious Diseases of Poverty*, *5*(1), 78. DOI: 10.1186/s40249-016-0164-3 PMID: 27488674

Tu, Y. (2011). The discovery of artemisinin (Qinghaosu) and gifts from Chinese medicine. *Nature Medicine*, *17*(10), 1217–1220. DOI: 10.1038/nm.2471 PMID: 21989013

Tu, Y. (2017). *From Artemisia annua L. to Artemisinins: The Discovery and Development of Artemisinins and Antimalarial Agents*. Academic Press.

Tzanova, M., Atanasov, V., Yaneva, Z., Ivanova, D., & Dinev, T. (2020). Selectivity of Current Extraction Techniques for Flavonoids from Plant Materials. *Processes (Basel, Switzerland)*, *8*(10), 1222. DOI: 10.3390/pr8101222

Tzvetkov, N. T., Kirilov, K., Matin, M., & Atanasov, A. G. (2024). Natural product drug discovery and drug design: Two approaches shaping new pharmaceutical development. *Nephrology, Dialysis, Transplantation*, *39*(3), 375–378. DOI: 10.1093/ndt/gfad208 PMID: 37708048

U.S. Food and Drug Administration. (n.d.). *How drugs are developed and approved*. Retrieved September 23, 2025, from https://www.fda.gov/drugs/development-approval-process-drugs/how-drugs-are-developed-and-approved

Ugbogu, E. A., Dike, E. D., Uche, M. E., Etumnu, L. R., Okoro, B. C., Ugbogu, O. C., Adurosakin, O. E., Chinma, C. E., Ohaeri, E., & Iweala, E. J. (2023). Ethnomedicinal uses, nutritional composition, phytochemistry, and potential health benefits of Carica papaya. Pharmacological Research. Modern Chinese Medicine, 7, 100266. doi:10.1016/j.prmcm.2023.100266DOI: 10.1016/j.prmcm.2023.100266

Ugwuibe, C. O., Onah, F. N., & Olise, C. N. (2021). Flood disasters in Aba North Local Government Area of Abia State, Nigeria: Policy options. In Economic effects of natural disasters (pp. 373-380). Academic Press. https://doi.org/doi:10.1016/B978-0-12-817465-4.00023-6DOI: 10.1016/B978-0-12-817465-4.00023-6

Ullah, A., Munir, S., Badshah, S. L., Khan, N., Ghani, L., Poulson, B. G., Emwas, A.-H., & Jaremko, M. (2020). Important Flavonoids and Their Role as a Therapeutic Agent. *Molecules (Basel, Switzerland)*, *25*(22), 5243. DOI: 10.3390/molecules25225243 PMID: 33187049

Umoh, U. F., Thomas, P. S., Essien, E. E., Okokon, J. E., De Leo, M., Ajibesin, K. K., Flamini, G., & Eseyin, O. A. (2021). Isolation and characterization of bioactive xanthones from Hippocratea africana (Willd.)Loes.ex Engl. (Celastraceae). Journal of Ethnopharmacology, 280, 114031. doi:10.1016/j.jep.2021.114031 PubMedDOI: 10.1016/j.jep.2021.114031 PMID: 33737141

United Nations. (2015). *Transforming our world: The 2030 Agenda for Sustainable Development*. Retrieved from https://sdgs.un.org

Upadhyay, S. K., & Singh, S. P. (2023). *Plants as bioreactors for industrial molecules*. John Wiley & Sons. DOI: 10.1002/9781119875116

Uwimana, A., Umulisa, N., Venkatesan, M., Svigel, S. S., Zhou, Z., Munyaneza, T., & Udhayakumar, V. (2021). Association of *Plasmodium falciparum* kelch13 R561H genotypes with delayed parasite clearance in Rwanda. *Nature Medicine*, *27*(2), 378–381. PMID: 33864801

Uzor, P. F. (2020). Alkaloids from Plants with Antimalarial Activity: A Review of Recent Studies. *Evidence-Based Complementary and Alternative Medicine : eCAM, 2020*(1), 8749083. DOI: 10.1155/2020/8749083 PMID: 32104196

Uzor, P. F., Prasasty, V. D., & Agubata, C. O. (2020). *Natural Products as Sources of Antimalarial Drugs*. Evidence-Based Complement Alternative Medicine., DOI: 10.1155/2020/9385125

Vaghela, U. P., Jani, B., Tank, T., Kalaria, K., Kanabar, V., Parekh, K., & Yadav, R. (2025). Antimalarial Potential of Medicinal Plants: Phytochemical Insights and Host-Directed Strategies. *The Journal of Communicable Diseases, 57*(3), 174–181. DOI: 10.24321/0019.5138.202584

van Agtmael, M. A., Eggelte, T. A., & van Boxtel, C. J. (1999). Artemisinin drugs in the treatment of malaria: From medicinal herb to registered medication. *Trends in Pharmacological Sciences, 20*(5), 199–205. DOI: 10.1016/S0165-6147(99)01302-4 PMID: 10354615

Van Andel, T., Onselen, S. B., Myren, B., Towns, A., & Quiroz, D. (2015). ?oThe medicine from behind ??: The frequent use of enemas in Western African traditional medicine. Journal of Ethnopharmacology, 174, 637 ?"643. doi:10.1016/j.jep.2015.06.040 PubMedDOI: 10.1016/j.jep.2015.06.040 PMID: 26133063

van der Pluijm, R. W., Amaratunga, C., Dhorda, M., & Dondorp, A. M. (2021). Triple artemisinin-based combination therapies for malaria–a new paradigm? *Trends in Parasitology, 37*(1), 15–24. DOI: 10.1016/j.pt.2020.09.011 PMID: 33060063

Vanaja, P., Moorthy, N. H. N., Rajpoot, V. S., Rao, H., Goswami, R. K., Subash, P., Khute, S., & Rao, K. S. (2025). Metabolite profiling, antimalarial potentials of Schleichera oleosa using LC-MS and GC-MS: In vitro, molecular docking and molecular dynamics. *Frontiers in Molecular Biosciences, 12*, 1543939. DOI: 10.3389/fmolb.2025.1543939 PMID: 40026697

Varghese, R., Shringi, H., & Efferth, T. (2025). Artificial intelligence driven approaches in phytochemical research: trends and prospects. Phytochemistry Reviews, February 27, 1–21. mdpi.com+9link.springer.com±9pmc.ncbi.nlm.nih.gov±9DOI: 10.1007/s11101-025-10096-8

Vij, I., & Pathania, A. (2023). An Overview- Advances in Chromatographic Techniques in Phytochemistry. *E3S Web of Conferences, 391*, 01038. Retrieved September 28, 2025, from https://www.e3s-conferences.org/articles/e3sconf/abs/2023/28/e3sconf_icmed-icmpc2023_01038/e3sconf_icmed-icmpc2023_01038.html

Vijayan, K., Wei, L., Glennon, E. K., Mattocks, C., Bourgeois, N., Staker, B., & Kaushansky, A. (2021). Host-targeted interventions as an exciting opportunity to combat malaria. *Chemical Reviews*, *121*(17), 10452–10468. DOI: 10.1021/acs.chemrev.1c00062 PMID: 34197083

Visser, B. J., van Vugt, M., & Grobusch, M. P. (2014). Malaria: An update on current chemotherapy. Expert Opinion on Pharmacotherapy, 15(15), 2219 ?"2254. doi:10.1517/14656566.2014.944499 PubMedDOI: 10.1517/14656566.2014.944499 PMID: 25110058

Vitale, S., Colanero, S., Placidi, M., Di Emidio, G., Tatone, C., Amicarelli, F., & D ?(tm)Alessandro, A. M. (2022). Phytochemistry and biological activity of medicinal plants in wound healing: An overview of current research. Molecules (Basel, Switzerland), 27(11), 3566. doi:10.3390/molecules27113566 PubMedDOI: 10.3390/molecules27113566 PMID: 35684503

Wang, Y., Michael, S., Yang, S. M., Huang, R., Cruz-Gutierrez, K., Zhang, Y., et al. (2022). Retro drug design: from target properties to molecular structures. Journal of Chemical Information and Modeling, 62(11), 2659–2669. premierscience.comDOI: 10.1021/acs.jcim.2c00123

Wang, C., Zhang, H., Wang, X., Wang, X., Li, X., Li, C., Wang, Y., & Zhang, M. (2024). Comprehensive review on fruit of Terminalia chebula: Traditional uses, phytochemistry, pharmacology, toxicity, and pharmacokinetics. *Molecules (Basel, Switzerland)*, *29*(23), 5547. DOI: 10.3390/molecules29235547 PMID: 39683707

Wangdi, K., Gatton, M. L., Kelly, G. C., & Clements, A. C. (2021). Cross-border malaria: A major obstacle for malaria elimination. *Advances in Parasitology*, *89*, 79–107. DOI: 10.1016/bs.apar.2015.04.002 PMID: 26003036

Wang, K., Huang, Y., Wang, Y., You, Q., & Wang, L. (2024). Recent advances from computer-aided drug design to artificial intelligence drug design. *RSC Medicinal Chemistry*, *15*(12), 3978–4000. pubs.acs.orgpubs.rsc.org. DOI: 10.1039/D4MD00522H PMID: 39493228

Wang, W., Rao, L., Wu, X., Wang, Y., Zhao, L., & Liao, X. (2021). Supercritical Carbon Dioxide Applications in Food Processing. *Food Engineering Reviews*, *13*(3), 570–591. DOI: 10.1007/s12393-020-09270-9

Ward, K. E., Fidock, D. A., & Bridgford, J. L. (2022). Plasmodium falciparum resistance to artemisinin-based combination therapies. *Current Opinion in Microbiology*, *69*, 102193. DOI: 10.1016/j.mib.2022.102193 PMID: 36007459

Weiss, D. J., Bertozzi-Villa, A., Rumisha, S. F., Amratia, P., Arambepola, R., Battle, K. E., & Bhatt, S. (2021). Indirect effects of the COVID-19 pandemic on malaria intervention coverage, morbidity, and mortality in Africa. *Nature Medicine*, *27*(3), 703–709. PMID: 32971006

Wen, M., Zeng, J., Qiu, F., Zhang, F., & Liao, Z. (2024). De Novo Synthesis of Anticholinergic Hyoscyamine and Scopolamine in Nicotiana benthamiana Based on Elucidating Tropane Alkaloid Biosynthetic Pathway of Anisodus luridus. *Agronomy (Basel)*, *14*(11), 2460. DOI: 10.3390/agronomy14112460

Wetzler, E. A., Marchesini, P., Villegas, L., & Canavati, S. (2022). Changing transmission dynamics among migrant, indigenous and mining populations in a malaria hotspot in Northern Brazil: 2016 to 2020. *Malaria Journal*, *21*(1), 127. DOI: 10.1186/s12936-022-04141-6 PMID: 35439994

Whitty, C. J., Ansah, E. K., & Reyburn, H. (2021). Malaria control in Africa: Progress but still much to do. *BMJ (Clinical Research Ed.)*, *375*(2434).

WHO. (2019). WHO global report on traditional and complementary medicine. https://www.who.int/publications/i/item/978924151536

WHO. (2021). *Malaria in the WHO South-East Asia Region 2000–2020*. World Health Organization. https://www.who.int [Access September 15, 2025]

WHO. (2022). Report on Malaria in Nigeria 2022. Pp 195. ISBN: 978-929023498-2

WHO. (2022). *World Malaria Report 2022*. World Health Organization. https://www.who.int [Access September 15, 2025]

WHO. (2023). *WHO's annual malaria report spotlights the growing threat of climate change*. World Health Organization. https://www.who.int[Access September 15, 2025]

WHO. (2024). *World Malaria Report 2024*. World Health Organization. https://www.who.int [Access September 15, 2025]

WHO. Fact sheet NA 134, (2008), https://www.who.int/mediacentre/factsheets/2003/fs134/en/

WHO. World Malaria Report (2023). Geneva, World Health Organization, 2023. https://www.who.int/teams/global-malaria-programme/reports/world-malaria-report-2023. Accessed: January 8, 2024.

Willcox, M., Graziose, R., & Bodeker, G. (2011). Traditional herbal medicines for malaria. *BMJ (Clinical Research Ed.)*, *343*, d7303. PMID: 15539672

Wondafrash, D. Z., Bhoumik, D., Altaye, B. M., Tareke, H. B., & Assefa, B. T. (2019). *Antimalarial Activity of Cordia africana (Lam.) (Boraginaceae) Leaf Extracts and Solvent Fractions in Plasmodium berghei-Infected Mice*. Evidence-Based Complement Alternative Medicine., DOI: 10.1155/2019/8324596

Woodruff, H. B. (1980). Natural products from microorganisms. *Science, 208*(4449), 1225–1229. DOI: 10.1126/science.7375932 PMID: 7375932

World Health Organization. (2002). WHO traditional medicine strategy 2002-2005. In the WHO traditional medicine strategy 2002-2005 (pp. 61-61).

World Health Organization. (2015). *Global Technical Strategy for Malaria 2016–2030*. WHO.

World Health Organization. (2025). *Malaria vaccines (RTS,S and R21): Questions and answers.* Retrieved from https://www.who.int/news-room/questions-and-answers/item/q-a-on-rts-s-malaria-vaccine [Access September 15, 2025]

Wu, J., Lv, S., Zhao, L., Gao, T., Yu, C., Hu, J., & Ma, F. (2023). Advances in the study of the function and mechanism of the action of flavonoids in plants under environmental stresses. *Planta, 257*(6), 108. DOI: 10.1007/s00425-023-04136-w PMID: 37133783

Wu, P., & Lu, J. M. (2019). Stability of Natural Products: Theory and Practice. *Journal of Natural Products, 82*(2), 267–276.

Wu, S., Nie, Q., Tan, S., Liao, G., Lv, Y., Lv, C., Chen, G., & Liu, S. (2023). The immunity modulation of transforming growth factor-β in malaria and other pathological process. *International Immunopharmacology, 122*, 110658. DOI: 10.1016/j.intimp.2023.110658 PMID: 37467691

Xiao, Z., Morris-Natschke, S. L., & Lee, K. H. (2016). Strategies for the Optimization of Natural Leads to Anticancer Drugs or Drug Candidates. *Medicinal Research Reviews, 36*(1), 32–91. DOI: 10.1002/med.21377 PMID: 26359649

Xia, X. (2017). Bioinformatics and drug discovery. *Current Topics in Medicinal Chemistry, 17*(15), 1709–1726. DOI: 10.2174/1568026617666161116143440 PMID: 27848897

Xu, K., Qu, L., Li, H., Ren, X., Yan, N., & Fu, X. (2024). Functional properties of dietary quercetin in cardiovascular health and disease. *Food Frontiers, 5*(5), 1951–1967. DOI: 10.1002/fft2.434

Xu, Q., Bauer, R., Hendry, B. M., Fan, T. P., Zhao, Z., Duez, P., & Robinson, N. (2013). The quest for modernisation of traditional Chinese medicine. *BMC Complementary and Alternative Medicine, 13*(1), 132. DOI: 10.1186/1472-6882-13-132 PMID: 23763836

Yang, W., Chen, X., Li, Y., Guo, S., Wang, Z., & Yu, X. (2020). Advances in Pharmacological Activities of Terpenoids. *Natural Product Communications, 15*(3), 1934578X20903555. DOI: 10.1177/1934578X20903555

Yang, J., Li, K., He, D., Gu, J., Xu, J., Xie, J., Zhang, M., Liu, Y., Tan, Q., & Zhang, J. (2020). Toward a better understanding of metabolic and pharmacokinetic characteristics of low-solubility, low-permeability natural medicines. *Drug Metabolism Reviews, 52*(1), 19–43. DOI: 10.1080/03602532.2020.1714646 PMID: 31984816

Yatoo, M. I., Dimri, U., Gopalakrishnan, A., Karthik, K., Gopi, M., Khandia, R., & Saxena, A. (2017). Beneficial health applications and medicinal values of Pedicularis plants: A review. *Biomedicine and Pharmacotherapy, 95*, 1301–1313. DOI: 10.1016/j.biopha.2017.09.041 PMID: 28938521

Yeh, Y. C., Huang, T. H., Yang, S. C., Chen, C. C., & Fang, J. Y. (2020). Nano-based drug delivery or targeting to eradicate bacteria for infection mitigation: A review of recent advances. *Frontiers in Chemistry, 8*, 286. DOI: 10.3389/fchem.2020.00286 PMID: 32391321

Yin, T., Panapitiya, G., Coda, E. D., & Saldanha, E. G. (2023). Evaluating uncertainty-based active learning for accelerating the generalization of molecular property prediction. Journal of Cheminformatics, 15(1), 105. medium.comDOI: 10.1186/s13321-023-00753-5

Yuan, H., Ma, Q., Ye, L., & Piao, G. (2016). The traditional medicine and modern medicine from natural products. *Molecules (Basel, Switzerland), 21*(5), 559. DOI: 10.3390/molecules21050559 PMID: 27136524

Yu-Ping, L., Mendonça, D., Sheng-Khai, L., Phan-Sing, Y. A., Chimplee, S., Chuprom, J., Boonhok, R., Mahboob, T., Oliveira, S. M., Rajagopal, M., Pereira, M. L., Girol, A. P., & Nissapatorn, V. (2024). Malaria – the importance of phytochemicals as sources of alternative medicines. *Indian Journal of Natural Products and Resources (IJNPR) [Formerly Natural Product Radiance (NPR)], 15*(2), 274–285. DOI: 10.56042/ijnpr.v15i2.11493

Yu, S., Wang, J., Luo, X., Zheng, H., Wang, L., Yang, X., & Wang, Y. (2022). Transmission-blocking strategies against malaria parasites during their mosquito stages. *Frontiers in Cellular and Infection Microbiology, 12*, 820650. DOI: 10.3389/fcimb.2022.820650 PMID: 35252033

Zahin, M., Aqil, F., & Ahmad, I. (2009). The in vitro antioxidant activity and total phenolic content of four Indian medicinal plants. *International Journal of Pharmacy and Pharmaceutical Sciences*, *1*(1), 88–95.

Zeka, K., Ruparelia, K., Arroo, R. R. J., Budriesi, R., & Micucci, M. (2017). Flavonoids and Their Metabolites: Prevention in Cardiovascular Diseases and Diabetes. *Diseases (Basel, Switzerland)*, *5*(3), 19. DOI: 10.3390/diseases5030019 PMID: 32962323

Zhang, Y. L., Sun, S. J., & Zeng, L. (2024). *Biological effects and mechanisms of dietary chalcones: Latest research progress, future research strategies, and challenges*. DOI: 10.1039/D4FO03618B

Zhang, C., & Hong, K. (2020). Production of Terpenoids by Synthetic Biology Approaches. *Frontiers in Bioengineering and Biotechnology*, *8*, 347. Advance online publication. DOI: 10.3389/fbioe.2020.00347 PMID: 32391346

Zhang, L., Ismail, M. M., Rocchetti, G., Fayek, N. M., Lucini, L., & Saber, F. R. (2022). The untargeted phytochemical profile of three meliaceae species related to in vitro cytotoxicity and anti-virulence activity against MRSA isolates. *Molecules (Basel, Switzerland)*, *27*(2), 435. DOI: 10.3390/molecules27020435 PMID: 35056761

Zhang, W., Zeng, Y., Jiao, M., Ye, C., Li, Y., Liu, C., & Wang, J. (2023). Integration of high-throughput omics technologies in medicinal plant research: The new era of natural drug discovery. *Frontiers in Plant Science*, *14*, 1073848. DOI: 10.3389/fpls.2023.1073848 PMID: 36743502

Zhang, Y., Alvarez-Manzo, H., Leone, J., Schweig, S., & Zhang, Y. (2021). Botanical medicines Cryptolepis sanguinolenta, Artemisia annua, Scutellaria baicalensis, Polygonum cuspidatum, and Alchornea cordifolia demonstrate inhibitory activity against Babesia duncani. *Frontiers in Cellular and Infection Microbiology*, *11*, 624745. DOI: 10.3389/fcimb.2021.624745 PMID: 33763384

Zhao, L., Zhu, Y., Jia, H., Han, Y., Zheng, X., Wang, M., & Feng, W. (2022). From plant to yeast—Advances in biosynthesis of artemisinin. *Molecules (Basel, Switzerland)*, *27*(20), 6888. DOI: 10.3390/molecules27206888 PMID: 36296479

Zheng, M., Zhu, Y., Zhuang, Y., Tan, K. B., & Chen, J. (2023). Effects of grape seed extract on the properties of pullulan polysaccharide/xanthan gum active films for apple preservation. *International Journal of Biological Macromolecules*, *241*, 124617. DOI: 10.1016/j.ijbiomac.2023.124617 PMID: 37119919

Zhu, Y., Ouyang, Z., Du, H., Wang, M., Wang, J., Sun, H., Kong, L., Xu, Q., Ma, H., & Sun, Y. (2022). New opportunities and challenges of natural products research: When target identification meets single-cell multiomics. *Acta Pharmaceutica Sinica. B*, *12*(11), 4011–4039. DOI: 10.1016/j.apsb.2022.08.022 PMID: 36386472

About the Contributors

Odangowei Inetiminebi Ogidi holds a Bachelor of Science degree in Biochemistry, Master of Science and Doctor of Philosophy degrees in Biotechnology at The Niger Delta University Wilberforce Island Bayelsa State, Nigeria and Federal University of Technology Owerri, Imo State, Nigeria respectively. He is a Lecturer, Sub-Dean, Faculty of Basic Medical Sciences, and Acting Head, Department of Biochemistry, Bayelsa Medical University, Yenagoa, Bayelsa State, Nigeria. He has also served as a Lecturer, Head of Departments of Science Laboratory Technology and Biochemistry, and Deputy Director, Centre for Continuing Education in Federal Polytechnic Ekowe, Bayelsa State. He has authored over 80 peer-reviewed academic articles in reputable local and international journals and presented over 35 conference papers. He has over 80 book chapters published in IGI Global Scientific Publishing, Elsevier, Springer Nature, CRC Press Taylor & Francis, Apple Academic Publishing and Wiley and Sons. He is currently editing 10 books in IGI Global Scientific Publishing, Springer Nature, CRC Press Taylor & Francis, Apple Academic Publishing, Bentham Science. He is a member of various Journal Editorial Boards. His research interest has been Environmental Biotechnology, Phytomedicine, Phytochemistry, Human and Environmental health risk assessments and ecotoxicology amongst others. Dr. Ogidi is a member of West Africa Society of Toxicology, Nigerian Society of Biochemistry and Molecular Biology, Foundation for African Development through International Biotechnology and Nigerian Environmental Society.

***

Testimonies Chikanka Adebayo-Olajide is a seasoned microbiologist with over eight years of academic and research experience. She holds a PhD in Microbiology and is widely recognized for her expertise in antibiotic resistance, environmental microbiology, and public health microbiology. Her scientific journey has been marked by a commitment to addressing some of the most pressing microbial threats to human health and the environment. Dr. Adebayo-Olajide has spent more than 8 years inspiring undergraduate students through her dynamic teaching, mentorship, and supervision of research. She is deeply involved in curriculum development and interdisciplinary scientific collaboration, with a passion for fostering critical thinking and practical laboratory skills in her students. Dr. Adebayo-Olajide's research centres on the mechanisms and transmission of antibiotic resistance in clinical and environmental settings, the role of microbial communities in water and soil ecosystems, and the intersection of microbiology and public health. Her work has significantly contributed to understanding how environmental reservoirs contribute to the spread of resistant pathogens. She has authored and co-authored over 20 peer-reviewed publications in high-impact international journals, including Annals of Clinical and Laboratory Research, International Journal of Pathogen Research, and American Chemical Society. Her research has been presented at conferences, earning her recognition and invitations to serve as peer reviewer. She continues to be a strong advocate for women in STEM, mentoring young scientists and promoting equitable access to scientific education and research opportunities in Nigeria.

Mary-Ibenreh Ogaboh Agba is an academic staff member in the Department of Botany, University of Calabar, Nigeria. She holds a Bachelor of Science (B.Sc.) in Botany, a Master of Science (M.Sc.) in Phytopathology, and a Doctor of Philosophy (Ph.D.) in Applied Mycology. A passionate scholar and researcher, Dr. Agba has extensive expertise in indigenous plants, fungal biology, and mushroom cultivation, with additional skills in molecular and computational biology. Her scientific curiosity and collaborative spirit have positioned her as a valuable team player in multidisciplinary research focused on sustainable agriculture, food security, and biotechnology. Her current research interests center on the domestication of indigenous mushroom species, establishing their phylogenetic relationships, and exploring their nutraceutical potentials. She is particularly interested in understanding the genetic basis of edible mushrooms to enhance domestication and productivity. Additionally, her work investigates pathogens that cause diseases in mushrooms during cultivation and seeks plant-based, eco-friendly solutions to control these diseases. Dr. Agba is widely regarded as a hardworking, trustworthy, and highly organized individual. Her long-term goal is to become a leading expert in her field, contributing to scientific innovation, food health improvement, and environmental sustainability. She believes that true progress comes from dedication, passion, and integrity—qualities she embodies in both her academic and personal pursuits.

Adinarayana Andy is a dedicated Pharmacy Manager with extensive experience in pharmacy management and drug discovery research. Licensed in Michigan and Ohio, Andy has accumulated over 16 years of experience working at independent pharmacies, leading national drugstore chains, and in pharmaceutical research organizations. His expertise includes navigating complex state and federal requirements, enhancing pharmacy performance metrics, and delivering patient-centered care. Education: Master of Business Administration (Project Management): University of the Cumberlands, Kentucky, USA (2017) Doctor of Philosophy (Biotechnology): Acharya Nagarjuna University, Guntur, India (2012) Master of Pharmacy (Pharmaceutical Analysis and Quality Assurance): Berhampur University, Orissa, India (2004) Bachelor of Pharmacy: Andhra University, Vishakhapatnam, India (2002) Licenses Michigan Pharmacist License Michigan Controlled Substance License Ohio Pharmacist License

Goddidit Enoze holds B.Sc. Biological Science, MSc Plant Biology and Biotechnology and PhD in Plant Biology and Biotechnology all from the University of Benin, Nigeria. She has numerous publications to her credit.

Vikas Balaramegowda is a biomedical science graduate with an MSc from Swansea University and a background in pharmacy. He has developed practical expertise in microbiology, biochemistry, and clinical diagnostics through his work across both NHS and industry settings. His experience spans quality control and production roles at Thermo Fisher Scientific and Medik8, as well as hands-on diagnostic support in NHS microbiology, where he gained valuable skills in aseptic techniques, autoclaving, contamination control, and LIMS data management. Alongside professional practice, Vikas has been active in academic research, including projects on nanoparticle effects on blood clotting using ROTEM, emerging biomarkers in Alzheimer's disease, and public and professional perceptions of pain management. These experiences have strengthened his interest in bridging laboratory science with real-world healthcare impact. He is a registered pharmacist in India and an active member of international scientific networks. His long-term ambition is to progress into a Biomedical Scientist role within the NHS, combining his diagnostic expertise with a passion for translational research to improve patient outcomes.

Darshan Balaramegowda is a clinical research professional and academic with expertise spanning clinical trials, patient recruitment, pharmacovigilance, and advanced data analytics. He holds a Doctor of Pharmacy (PharmD) from S J M College of Pharmacy, under Rajiv Gandhi University of Health Sciences, Karnataka, India, and a Master of Research (MRes) in Clinical Science from Norwich Medical School, under the University of East Anglia (UEA), England,

United Kingdom. His research has focused on drug safety, pharmacoepidemiology, pre-clinical pharmacology, and neurocognitive health, with publications addressing adverse drug reactions, antibiotic safety, and self-medication practices. Darshan has conducted large-scale data analyses using international databases such as FAERS and CPRD, applying advanced statistical methods in SPSS, STATA, and R to generate actionable insights for clinical safety and epidemiology. In recognition of his outstanding research contributions, he was awarded the prestigious Susan Marmor Prize at UEA (2024 - 2025) for achieving the highest dissertation score in Clinical Science. His award-winning project on brain health earned a £2,500 cash prize, followed by a feature interview published across the University of East Anglia and Norwich Medical School websites and media platforms. The full story can be accessed here: Susan Marmor Prize – UEA. Beyond research, Darshan has served as an Assistant Professor in the Pharmacy Practice Department at S J M College of Pharmacy, mentoring PharmD and BPharm students in clinical pharmacology, research methodology, and pharmacotherapeutics. He is also a peer reviewer for the International Journal of Emerging Trends in Pharmacy and Medicine, contributing to quality assurance in scientific publishing. Darshan continues to advance research at the intersection of clinical trials, data science, and translational medicine, with a strong commitment to improving patient outcomes through evidence-based practice and innovation.

Effiom Eyo Ita is a Plant Biotechnologist with a Ph.D. in Plant Biotechnology from The University of Calabar, Nigeria. He was a visiting research scientist for two years at the Laboratory of Plant Cell Technology, Graduate School of Horticulture, Chiba University, Japan. After his Ph.D. research in Japan, Effiom returned to the University of Calabar, where he currently teaches and conducts research in the Department of Genetics and Biotechnology. As an instructor, Effiom teaches courses in molecular genetics and biotechnology at the undergraduate and postgraduate levels and supervises students' research projects. Also, Effiom is a recipient of the Plant Breeding Academy of the University of California (UC) Davis fellowship for the Africa Plant Breeding Academy (AfPBA) CRISPR course (first cohort), 2023. His research interest includes collection, characterization and conservation of neglected and underutilized plant species (NUS), genetic engineering of plants for stress resistance and increased productivity, regulation of gene expression by small RNAs, CRISPR/Cas9 genome editing for biotic and abiotic stress resistance and increased nutritional value. Through his experience and skills, Effiom has published a book chapter, several peer reviewed articles and conference papers.

T.C. Manjunath was born on 6th February 1967. He did his B.E. from RV College of Engg. in 1989 (B'lore Univ), M.E. in Robotics & Automation from Govt.'s LD College of Engg., (Gujarat Univ., Ahmedabad) in 1992 with FCD-First Rank & PhD in Systems & Control Engg. from IIT Bombay in the year 2007, got best research scholar award for the entire IITB. He is currently working as the Dean Research (R & D) and as Professor in Dept. of Computer Science & Engg. with specialization in IoT, Cyber Security, Blockchain Technology in Rajarajeswari College of Engineering, Bengaluru, Karnataka. He has got a teaching (academic), research & administrative experience of more than 35+ years (10 years as Principal & 8 years as HoD, 1 year as Dean Research & rest as faculty) and has published more than 1500+ research papers in various national & international journals & conferences, with 175+ patents, 100+ book-chapters, 25 awards, 100s of Keynote talks and also published 25 text books in various field of science, engineering & technology, completed projects worth Rs. 9 Crores till date & guided 10 PhD scholars in VTU. He is a member of 30 Professional Society Chapters and is a fellow of IE, IETE, AMIEE, Sr. Member of IEEE and a chartered engineer.

P. Selvakumar is currently an Associate Professor in the Department of Science and Humanities at Nehru Institute of Technology, Coimbatore, Tamil Nadu, India. Prior to joining Nehru Institute of Technology, he held positions as an Assistant Professor in the Department of Science and Humanities various engineering colleges in Coimbatore, Tamil Nadu, India, spanning from 2011 to 2023. Dr.P. Selvakumar's academic and research interests lie primarily in the field of phytochemistry. He has made significant contributions to his field, with an impressive record that includes 30 journal publications, 12 patents, and 20 conference papers. Additionally, he has organized 5 seminars and conferences, further demonstrating his commitment to academic and scientific exchange. Throughout his career, Dr. P.Selvakumar has been recognized for his dedication and excellence in teaching, having been honored with several awards, including the Best Teacher Awards. He holds a prominent position in the academic community, contributing actively to research.

Dhanalakshmi Perumal Since joining Dr. MGR Educational and Research Institute, Dr. Dhanalakshmi has been actively involved in teaching and mentoring students in the areas of clinical pharmacy, pharmacovigilance, medicinal chemistry, and drug formulation. She has over three years of experience as an Assistant Professor, along with serving as a hospital preceptor to guide students in patient-centered pharmacy practice. In addition to her teaching and clinical training responsibilities, she is currently pursuing a PhD focused on hypertensive disorders of pregnancy, reflecting her commitment to advancing research and improving maternal healthcare outcomes.

Julius Oyohosuho Phillip is a dedicated lecturer at the Department of Genetics and Biotechnology, University of Calabar, Nigeria. His academic interests centre on plant immunity and metabolomics, where he explores the intricate biochemical networks that underpin plant defense mechanisms. With a passion for advancing agricultural resilience through molecular biology, Julius contributes to both teaching and research, inspiring the next generation of scientists.

Aman Suresh Tharayil is an Assistant Professor in the Faculty of Pharmacy at Dr. M.G.R. Educational and Research Institute, Chennai, where teaching and research focus on Pharmacy Practice, pharmacoepidemiology, and patient-centered outcomes across vector-borne and chronic diseases. Training includes a Doctor of Pharmacy (Pharm-D) from SJM College of Pharmacy, RGUHS, and ongoing doctoral studies (PhD) in Pharmacy Practice at SIMATS, Chennai, integrating clinical inquiry with methodological rigor in study design, biostatistics, and research governance. Academic appointments span SJM College of Pharmacy (Karnataka) and Sandip Institute of Pharmaceutical Sciences (Maharashtra) prior to the current role, with teaching across B.Pharm, D.Pharm, and Pharm.D curricula—covering Pharmacy Practice, Pharmacoepidemiology, Pharmacoeconomics, Pharmacotherapeutics, Biostatistics, and Research Methodology—alongside mentorship of Pharm.D projects.

Peggy Willie Obaseojei is a Senior lecturer in the Department of Genetics and Biotechnology at the University of Calabar, Nigeria. She teaches undergraduate and postgraduate courses including Introduction to Genetics, Molecular Biology, Cytogenetics, and Research Techniques in Biotechnology. Her research focuses on genome editing in indigenous African crops such as African yam bean and cowpea, aimed at improving productivity and disease resistance. She also maintains a strong interest in medicinal plants research, exploring their bioactive properties and applications in primary healthcare. Dr. Willie holds a Ph.D. in Plant Biotechnology and is a graduate of the second cohort of the African Plant Breeding Academy (AfPBA)/CRISPR course, a prestigious fellowship offered by the University of California, Davis. She has extensive experience in molecular biology, cell and tissue culture, and plant gene transfer techniques. A passionate educator and mentor, she has supervised numerous undergraduate research projects and contributed to scholarly publications in her field. Her academic and research efforts are driven by a commitment to advancing agricultural biotechnology and harnessing plant science innovations for sustainable development in Africa.

Young Ibiang holds a first degree in Genetics, and M.Sc. in Environmental Biotechnology both from the University of Calabar, Nigeria. He obtained a PhD in Environmental Horticulture from Chiba University, Japan, in 2018. His research interests include Environmental toxicology, physiology and biotechnology; heavy metal stress tolerance, soil-plant-microbes interaction, plant nutrition, bio-fertilizer, bio-protection, and bioresources utilization. He has published in local and international journals.

Index

A

B

C

D

E

F

G

www.ingramcontent.com/pod-product-compliance
Lightning Source LLC
LaVergne TN
LVHW060002031026
849161LV00025B/1302